DATE DUE

DEMCO, INC. 38-2931

NEUROMETHODS ☐ 15

Neurophysiological Techniques

NEUROMETHODS

Program Editors: Alan A. Boulton and Glen B. Baker

1. **General Neurochemical Techniques**
   Edited by *Alan A. Boulton and Glen B. Baker,* 1985
2. **Amines and Their Metabolites**
   Edited by *Alan A. Boulton, Glen B. Baker, and Judith M. Baker,* 1985
3. **Amino Acids**
   Edited by *Alan A. Boulton, Glen B. Baker, and James D. Wood,* 1985
4. **Receptor Binding Techniques**
   Edited by *Alan A. Boulton, Glen B. Baker, and Pavel D. Hrdina,* 1986
5. **Neurotransmitter Enzymes**
   Edited by *Alan A. Boulton, Glen B. Baker, and Peter H. Yu,* 1986
6. **Peptides**
   Edited by *Alan A. Boulton, Glen B. Baker, and Quentin Pittman,* 1987
7. **Lipids and Related Compounds**
   Edited by *Alan A. Boulton, Glen B. Baker, and Lloyd A. Horrocks,* 1988
8. **Imaging and Correlative Physicochemical Techniques**
   Edited by *Alan A. Boulton, Glen B. Baker, and Donald P. Boisvert,* 1988
9. **The Neuronal Microenvironment**
   Edited by *Alan A. Boulton, Glen B. Baker, and Wolfgang Walz,* 1988
10. **Analysis of Psychiatric Drugs**
    Edited by *Alan A. Boulton, Glen B. Baker, and Ronald T. Coutts,* 1988
11. **Carbohydrates and Energy Metabolism**
    Edited by *Alan A. Boulton, Glen B. Baker, and Roger F. Butterworth,* 1989
12. **Drugs as Tools in Neurotransmitter Research**
    Edited by *Alan A. Boulton, Glen B. Baker, and Augusto V. Juorio,* 1989
13. **Psychopharmacology**
    Edited by *Alan A. Boulton, Glen B. Baker, and Andrew J. Greenshaw,* 1989
14. **Neurophysiological Techniques: Basic Methods and Concepts**
    Edited by *Alan A. Boulton, Glen B. Baker, and Case H. Vanderwolf,* 1990
15. **Neurophysiological Techniques: Applications to Neural Systems**
    Edited by *Alan A. Boulton, Glen B. Baker, and Case H. Vanderwolf,* 1990
16. **Molecular Neurobiological Techniques**
    Edited by *Alan A. Boulton, Glen B. Baker, and Anthony T. Campagnoni,* 1990
17. **Neuropsychology**
    Edited by *Alan A. Boulton, Glen B. Baker, and Merrill Hiscock,* 1990

NEUROMETHODS

Program Editors: Alan A. Boulton and Glen B. Baker

NEUROMETHODS □ 15

Neurophysiological Techniques
Applications to Neural Systems

Edited by

Alan A. Boulton

University of Saskatchewan, Saskatoon, Canada

Glen B. Baker

University of Alberta, Edmonton, Canada

and
Case H. Vanderwolf

University of Western Ontario, London, Canada

Humana Press • Clifton, New Jersey

Library of Congress Cataloging in Publication Data

Main entry under title:
Neurophysiological techniques. Applications to neural systems /
   edited by Alan A. Boulton, Glen B. Baker, and Case H. Vanderwolf.
      p.   cm. — (Neuromethods : 15)
   Includes bibliographical references and index.
   ISBN 0-89603-185-3
      1. Neurophysiology—Research—Methodology.   2. Electrophysiology-
-Research—Methodology.   3. Evoked potentials (Electrophysiology)
I. Boulton, A. A. (Alan A.)   II. Baker, Glen B., 1947-
III. Vanderwolf, C. H.   IV. Series.
      [DNLM: 1. Electrophysiology—methods.   2. Nervous System-
-physiology.   3. Neurophysiology—methods.   W1 NE337G v. 15 / WL
102 N49579]
QP356.N48283   1990
591.1'88—dc20
DNLM/DLC
for Library of Congress   90-44264
                                                                                        CIP

© 1990 The Humana Press Inc.
Crescent Manor
PO Box 2148
Clifton, NJ 07015

Printed in the United States of America

Preface to the Series

When the President of Humana Press first suggested that a series on methods in the neurosciences might be useful, one of us (AAB) was quite skeptical; only after discussions with GBB and some searching both of memory and library shelves did it seem that perhaps the publisher was right. Although some excellent methods books have recently appeared, notably in neuroanatomy, it is a fact that there is a dearth in this particular field, a fact attested to by the alacrity and enthusiasm with which most of the contributors to this series accepted our invitations and suggested additional topics and areas. After a somewhat hesitant start, essentially in the neurochemistry section, the series has grown and will encompass neurochemistry, neuropsychiatry, neurology, neuropathology, neurogenetics, neuroethology, molecular neurobiology, animal models of nervous disease, and no doubt many more "neuros." Although we have tried to include adequate methodological detail and in many cases detailed protocols, we have also tried to include wherever possible a short introductory review of the methods and/or related substances, comparisons with other methods, and the relationship of the substances being analyzed to neurological and psychiatric disorders. Recognizing our own limitations, we have invited a guest editor to join with us on most volumes in order to ensure complete coverage of the field. These editors will add their specialized knowledge and competencies. We anticipate that this series will fill a gap; we can only hope that it will be filled appropriately and with the right amount of expertise with respect to each method, substance or group of substances, and area treated.

Alan A. Boulton
Glen B. Baker

Preface

The development of neurophysiology, the study of the activity of living nervous tissue, has relied heavily on the techniques of electrophysiology. This emphasis is revealed in volumes 14 and 15 of this series, which show how electrophysiological techniques can be applied to research topics ranging from ion channels to human behavior. Kitai and Park show how cellular neurophysiology can be related to classical neuroanatomy, an important basis for any type of functional analysis. Wonderlin, French, Arispe, and Jones describe new (single channel) and more traditional (whole cell) techniques for studying the role of ion channels in cellular processes, a field that is currently developing very rapidly. An exciting nontraditional approach to the study of cellular electrophysiology is discussed by Hopp, Wu, Xiao, Rioult, London, Zecevic, and Cohen in their paper on optic measurement of membrane potentials. Humphrey and Schmidt offer a thoughtful review of the uses and limitations of the technique of recording extracellular unit potentials in the brain. Hoffer presents an introduction to a field that is of great interest but is technically very difficult—the recording from cells and axons in the spinal cord and peripheral nervous system in freely moving animals. An electrophysiological approach to the analysis of the neural mechanisms of normal behavior is presented by Halgren in a wide-ranging review of the field of evoked potentials in humans. The papers by Carlini and Ransom (ion-selective electrodes) and Maidment, Martin, Ford, and Marsden (in vivo voltammetry) describe techniques that could be said to lie at the border between neurophysiology and neurochemistry, and that promise new insights into the dynamics of neurochemically defined classes of neuronal activity. Finally, Leung discusses the increasing use and sophistication of computational techniques in the analysis of neurophysiological data.

Not all readers will agree with my selection of topics. However, I think that all will agree that the contributors have presented excellent discussions of their respective fields that will be of wide and enduring interest. For this, I thank the contributors most heartily.

C. H. Vanderwolf

Contents

Preface to the Series v
Preface vi
List of Contributors xiii

EXTRACELLULAR SINGLE-UNIT RECORDING METHODS
Donald R. Humphrey and Edward M. Schmidt

1. Introduction 1
   1.1. Some Definitions 2
2. Extracellular Fields of Single Neurons 3
   2.1. Amplitude and Duration of Single-Unit
        Spikes 3
   2.2. Spike Configuration and Polarity 3
   2.3. Dependence of Field Parameters on Cell
        Geometry and Size 9
   2.4. Extracellularly Recorded Axon or Fiber
        Spikes 14
3. Recording Methods 16
   3.1. Construction and Electrical Properties
        of Extracellular Microelectrodes 16
   3.2. Recording Circuits and Amplifiers 34
   3.3. Microdrives 36
   3.4. Improvement of Recording Stability 36
   3.5. Electrode Insertion and Advancement 39
   3.6. Isolating Single Units 41

3.7. Distinguishing Antidromically from
Orthodromically Evoked Responses 46
4. Sampling Single-Neuron Activity 51
4.1. How Sampling Biases Can Arise from
Variations in Cell Size 54
References 59

TECHNIQUES TO STUDY SPINAL-CORD, PERIPHERAL
NERVE, AND MUSCLE ACTIVITY IN FREELY MOVING
ANIMALS
Joaquín Andrés Hoffer

1. Introduction 65
2. Floating Microelectrodes for Recording from
Single Neurons 66
2.1. Microelectrode Design: Theoretical and
Practical Considerations 68
2.2. Fabrication of Floating Microelectrodes 71
2.3. Surgical Implantation of Floating Microelectrodes in Ventral Roots, Dorsal Root
Ganglia, or Spinal Cord 72
2.4. Connectors 74
2.5. Amplification, Discrimination, and Record-
ing of Single-Unit Potentials 75
2.6. Minimization of Noise Pickup and Move-
ment Artifact 76
2.7. Criteria for the Identification of Recorded
Neurons 77
3. Peripheral Nerve Cuff Electrodes 78
3.1. Nerve Cuff Recording Electrodes: Theoretical and Practical Considerations 79
3.2. Fabrication of Nerve Cuff Recording Electrodes 83
3.3. Surgical Implantation of Nerve Cuff Electrodes 87
3.4. Recording and Processing of Nerve Cuff
Signals 87

3.5. Estimation of Axonal Conduction Velocity of a Recorded Neuron Using the Spike-Triggered Averaging Technique 91
3.6. Peripheral Nerve Stimulating Electrodes 93
3.7. Peripheral Nerve Blocking Cuffs 98
3.8. Applications of Nerve Cuffs to the Study of Other Systems 103
3.9. Spinal Cord ENG Electrodes 106
4. EMG Electrodes 107
   4.1. EMG Recording: Theoretical and Practical Considerations 107
   4.2. Fabrication and Surgical Implantation of EMG Electrodes 110
   4.3. EMG Signal Recording and Processing 110
   4.4. Determination of the Target Muscle of a Recorded Motoneuron Using Spike-Triggered Averaging 111
5. Tendon Force Transducers 113
   5.1. Fabrication and Surgical Implantation of Tendon Force Transducers 113
   5.2. Tendon Force Signal Recording and Calibration 115
6. Muscle and Tendon Length Transducers 116
   6.1. Length Measurements: Theoretical and Practical Considerations 116
   6.2. Fabrication and Surgical Implantation of Distensible Length Transducers 119
   6.3. Measurement of Whole Muscle Length with Distensible Length Transducers 120
   6.4. Fabrication and Surgical Implantation of Piezoelectric Transducers 121
   6.5. Measurement of Tendon Length, Muscle Fiber Length, and Pinnation Angle 123
7. Selection, Training, and Care of Implanted Animals 126
   7.1. Implanted Venous Catheter 127
8. Limitations of Chronic Recording Techniques 128
   8.1. Assessment of Chronic Damage Caused by Implanted Devices 128

8.2. Expected Functional Longevity of Implanted
Devices 133
9. Clinical Applications of Chronic Recording Techniques 134
References 136

HUMAN EVOKED POTENTIALS
Eric Halgren

1. Introduction 147
1.1. Organization and Scope of This Review 147
1.2. History 148
1.3. Components 149
2. Methodology 154
2.1. Recordings 154
2.2. Analysis 161
2.3. Generator Localization 167
3. Sensory EPs 176
3.1. Auditory Evoked Potentials (AEP) 176
3.2. Somatosensory Evoked Potentials (SEP) 181
3.3. Visual EPs 185
4. Movement Potentials 190
4.1. Methods 190
4.2. Components 190
4.3. Topography 192
4.4. Generators—P1/N2/P2/P3 193
4.5. Generators—RP, NS' 195
4.6. Cognitive Correlates—RP 197
5. Cognitive EPs 200
5.1. Methods and Components 200
5.2. Cognitive Correlates of the N4 202
5.3. Cognitive Correlates of the P3 205
5.4. Generation of the P3 207
5.5. Generation of the N4 214
5.6. Contingent Negative Variation 215
5.7. Interpretation of Cognitive EPs 220
6. Uses of EPs 223
References 228

FIELD POTENTIALS IN THE CENTRAL NERVOUS SYSTEM—
RECORDING, ANALYSIS, AND MODELING
Lai-Wo Stan Leung

1. Introduction 277
2. Field Potential Theory 278
   2.1. General 278
   2.2. Principles of Current Flow 279
   2.3. Equations for Current Flow 281
   2.4. Qualitative Properties of Field Potentials 287
   2.5. Simulation of Field Potentials 291
3. Techniques in Field Potential Recording and
   Analysis 294
   3.1. Field Potential Mapping (Laminar Analysis) 294
   3.2. Measurements of Conductivity 296
   3.3. The Current Field 298
   3.4. Current-Source-Density Analysis 299
4. Interpretation of Field Potentials 304
   4.1. General Principles 304
   4.2. Examples 305
   Appendix: Multiple Electrode Arrays 309
   References 309

COMPUTER TECHNIQUES IN NEUROPHYSIOLOGY
Lai-Wo Stan Leung

1. Introduction 313
   1.1. General Introduction 313
   1.2. A Microcomputer System 315
2. The Computer in a Neurophysiological Labora-
   tory 324
   2.1. Recording of Neurophysiological Signals 324
   2.2. Manipulation and Analysis of Data 343
   2.3. Control and Output Functions 354
3. Behavioral Analysis Using a Microcomputer 358
   3.1. General 358
   3.2. The Video Signal 359

3.3. Analysis of the Video Signal 359
3.4. Other Movement Analysis Systems 361
References 362
Appendix: Glossary and Acronyms 365
Index **371**

Contributors

GLEN B. BAKER • *Neurochemical Research Unit, Department of Psychiatry, University of Alberta, Edmonton, Alberta, Canada*

ALAN A. BOULTON • *Neuropsychiatric Research Unit, University of Saskatchewan, Saskatoon, Saskatchewan, Canada*

ERIC HALGREN • *VA Southwest Regional Epilepsy Center, Wadsworth VAMC, W. Los Angeles, California and Department of Psychiatry and Brain Research Institute, University of California at Los Angeles*

JOAQUÍN ANDRÉS HOFFER • *Departments of Medical Physiology and Clinical Neurosciences, University of Calgary, Calgary, Alberta, Canada*

DONALD R. HUMPHREY • *Department of Physiology, Emory University School of Medicine, Atlanta, Georgia*

LAI-WO STAN LEUNG • *Department of Clinical Neurological Sciences and Physiology, University of Western Ontario, London, Canada*

EDWARD M. SCHMIDT • *Laboratory of Neural Control, National Institutes of Health, Bethesda, Maryland*

CASE H. VANDERWOLF • *University of Western Ontario, London, Canada*

Extracellular Single-Unit Recording Methods*

Donald R. Humphrey and Edward M. Schmidt

1. Introduction

Since their refinement in the early 1950s, extracellular, single-unit recording methods have been used to obtain a wealth of data about the properties of CNS structures. The applications of the technique have been diverse: extracellular microelectrodes have been used to map the potential fields of single discharging neurons in order to answer fundamental questions about the excitability of CNS dendrites (Frank and Fuortes, 1955; Fatt, 1957; Nelson and Frank, 1964), and more recently they have been used to study the behaviorally related discharge patterns of CNS neurons in the awake, moving animal (e.g., Evarts, 1968; Mountcastle et al., 1975). To an appreciable extent, the exciting new neuroanatomical tracing methods that have been developed over the past decade (cf Jones and Wise, 1977) have supplanted extracellular recording methods as a technique for tracing CNS connectivity patterns. However, the single-unit recording method is the technique of choice for studies of the responses of central neurons to sensory stimuli and of their behaviorally related firing patterns in the alert, moving animal. Moreover, many applications remain for the tracing of functional network connections on a microanatomical scale.

It is the purpose of this chapter, therefore, to outline certain basic principles concerning the extracellular potential fields of single, active neurons, and the techniques for recording their action potentials extracellularly. It is hoped that this material will be useful to investigators who are currently using this technique, or who plan to use it, within their own laboratories. Some of the material that is presented here is new, but much of it is similar to that found in a number of previous excellent discussions of the

*With special reference to those used in the mammalian CNS.)

1

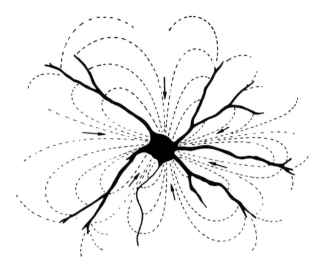

Fig. 1. Direction of lines of current flow around a stellate-shaped neuron during an action potential in its soma. Intracellularly, current flows radially outward from the soma into the dendritic tree. Extracellularly, it flows, in general, radially inward from dendritic "sources" to a somatic "sink" (from Humphrey, 1976).

extracellular recording method, which may be consulted for additional details (e.g., Towe, 1973; DeValois and Pease, 1973; Snodderly, 1973).

1.1. Some Definitions

The following terms will be used extensively in this chapter, and it is useful to define them at this point.

> *Extracellular potential field*—When a neuron discharges
> (i.e., generates an action potential), it undergoes an
> increase in conductivity over excitable regions of its
> membrane; usually, at the axon hillock and/or soma.
> The current that flows into the cell across this increased
> membrane conductance will flow along the core of the
> cell, and then exit at various regions of adjacent, in-
> active membrane to return to the site of current entry by
> way of diverse paths through the extracellular medium
> (*see* Fig. 1). The flow of current across this resistive

medium generates a complex potential field around the neuron; the properties of this field depend on the size and geometry of the cell, and the location and time-course of the membrane conductance increase. The terms *extracellular field* or *spike potential field* will be used here to refer to the complex field around a discharging neuron.

Extracellular spike—the time-varying potential that is recorded at a single locus within the extracellular field of a single neuron during one of its action potentials.

Single unit—a single, discharging neuron, the spikes of which are clearly discriminated or isolated by a recording microelectrode.

2. Extracellular Fields of Single Neurons

2.1. Amplitude and Duration of Single-Unit Spikes

As can be seen in Fig. 2, single-unit spike potentials are considerably shorter in duration and, on the average, larger in amplitude than potentials that are recorded from the surface or within the depths of the brain with *macro*electrodes. One reason for such differences in amplitude is that the largest potentials that are generated by a neuron will be in the immediate vicinity of the site of the membrane conductance change. In order to record these potentials in full amplitude, an electrode is required with exposed tip dimensions that are small when compared to those of the steepest portion of the active neuron's extracellular potential field. For cortical neurons, these dimensions may be on the order of as little as 20 μm. Electrode tips with dimensions approaching this value, when placed adjacent to a small, discharging neuron, may present an isopotential surface that effectively "shorts out" the cell's potential field. It is perhaps for this reason that *macroelectrodes* or gross recording electrodes are inappropriate for recording single-unit spikes.

2.2. Spike Configuration and Polarity

Unlike intracellularly recorded action potentials, extracellular spikes may vary markedly in configuration and even in polarity, depending on the geometry of the cell and the location of the

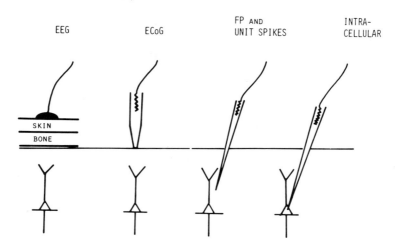

Fig. 2. A comparison of the amplitudes and durations of electric potentials recorded from the scalp (electroencephalogram or EEG) or surface of the cortex (electrocorticogram or ECoG) with *macro*electrodes, or adjacent to or within single neurons with *micro*electrodes. The potentials detected with macroelectrodes tend to be dominated by extracellular currents arising from comparatively long duration (10–1000 ms) postsynaptic potentials in neurons or events of similar duration in glial cells, whereas microelectrodes can also detect rapid changes in membrane potential in adjacent neurons or axons, such as action potentials or unit "spikes." (For an explanation of the physics underlying these differences *see* Humphrey, 1968).

	EEG	ECoG	Extracell. microelec.	Intracell. microelec.
Area of recording surface	2–10 mm²	1–3 mm²	2–50 μm²	0.4–3.0 μm²
Amplitude of recorded potentials, mV	0.01–0.2	0.05–1.0	0.05–5.0	0.1–100.0
Duration of dominant potentials, ms	15–1000	15–1000	0.3–1000	0.8–dc[a]

([a]dc = direct current, or sustained membrane potential)

recording electrode. In many cases, such variations are of little interest to the investigator, with the simple occurrence of an evoked spike or some parameter of the spike train being the only variables of interest. Variations in spike shape are often helpful in guiding microelectrode placement, however, and may in addition provide valuable information about the probable geometry, and hence type, of the cell recorded from (e.g., whether it is pyramidal or stellate in shape). It may be helpful, therefore, to review briefly information about the dependence of recorded spike shape on cell geometry and electrode location. However, in order to understand how such variations arise, first let us consider the following simple example.

Imagine a simple, spherical neuron (such as the model ganglion cell in Fig. 3) that undergoes a spike-generating conductance change over only a portion of its soma. During the action potential, the current (J_m) that flows out of the cell across the inactive region of membrane will consist of both capacitive and resistive components:

$$J_m = J_{capac.} + J_{res.} \qquad (1)$$
$$= C_m \, (dV_m/dt) + G_m V_m$$

where V_m is the transmembrane potential, C_m is the membrane capacitance and G_m is the conductance of the inactive region of membrane. As can be seen in Fig. 3A, the capacitive component of the membrane current may be biphasic, being first outward across the inactive portion of membrane during the intracellular action potential's rise and then inward during its declining phase. Since (a) the capacitive component may dominate the membrane current during the action potential and (b) the time-course of the *extracellular* spike will depend on that of the membrane current rather than the membrane potential, it can be seen that the extracellular spike may be biphasic.

Consider now spike polarity. From an extracellular "observation" or recording point, current that flows out of a cell across some portion of its membrane will appear to be a current *source*, whereas current that flows into a cell over another portion of its membrane will appear to be a current *sink*. At distances greater than two to three soma diameters from a simple spherical neuron such as that shown in Fig. 3, the field that it generates will be similar to that of a

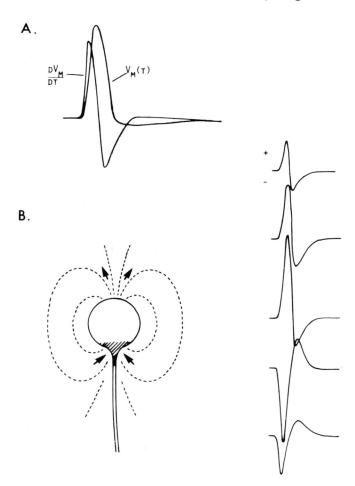

Fig. 3. Some determinants of spike configuration and polarity. (A) Membrane current flow during the spike involves a capacitative component that is proportional to dV_m/dt and is thus biphasic. Since the shape of the extracellular spike depends strongly on the time-course of membrane current, it also may be biphasic. (B) Hypothetical lines of current flow around a simple ganglion cell during an action potential at its axon hillock (dashed area). The sequence of spikes that would be recorded by an electrode passing such a cell from above is shown on the right. *See* text for additional details.

current dipole whose source is located at the center of the cell portion where current flows outward across the membrane and whose sink is located at the center of the region where the membrane current flows into the cell. In a conducting medium of average or bulk conductivity σ, the potential that would be generated at any point by such a current dipole would be given (from the superposition principle) by

$$V_e = \frac{1}{4\pi\sigma} \left(\frac{J^+}{r^+} - \frac{J^-}{r^-} \right) \tag{2}$$

where V_e = the (instantaneous) extracellular potential; J^+ = the (instantaneous) intensity of the current source; J^- = the intensity of the current sink; r^+ = the distance from the source to the extracellular recording position; and r^- = the distance from the sink to the recording position.

Since the inwardly and outwardly directed membrane current must at all times be equal in magnitude, Eq. (2) reduces to

$$V_e = \frac{J}{4\pi\sigma} \left(\frac{1}{r^+} - \frac{1}{r^-} \right) \tag{3}$$

Thus, the polarity of the recorded potential (with respect to a distant reference electrode) will be positive if the electrode is nearer the site of outward current flow and negative if it is nearer the site of inward current flow.

Even this simple example illustrates, therefore, how a biphasic extracellular spike may be generated and how spike polarity may vary with electrode location. With neurons of more complex geometry embedded in a nonhomogeneous medium, the variations in spike shape will be more complex, for the membrane sources and sinks are distributed, and their amplitudes at any time-point will depend on the cable or core conductor properties of the neuron. Nonetheless, the simple equations given above can aid in providing intuitive explanations, on condition that they are extended to the distributed case. In the somewhat more complicated case illustrated in Fig. 4, for example, it can be seen that the dipole has been replaced by a single sink and a distributed source, corresponding to a somatic action potential in a cell with one major dendrite. In this case, the extracellular potential is given by

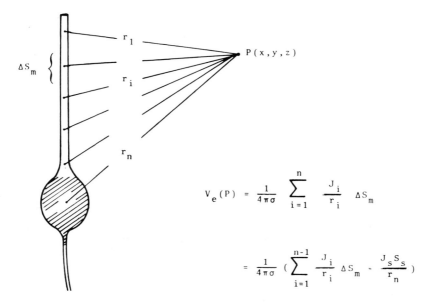

$$V_e(P) = \frac{1}{4\pi\sigma} \sum_{i=1}^{n} \frac{J_i}{r_i} \Delta S_m$$

$$= \frac{1}{4\pi\sigma} \left(\sum_{i=1}^{n-1} \frac{J_i}{r_i} \Delta S_m - \frac{J_s S_s}{r_n} \right)$$

Fig. 4. Variables relating the cell's distribution of membrane current to the potential at an extracellular point. During an action potential in the cell's soma (hatched region), current flows inward across the membrane, along the dendritic core, and outward at various regions along the dendrite. Extracellularly, the cell appears electrically as a concentrated sink at the soma, with a distributed current source along the dendrite. A first approximation of the potential at a point P is given by the expressions shown. J_s = instantaneous current density over the soma; S_s = somatic surface area; J_i = current density over the ith segment of surface area ΔS (*see* Humphrey, 1968).

$$V_e = \frac{1}{4\pi\sigma} \sum_{i} (J_{m,i}/r_i) \, \Delta S_m \qquad (4)$$

where ΔS_m is a differential element of membrane surface area, over which the current density is $J_{m,i} \cdot J_{m,i}$ will vary in intensity over the surface of the cell, and is defined as positive for outwardly directed current. In the continuous case, this sum is of course replaced by a surface integral,

$$V_e = (1/4\pi\sigma) \int_{S_m} (J_m/r) \, dS_m \qquad (5)$$

2.3. Dependence of Field Parameters on Cell Geometry and Size

2.3.1. Cell Geometry

The sequence of extracellular spikes that is recorded as an electrode is moved through the field of an antidromically activated *pyramidal cell* along a track parallel to its apical dendrite is shown in Fig. 5. At points superficial to the apical dendrite, the spike is negative, usually of 40-100 μV in amplitude when first clearly detected, and 0.5–0.8 ms in duration. At points nearer the apical dendritic trunk, the spike is positive-negative, reversing again to a negative potential (often of surprisingly small amplitude) as the apparent region of the soma is passed; if the electrode encounters the soma, a somewhat different sequence is seen, as is described below. Sequential recordings of this type have been obtained from antidromically activated cat pyramidal tract (PT) cells (Rosenthal *et al.*, 1966; Humphrey, 1968), and the sequence is at least partially predictable from core and volume conductor theory (Lorente de Nó, 1947; Rall, 1962; Humphrey, 1968). The sequence is somewhat different for antidromically activated PT cells in the monkey, with the negative phase being more prominent and the positive-negative phase less pronounced as the electrode is advanced through the cell's field (Humphrey, 1979).

Figure 6A shows, on the other hand, the sequence of extracellular spikes that is recorded as a microelectrode passes through the field of a *stellate shaped*, spinal motorneuron. Again the potentials that are shown are those that are recorded when the electrode does not encounter and penetrate the soma. In this case, the spikes are everywhere negative–positive, a result that has also been predicted for neurons of this shape with core and volume conductor theory (Rall, 1962; Humphrey, 1976). Indeed, the theoretical predictions are surprisingly accurate, as can be seen by comparing Figs. 6A and 6B. This is so despite the many simplifying assumptions about the spatial extent and homogeneity of the conducting medium that are necessary for computations of this type (*see* Humphrey, 1968).

Prior to use of the appropriate quantitative theories (Rall, 1962), it was believed that such differences in spike polarity and configuration resulted from differences in the degree of active invasion of the cell's dendrites by a propagating action potential (e.g., Fatt, 1957; Nelson and Frank, 1964); examples of such inva-

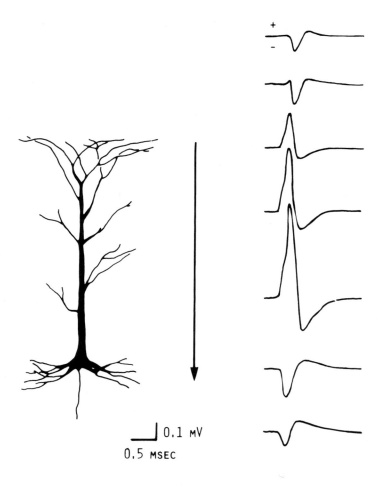

Fig. 5. Sequence of extracellular spike waveforms observed as an electrode passes through the field of a pyramidally shaped neuron in the direction shown. The spikes are plotted approximately at the depths in relation to the cell body at which they would be recorded. *See* text for further details.

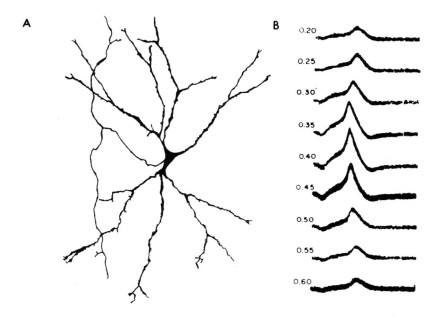

Fig. 6A. (Left) A camera lucida tracing of a stellate-shaped spinal motorneuron. (Right) Sequence of potentials recorded as a microelectrode passes through the field of an antidromically activated motorneuron. The numbers represent readings in millimeters relative to an arbitrary zero point. *Negativity is shown in this figure and 6B only as an upward deflection* (from Fatt, 1957 and Humphrey, 1976).

sion have in fact been found in other cells (e.g., cerebellar Purkinje cells). However, it is now known that differences in spike potentials of the type shown in Fig. 5 and 6 can be accounted for solely on the basis of differences in cell geometry, with active spike generation occurring only at the axon hillock (pyramidal cell) and/or soma (stellate cell).

In the case of the *pyramidal* cell, for example, a concentrated current sink exists at the hillock during the peak of the action potential, whereas the apical and basal dendrites appear extracellularly as distributed current sources. At points distant from the dendrites, the contribution to the recorded potential from the concentrated sink at the hillock dominates, and the spike is negative in polarity. As the electrode approaches the apical dendrite, however, the contribution from the outwardly directed membrane

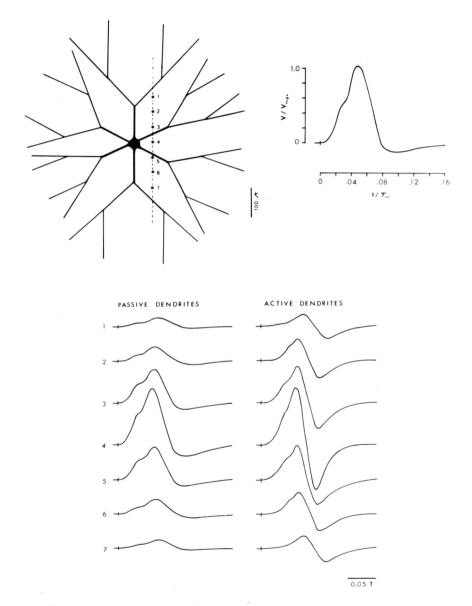

Fig. 6B. Computed extracellular potentials around an anti-dromically activated, stellate-shaped cell, assuming passive dendrites (lower figure, left) and active dendrites (right column of tracings). The

current dominates, and the spike is positive-negative. At points ventral to the soma, the contribution from the somatic sink again dominates, and the spike is again negative.

In the case of the *stellate* cell, the dendritic sources are much more diffuse and distributed, so that the concentrated sink at the soma dominates the recorded potential everywhere, except immediately adjacent to each dendrite (Rall, 1962). Consequently, the spike is negative at all points that are not immediately adjacent to a region of membrane with outwardly directed current.

One final case should be mentioned. If the recording tip approaches and abuts against the soma or a proximal dendritic trunk, the recorded potential is different from those illustrated above. In this case, a large monophasic positive spike is recorded, the amplitude of which may approach 5–10 mV. Such potentials have been termed "giant extracellular spikes" by some investigators (Freygang and Frank, 1959), and they appear to be generated by current directed outwardly across the membrane and across an extracellular resistance made higher by the presence of the electrode tip; the portion of the membrane recorded from may also have been made inactive by pressure from the recording tip. A more detailed discussion of this phenomenon may be found elsewhere (Freygang and Frank, 1959).

2.3.2. Cell Size

Using a lumped circuit analog, the peak membrane current (I_m) that flows into (and out of) a cell during its discharge will be given by the following formula:

$$I_m = (\Delta V_m / Z_{in}) \tag{6}$$

where ΔV_m = the amplitude of the transmembrane action potential when measured from the resting potential and Z_{in} = the neuron's input impedance when viewed from the site of the conductance increase.

←—————————————————————————————————

assumed model cell had six major dendrites, with secondary and tertiary branches; a drawing of its geometry is shown at the upper left. The assumed intrasomatic action potential shape at the soma is shown at the upper right. Time is in units of $T = t/\tau_m$, where t = time and τ_m = the membrane time constant. A modified form of Eq. (5) was used with core conductor theory to compute the potentials (from Humphrey, 1976).

The transmembrane action potentials of large (20–50 μm soma diameter) and small (10–20 μm) neurons do not appear to differ significantly, being on the order of 70–90 mV in cells of each size when comparable measurements have been obtained (e.g., Takahashi, 1965; Kernell, 1966). Since the input impedance of a large neuron will be *less* than that of a smaller cell, it follows that the discharge of the large cell will involve a greater peak flow of membrane current. Since the amplitude of the extracellular spike will vary directly with the magnitude of this current, it also follows that larger neurons will generate larger spikes than will small cells, and that their potential fields will be detectable over greater distances.

Data that illustrate this point are shown in Fig. 7. The curves in this figure show average extracellular-spike amplitudes as functions of distance (from the point of maximum recorded amplitude) for fast (large) and slowly conducting (small) PT cells in the monkey. The average spike amplitudes recorded from the fast cells, as well as the spatial spread of their potential fields, are clearly larger than the corresponding measurements from the smaller slow cells. Such differences are not simply the result of differences in electrode distance from fast and slow cells, for any systematic variation of this type would cancel out over a number of neurons. Moreover, in this case all electrode tracks were parallel to the fifth cortical layer, where fast and slow PT cells are intermingled (Humphrey and Corrie, 1978).

As will be further discussed below, such differences in the amplitudes and the spatial spread of the extracellular spikes of large and small cells introduce a systematic sampling bias that favors the isolation—by microelectrodes—of large neurons. Such biases must be corrected for if unit population data are to be used to estimate the functions of tissue that contains cells that have different response properties and that also differ in size.

2.4. Extracellularly Recorded Axon or Fiber Spikes

Despite their small diameter, it is not uncommon to record the extracellular action potentials of single fibers when a microelectrode is advanced into a tract or into the subcortical white matter. Single-fiber spikes may often be distinguished from the spikes generated by neuronal cell bodies on the basis of their shape and duration. As can be seen in Fig. 8, for example, cell body spikes—

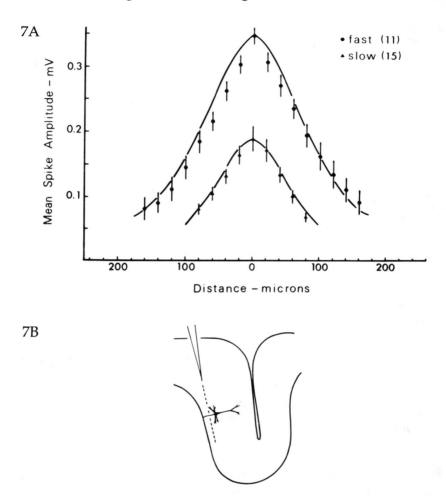

Fig. 7. (A) Average extracellular spike amplitude as a function of distance from the point of maximum recorded amplitude for 11 fast and 15 slow PT neurons. Each vertical bar represents ± one SE. (B) The cells were located in the anterior bank of the central fissure of the monkey's cortex, so that the fields were measured in a radial direction around pyramidally shaped neurons, i.e., along a direction perpendicular to the apical dendrite. Note in panel A the much larger maximum spike amplitudes for the fast (large) cells, and the considerably greater radial distance over which their spikes exceed the recording noise level ($\simeq$ 40 μV) (from Humphrey et al., 1978a).

whether the positive-negative spikes of pyramidal cells or the negative-positive spikes of stellate cells—are generally characterized by an inflection on the rising phase of the initial component of the spike; this inflection is thought to represent the transition from the axon hillock to the somatic spike, and is present with both anti- and orthodromic activation (Fuortes et al., 1957; Towe, 1973; Humphrey, unpublished observations); it is accentuated during high-frequency (usually antidromic) activation of the neuron. No such inflection is detectable on the rising phase of a fiber or axon spike (cf Fig. 8). In addition, although an axon spike may be bi- or triphasic, depending on whether or not propagation is only toward or actually past the electrode, the second (usually negative) phase is less pronounced than the second phase of a biphasic cell body spike. Finally, axon spikes are typically of shorter duration than cell body spikes, being on the order of only 0.4–0.5 ms in duration. Cell body spikes, on the other hand, are on the order of 0.7–1.0 ms in duration if both phases are measured.

3. Recording Methods

3.1. Construction and Electrical Properties of Extracellular Microelectrodes

The extracellular microelectrodes that are currently in use are of two basic types: (a) micropipets, filled with an appropriate electrolyte and coupled to the amplifier input stage with a Ag/AgCl or platinum wire; and (b) metal electrodes, electrolytically sharpened to micron tip dimensions and coated except at the tip with glass, varnish, or long-chain polymers that are deposited by vaporization (e.g., Parylene; cf Loeb et al., 1977). The electrical properties of these two types of electrode differ significantly, as do their construction methods; they will therefore be discussed separately.

3.1.1. Glass Microelectrodes

The glass micropipet, with a tip diameter on the order of 1 μm and filled with a 2*M* NaCl solution, is perhaps the most widely used microelectrode for recording extracellularly from single units within brain structures that are less than 6–7 mm from the surface of the brain, and in acute preparations where the dura mater can be

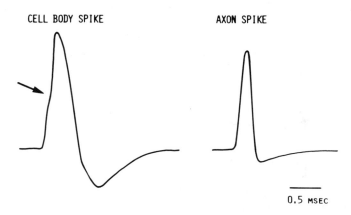

CELL BODY SPIKE   AXON SPIKE

0.5 MSEC

Fig. 8. Shapes of extracellularly recorded cell-body and axon spikes. Note the inflection on the rising phase of the cell-body spike (arrow), its more pronounced second phase, and its longer duration.

reflected. The electrodes are easy to construct and are capable of yielding recordings of comparatively low noise and high quality.

A drawing of a glass microelectrode is shown in Fig. 9, with the various portions of the electrode being labeled. In order to minimize tissue damage from electrode penetration, it is desirable to have the shank as long as the additional requirements of rigidity and mechanical stability will allow. Typical electrodes for single-unit recording in cortex and brain stem have shank lengths on the order of 10 mm, and tip diameters of 0.5–1.0 μm.

As is well known, micropipets are formed by electrode pullers, which are nothing more than devices for heating the center of a section of glass tubing for a length of 5–10 mm while applying a longitudinal stretching force to the two ends. With the correct combination of glass properties, localized heating, and pulling force, the tubing elongates smoothly, becoming thinner in diameter along the heated portion, but maintaining a constant ratio of wall thickness to lumen diameter along this same constricting region. Finally, the tubing ruptures at its thinnest region, yielding two (not necessarily identical) micropipets with open tips, the diameters of which are typically 0.5 μm or less.

A number of excellent electrode pullers are available commercially. Moreover, an excellent discussion of electrode pullers,

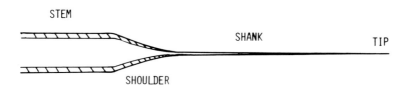

Fig. 9. Nomenclature for various portions of a microelectrode (from Frank and Becker, 1964).

the effects of heating temperature and pulling force on electrode shape, and microelectrode techniques in general may be found in an authoritative chapter by Frank and Becker (1964). Here we will present only a brief "recipe" for the construction of extracellular micropipets, which have been found to be suitable for recording from single units with a wide range of axonal conduction velocities and presumed sizes (e.g., Humphrey and Corrie, 1978).

Glass capillary tubing 1.0–1.2 mm od (e.g., borosilicate capillary tubing, or microfilament capillary tubing that has a glass fiber along one side of its lumen) is cleaned thoroughly and cut to 12–15-cm lengths by scoring the glass at the desired depth with a small needle file, and breaking it cleanly at this point. Micropipets are then pulled from these blanks, with heating coil current and solenoid pulling force being adjusted to yield an electrode with a shoulder that is approximately 3 mm long, a shank 10 mm in length, and a tip diameter of 0.5–1.0 μm.[†] If desired, the tip diameter can be enlarged to 1.0–1.5 μm in one of two ways: (a) by gently bumping the tip against the end of a fire-polished glass rod under both micrometer and microscopic control; or (b) by gently beveling the tip with a fine-grain, eccentric grinding wheel in the general manner described by Barrett and Graubard (1970) or by Brown and Flaming (1974). If microfilament capillary tubing is used, such enlargement is usually unnecessary for electrodes of optimum tip size (0.5 μm or so), and acceptably low resistance (7–10 MΩ when filled with 2–3M NaCl) may usually be obtained by

[†]This diameter approaches the limit of resolution in the light microscope. Tips smaller than 0.5 μm or so in diameter will have diffraction lines on either side when viewed under the microscope, so that their precise diameters cannot be measured using light microscopy.

simply varying the puller coil temperature and force values slightly.

The pipets are now ready for filling with an appropriate electrolyte. For extracellular recording, we prefer a 2–3M NaCl solution, since it contains the major ions found in the extracellular medium, albeit in considerably higher concentrations. If one desires to mark recording positions, the electrolyte may also be saturated with an appropriate dye, which can then be deposited at recording sites iontophoretically. At present, there are fewer satisfactory dye-marking methods for extracellular than for intracellular applications (*see,* for example, the excellent review by Tweedly, 1978). However, Fast Green FCF (Thomas and Wilson, 1965), Alcian Blue (Lee and Stean, 1969), Crystal Violet (MacNichol and Svaetichin, 1958), and Procion Brown (Freeman and Nicholson, 1975) dyes have all been used with moderate success, as has been the potassium-ferrocyanide Prussian Blue method (Bultitude, 1958; Humphrey, 1966). The original papers may be consulted for details.

The filling procedure is simplest for pipets pulled from microfilament capillary tubing. The electrolyte is simply injected from the butt end into the shoulder of the pipet with a 30-gage needle. The tip then fills by capillary action, with movement of the fluid being aided by the inner glass rod along the wall of the lumen. The stem may then be backfilled by injecting electrolyte as the needle is slowly withdrawn. This method is nearly foolproof, and the electrode can be filled with the desired electrolyte in a few seconds. Nonetheless, it is wise to examine the shank-tip region microscopically before use, to ensure that no air bubbles have been trapped during the filling procedure. If the pipets have been pulled from standard borosilicate tubing, they may also be filled by capillary action and backfill-injection; however, the movement of fluid from the tip inward requires several hours, and the electrodes must be kept with tips stored in the electrolyte, usually under a heat lamp so that the filling process is facilitated. Alternatively, they may be filled first with 95% ethyl alcohol by gently boiling them while they are immersed in an appropriate container in the alcohol, under reduced pressure (produced by a vacuum pump or line). Descriptions of these two methods may be found in Nastuk (1953). Obviously, the use of microfilament capillary tubing greatly simplifies the filling process.[‡] Moreover, micropipets with specifiable geometry and tip size, constructed from microfilament capillary tubing, are commercially available. Once filled, the electrodes are stored immersed in the electrolyte in a refrigerator in order to retard clogging of the tips by bacteria.

Electrodes that are prepared in this way have impedances of 6–10 MΩ when tested with a 1-kHz sine wave in saline. A simple circuit that is suitable for testing electrode impedance is shown in Fig. 10. In reality, micropipet impedance depends on the direction, frequency characteristics, and amplitudes of the currents carried by the tip; moreover, measured impedances in vivo may change markedly during electrode advancement, as the tip encounters and is infolded within neuronal and glial membranes. However, when tested in saline reproducible impedances may be obtained if small currents (10^{-9}–10^{-8} amps) are used; moreover, the appropriate test frequency for electrodes to be used for extracellular, single-unit recording is that in the neuronal spike range (1 kHz).

An additional, miscellaneous point or two should be made about the properties of glass microelectrodes. First, the minimum noise voltage that one would expect to be generated across a microelectrode of resistance R will be given by

$$V_{rms} = (4kTR\Delta F)^{1/2} \qquad (7)$$

where k is Boltzmann's constant, T is the temperature in degrees Kelvin, and ΔF is the recording bandwidth in Hz (Frank and Becker, 1964; Schoenfeld 1964). At room to body temperature

$$V_{rms} \simeq (2 \times 10^{-20} R \, \Delta F)^{1/2} \qquad (8)$$

Thus, with a 10-MΩ electrode and a recording bandpass of 5–10 kHz, one would expect minimum noise levels on the order of 20–40 μV rms. It is for this reason that recording microelectrodes should be constructed and filled with solutions of the highest reasonable conductivity, in such a way as to minimize electrode resistance. Indeed, contrary to popular myth, which views electrodes of high

[‡]*See also* Tasaki et al. (1968) for a description of the use of small glass fibers, introduced into the pipet before it is pulled, for enhancement of filling by capillary action. The principle is the same as that on which the Omega Dot™ tubing is based.

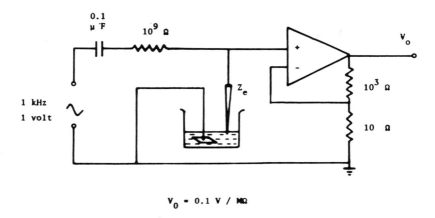

$$V_0 = 0.1 \text{ V} / \text{M}\Omega$$

Fig. 10. Simple circuit for testing microelectrode impedance in the spike frequency range. The amplifier is an FET operational amplifier with external circuitry for producing an overall gain of 100×. The electrode tip is immersed in agar–saline gel. The $10^9 = \Omega$ resistor is glass-enclosed (commercially available) to prevent leakage. With this circuit (and an electrode of 20 MΩ impedance or less), a current of 10^{-9} amps is injected through the microelectrode. With an amplifier gain of 100×, an output signal (V_o) is obtained, such that each 0.1 V of signal = 1 MΩ of electrode (and parallel shunt) impedance. *See* Frank and Becker (1964) for an alternate circuit.

resistance as "optimal" for recording from small units, the ideal electrode would be one with infinitely small tip dimensions and zero resistance. Unfortunately, this is impossible to achieve with either micropipets or metal electrodes, and small tips are to a certain extent necessarily correlated with high impedances. As we will indicate below, it is possible to correct this situation to a certain extent in metal electrodes with appropriate plating procedures.

A second point concerns the electrical properties of glass microelectrodes. These electrodes have a very high core resistance over the first few microns of the tip-shank region. In addition, the immersed portion of the pipet forms a cylindrical capacitor, with the capacitative "plates" being the inner and outer conducting media, and the wall of the pipet being the central dielectric. Although the most accurate circuit representation of a pipet in solution would be a distributed network, we can for present pur-

GLASS   MICROELECTRODE

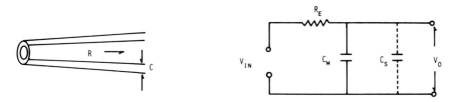

Fig. 11. Electrical properties of glass microelectrodes filled with a conducting electrolyte. (Left) The electrolyte in the core of a glass micropipet has a longitudinal resistance/unit length (R), and the glass wall of the pipet a capacitance/unit length (C) that affect the recorded signal. The core resistance is significant only near the small-diameter tip, and the wall capacitance only for the length of electrode that is immersed in the conducting medium. (Right) Lumped-circuit representation of the electrical properties of the micropipet. R_E is the total electrode core resistance, and C_W is the total capacitance across the wall of the immersed portion. Adding to C_W is the shunt capacitance, C_S, of the recording circuit. V_{1N} is the biological input signal, and V_o is the signal detected at the input of the amplification system. The absolute value or amplitude of V_o is given by

$$|V_o| = \frac{|V_{1N}|}{(1 + R_E^2 \, C^2 \, \omega^2)^{1/2}} \qquad (9)$$

where $C = (C_W + C_S)$, $\omega = 2\pi f$, and f is the frequency or major frequency component of the input signal in Hz. Thus, the glass microelectrode acts as a low-pass filter, tending to pass lower frequencies with little attentuation (and phase shift), and to attenuate higher frequencies. Eq. (9) relates the frequency of the input signal at which an attenuation of 30% occurs to the values of R_E and C_W.

poses represent the electrode by the simple lumped circuit in Fig. 11. Here R_E is the core resistance of the microelectrode in the region of the tip, and C_W is the shunt capacitance to ground across the wall of the immersed portion of the electrode. This circuit is, of course, that of a simple low-pass filter. Consequently, the input signal to the recording amplifier will decrease as the high-frequency content of the biological signal increases. For the simple lumped circuit shown, the input signal will be attenuated to 0.7× that of the biologic input signal at a frequency (*f*) of

$$f = 1/2\pi R_E C \tag{10}$$

Moreover, it will lag the input signal by a phase angle that also increases with signal frequency. The capacity of a glass microelectrode is on the order of 1.0 pF/mm of immersion (Frank and Becker, 1964; Schanne et al., 1968). Thus, with 10 mm of immersion, a 30% attenuation in signal amplitude will occur with a 10-MΩ electrode at a frequency of only 1.6 kHz, a value precisely within the range of the major frequency components of the action potential. Thus, appreciable signal distortion may occur if recordings are to be made from deep structures. This is a particular problem when attempting to record, for example, from deep diencephalic structures using a dorsoventral approach. Not only is the cumulative electrode capacitance substantial, but the cells are small, with small extracellular action potentials. In such cases, a capacity neutralization amplifier might prove helpful (Bak, 1958; Amatnieck, 1958), although such help comes at the expense of increased recording noise (cf Frank and Becker, 1964).

3.1.2. Metal Microelectrodes

In the literature there are dozens of "recipes" that describe techniques for constructing metal microelectrodes. Many of these are variations of and/or improvements on the methods described by Hubel (1957), Green (1958), and Wolbarsht et al. (1960) for constructing tungsten, stainless steel, or glass-coated platinum/ iridium microelectrodes, respectively. References to a number of the preparation and insulating techniques can be found in a paper by Loeb et al. (1977). The excellent papers by Gesteland et al. (1959) and Robinson (1968) should also be consulted for information concerning the electrical properties of metal microelectrodes. Here, we will consider only an outline of metal microelectrode "methodology."

3.1.2.1. WHY METAL MICROELECTRODES?   There are three major advantages offered by metal microelectrodes for extracellular, single-unit recording experiments. First, for signals in the spike frequency range, their impedance may be only 0.1–0.5× that of a glass microelectrode with equivalent unit-isolation properties; this is particularly true when the tip of the electrode is plated with platinum black (cf Wolbarsht et al., 1960). Thus, for this frequency range of signals, a metal microelectrode may offer superior (lower) noise characteristics. Second, when constructed of stainless steel, tungsten, or iridium, the electrode will have sufficient mechanical rigidity for puncturing (unscarred or moderately scarred) dura mater or other biological layers, with stem diameters of only 125–250 μm. Clearly, an electrode shaft of such small diameter is desirable when one must penetrate mechanically resistant tissue, or when the electrode traverses—in multiple penetrations—a region where minimal damage is desired. Finally, metal microelectrodes of desirable tip shape and size may be prepared in large quantities with comparable ease.

3.1.2.2. MATERIALS.   The majority of metal microelectrodes in use today are constructed of stainless steel, Elgiloy™, tungsten, platinum/iridium (10–30%), or pure iridium. Stainless steel microelecrodes (constructed from commercially available insect pins; cf Green, 1958) and Elgiloy™ (Suzuki and Azuma, 1976) have the advantage that recoding positions may be clearly marked by the Prussian Blue method (Green, 1958, Suzuki and Azuma, 1987), although at the expense of destroying the electrode tip. Marking lesions may also be made with other metal electrodes (usually by passing 10–20 μA for 20 s, electrode negative), but at the expense of blowing off insulation at the tip.

Platinum electrodes have the advantage of low noise characteristics (although these are not significantly better than those of other metals plated with platinum black) (cf Wolbarsht et al., 1960). However, for adequate rigidity they must be insulated with glass, a procedure that often yields an electrode with an od that is unacceptably large for deep and/or multiple penetrations.

Iridium and tungsten are both of sufficient rigidity to allow construction of extracellular electrodes of the type necessary for the penetration of dura and other tough membranes, yet with shaft diameters in range of only 150–300 μm when insulated. Moreover, tungsten microelectrodes may also be gold-plated and then platinized at the tip, yielding electrodes of great tensile strength and acceptably low noise (e.g., Baldwin et al., 1965; Merrill and Ainsworth, 1972). The impedance of iridium electrodes can be reduced by forming an iridium oxide film on the surface of the electrode. The oxide film is formed by potentiometric cycling of the electrode while it is immersed in a solution of sulfuric acid or saline. Nearly a tenfold reduction in impedance occurs at 1 kHz (Gielen and Bergveld, 1982) when the oxide is formed.

3.1.2.3. ELECTRODE SHARPENING.   The majority of metal microelectrodes in use today are sharpened to micron tip dimensions electrolytically, i.e., by passing an alternating or direct current through the electrode and a return lead (usually a carbon rod) in an appropriate etching solution. The metal is gradually etched away by electrolysis, and the taper and geometry of the electrode tip and shank may be manipulated within certain limits by varying the etching current and the dipping motion as the electrode is moved into and out of the etching solution. The articles referred to above may be consulted for details about appropriate solutions and currents. In addition, the paper by Freeman (1969) should be consulted for a mechanized method of slowly rotating a number of electrodes through an etching solution, so that large quantities may be etched in a uniform and reproducible way. Alternate methods of producing sharp tips on microelectrodes are grinding (Kaltenbach and Gerstein, 1986) and flame sharpening (cf Braga et al., 1977).

3.1.2.4. INSULATION AND ITS REMOVAL FROM THE ELECTRODE TIP.   This is a problem area in the construction of metal microelectrodes. Studies of the "sampling properties" of microlectrodes in cat retina, where three classes of ganglion cells with different properties and sizes have been identified, have suggested that glass-coated tungsten electrodes record successfully from the smallest cells only when the exposed tip dimensions are on the order of those shown in Fig. 12 (Stone, 1973; Levick and Cleland, 1974). When tested at 50 Hz, such electrodes have an impedance of 10–12 MΩ a value that would be expected to drop to 2–4 MΩ at 1 kHz; tip capacitance, tested at 135 kHz (cf Bak, 1967), is on the order of 5–10 pF. With considerable labor, electrodes with such tip dimensions may be constructed by following the procedure outlined by Levick (1972). In this case, a preetched fine tungsten wire is inserted into a pulled micropipet and cemented at the butt end. The tip may then be etched back under microscopic control, using a meniscus of etching solution trapped in a small platinum loop.

This procedure yields a microelectrode with the shank and shoulder dimensions of a glass microelectrode, with however, the attendant disadvantages of in-depth recording. Moreover, if a varnish is used as an insulating material instead of glass, it is difficult to obtain a cleanly exposed tip either by letting the varnish flow back from the tip under the influence of gravity or surface tension (cf Hubel, 1957) or by blowing it away by passing direct current through the electrode (electrode negative, 1–2 μA) while the tip is immersed in a conducting solution.

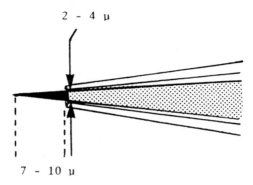

2 - 4 µ

7 - 10 µ

Fig. 12. Maximum tip dimensions found by Stone (1973) and Levick and Cleland (1974) to be suitable for recording from the smallest retinal ganglion cells. Similar dimensions should apply whether the electrode is insulated with glass or varnish, as long as the tips are cleanly exposed.

Loeb et al. (1977) have described an insulating material (Parylene) for metal electrodes, which shows great promise both for short-term, acute experiments and (in particular) for long-term implants (Schmidt et al., 1988). A high-voltage arcing procedure was described by Loeb et al., (1977) for cleanly exposing the tip of a completely insulated electrode; a modified form of this procedure is described below. Unfortunately, Parylene must be applied in an expensive vapor deposition process, making the technique un-available to most laboratories. On the other hand, Parylene-coated tungsten microelectrodes with specified tip dimensions are cur-rently available commercially, as are metal microelectrodes that have specified impedances and that are insulated with more tradi-tional epoxy varnishes.

3.1.2.5. ELECTRICAL PROPERTIES.   When a metal electrode is im-mersed in an electrolyte, chemical reactions occur at the interface. If the metal is partly soluble in the solution, its own ions may be involved in these reactions; if not (for example, as with inert metals, such as platinum), it may donate or receive electrons. As the reactions proceed, an electric gradient forms at the interface, which opposes further movement of (a net) charge. Charges that have already been transferred become trapped at the interface, forming an electric double layer. In brief, an *electrolytic capacitor* is formed at the exposed electrode tip–electrolyte interface. The value of this capacitance for bright platinum in saline, for example, is estimated to be on the order of 0.2 pF/μm^2 when tested at 1 kHz (Robinson, 1968). Because there will be some leakage resistance across this double layer, the tip of a metal electrode in an electrolyte may be represented electrically as a parallel resistance (R_T) and capacitance (C_T), as shown in Fig. 13. (Experimentally, it has been found that both C_T and R_T are not constant, but vary as $1/(2\pi f)^{1/2}$, where f is the applied signal frequency; R_T is also a function of the magnitude of the applied voltage. Thus, it is clear that this circuit representation is a crude approximation at best; cf Gesteland et al., 1959; Robinson, 1968). As with the glass pipet, a shunt capacitance to ground exists along the immersed portion of the shank and stem, the dielectric in this case being the electrode varnish or glass insulation. At immersion depths of 2–3 cm, this shunt capacitance may have a reactance at 1 kHz of only 2–3 MΩ; if the electrode tip impedance is of the same order or higher, it can be seen that considerable signal loss can occur.

For the simple circuit shown, the magnitude of the equivalent *tip* impedance ($|Z_e|_{tip}$) is

$$|Z_e|_{tip} = \frac{R_T}{[1 + (R_T C_T 2\pi f)^2]^{1/2}} \tag{11}$$

When tested in saline, it has been shown that the input–output phase angle for various metal microelectrodes is on the order of 45° over the frequency band of interest (0.1–10 kHz). This implies that the magnitudes of the capacitative reactance ($|X| = 1/C_T 2\pi f$) and resistance (R_T) are approximately equal. Thus, $R_T C_T 2\pi f \simeq 1.0$, and

$$|Z_e|_{tip} = R_T/2^{1/2} = (1/C_T 2\pi f)/2^{1/2} \tag{12}$$

For an exposed, conical tip having a length of 10 μm and a base radius of 2 μm (*see* Fig. 12), $C_T = 12$ pF, assuming a specific capacitance on the order of 0.2 pF/μm^2 (cf Robinson, 1968). Thus, at a frequency of 1 kHz, $|Z_{tip}| \simeq 10$ MΩ. Empirically measured tip impedances for platinum or tungsten microelectrodes with exposed tip dimensions of this order are actually lower than the theoretical value just computed. For example, a tungsten microelectrode with such tip dimensions may have a tip impedance at 1

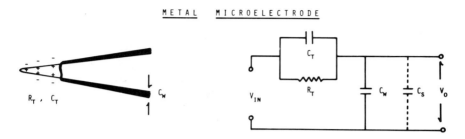

Fig. 13. Electrical properties of metal microelectrodes. (Left) An electrical double layer forms at the tip (*see* text), which has both a resistance (R_T) to current flow and an effective capacitance (C_T). The immersed, insulated portion of the electrode has a capacitance, C_W. (Right) Lumped-circuit representation of the electrical properties of a metal electrode. The tip resistance and capacitance (R_T, C_T) act as a high-pass filter in series with the input signal, V_{IN}, and the wall capacitance, C_W, as a shunt to the recording ground. DC or low-frequency signals are attenuated by the parallel combination of R_T and C_T, whereas high-frequency signals are attenuated by C_W. As shown in the text, the effective input impedance of the electrode is a decreasing function of the input signal frequency.

kHz of only 1–2 MΩ (Merrill and Ainsworth, 1972; Loeb et al., 1977). One reason for this discrepancy between experiment and theory is that the exposed metal surface is rough, which increases the real surface area of the electrode and reduces the impedance.

A metal electrode in an electrolyte behaves essentially as a capacitive element, with a tip impedance that is a decreasing function of applied signal frequency; in this respect, the equivalent circuit shown above is qualitatively correct. Moreover, it is clear that the tip impedance may be reduced to only 1/10–1/20 of that of an unplated tip by applying a layer of platinum black (cf Wolbarsht et al., 1960; Robinson, 1968; Merrill and Ainsworth, 1972). This spongy deposit greatly increases tip surface area by virtue of its surface invaginations, without greatly increasing the linear length and diameter of the envelope of the exposed tip region. Thus, tip capacitance is markedly increased and impedance lowered, with no marked impairment of the electrode's ability to record from small elements. Indeed, because of its superior noise characteristics, an electrode with platinum-black tip appears to be preferred for such applications. The references given immediately above should be consulted for the details of the platinizing process. When tungsten is used, an intermediate gold-plating step is also necessary (cf Merrill and Ainsworth, 1972).

In summary, metal microelectrodes suitable for recording from smaller cells within the CNS should have exposed (conical) tip dimensions no larger than 8–10 μm in length and 3–4 μm in diameter at the base. Unplated tungsten tips of this dimension usually yield capacitance values, when tested at 135 kHz with the Bak method (1967), of 6–10 pF; impedances at 1 kHz are on the order of 3–6 MΩ (with somewhat lower values if high-voltage arcing is used to expose the tip, which in turn roughens the exposed metal surface; cf Loeb et al., 1977). Electroplating the tip with platinum black increases tip capacitance several times, and can lower tip impedance, along with electrode noise, by a factor of 10. With iridium electrodes, the tip impedance and electrode noise can be reduced by forming an iridium oxide film on the exposed metal surface.

3.1.2.6. A RECIPE FOR EPOXYLITE-INSULATED TUNGSTEN MICROELECTRODES. The technique for making tungsten microelectrodes is similar to that described by Merrill and Ainsworth (1972), with the exception that, rather than collapsing a glass capillary tube onto the tungsten as insulation, 3–5 coats of baked Epoxylite are applied, so that the electrode is entirely insulated. The insulation is then removed from the tip with a high-voltage arcing procedure similar to that described by Loeb et al. (1977). Briefly, the procedure is as follows:

Prestraightened tungsten wire (0.010 in. diameter, 3–4 cm length) is cleaned in acetone with ultrasonic agitation. Each blank is then inserted into a length of similarly cleaned stainless-steel (SS) tubing, 4–5 cm in length (.022 in. od, .005 in. wall thickness; Small Parts, Inc., Miami, FL), and locked into position by gently crimping the tubing, or by applying SS flux and solder at the wire–tubing junction. The crimp must be applied lightly and at several points along the length of the tubing to prevent the latter from bending.

Ten to twelve electrodes are then etched simultaneously by rotating them through a 2–3M KNO_2 solution, using an apparatus similar to that described by Freeman (1969). Etching voltages of 4–8 V are employed.

The electrodes are then dipped in Epoxylite of moderate consistency (*see* Snodderly, 1973) and withdrawn smoothly with a small motorized rack and pinion assembly. The rate of withdrawal is controlled by varying motor speed, so that the height of the meniscus at the electrode–varnish interface is 0.5 mm or less. The electrodes are dipped twice in this manner, and are then allowed to dry in a dust-protected area (e.g., an unheated oven) for at least an hour. They are then baked at 120°C for 1 h. During both of these steps, the tips are kept pointed *downward*, so that the insulation does not flow back from the tip region. This entire dipping, drying, baking process is then repeated two additional times. (The intermediate air-drying step prevents formation of bubbles and drops at the tip.)

The electrodes are now ready for removal of the insulation from the tip. A single electrode is placed in a small plastic block that clamps it parallel to the X-axis of a microscope stage and allows it to be advanced along this direction by micrometer adjustment. A polished brass or stainless-steel rod (3–4-mm diameter, 10-cm length, with banana clip adaptor on one end) is positioned so that its smoothly rounded tip fills one-half of the microscope's field of view at a magnification of 100×. The electrode is positioned with the micrometer stage so that its tip is 50–200 μm from the tip of the rod. A high-voltage pulse (300–600 V, 0.25-ms duration) is then applied between the electrode and the rod. If the electrode is negative with respect to the rod, a "cone" of insulation is blown cleanly away from the tip over a length of 10–12 μm. The length of insulation removed is dependent in part on the electrode–rod distance, being greater for greater distances (*see also* Table II in Loeb et al., 1977). A single pulse is usually sufficient. If one is willing to sacrifice the very end of the sharpened tip, however, the electrode may be made positive with respect to the rod, and the insulation *and* the metal at the tip will be blown away *just at the tip region*. This latter method produces an electrode with a clean exposed tip of small surface area (10–20 μm^2). Tip capacitance readings at 135 kHz (Bak, 1967) are on the order of 10–20 pF, a value larger than expected when compared to those of electrodes whose tips have been exposed by current passage in saline or by retraction as a result of surface tension during drying. Apparently, the high-voltage arcing method produces a cleaner tip with a resulting higher capacitance/unit area. Impedances at 1 kHz are on the order of 1–2 MΩ. These electrodes are quite suitable for single-unit recording without further treatment, but platinizing will reduce impedances and noise levels even further. A diagram of the simple circuit used in the insulation-removal process is shown in Fig. 14.

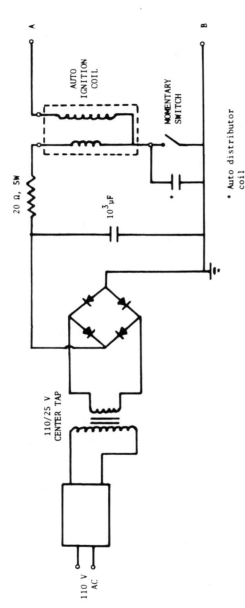

Fig. 14. Simple circuit for removing the insulation from the tip of a coated microelectrode by a high-voltage arcing technique. If terminal A is connected to the microelectrode, it becomes negative with respect to ground when the momentary switch is released. This voltage pulse blows the insulation away over a conical area, some 10–20μm in length, but does not destroy the tip. When B is connected to the microelectrode, it becomes positive with respect to the rod, and the tip and insulation in the tip region are blown away when the switch is released. A variac setting of 10–20 V and a rod–microelectrode distance of 50–100μm is typically employed. The auto ignition coil is a simple universal replacement coil (Sears and Co.).

Electrodes that are prepared in this manner seldom have insulation breaks, except at the tip. They may be checked for such breaks, however, by slowly immersing them, with a microdrive, tip first into saline, while checking electrode capacitance readings in the manner described by Bak (1967).

If desired, the electrode tips may be gold-plated and then platinized just before use in the manner described by Baldwin et al. (1965) and by Merrill and Ainsworth (1972). This yields a tough, low-noise electrode that is capable of penetrating dura and other dense tissue, and of recording from small neurons.

3.1.2.7. "FLOATING" MICROELECTRODES.   Some progress has been made recently in the development of miniature microelectrodes, which appear to be of greatest use for recording from reasonably superficial structures (e.g., the cerebral cortex). Such electrodes consist of very short lengths (2–3 mm) of iridium, platinum/iridium, or tungsten etched in the manner described above, insulated with Parylene, and then connected with very fine and flexible gold leads to a recording plug on the animal's skull or vertebral column. The electrodes are thus free to "ride" with tissue movements, and units may be recorded with them in a freely moving animal for relatively long periods of time. Fabrication and implantation of these electrodes have been described by Salcman and Bak (1976) and Schmidt et al. (1976).

3.1.2.8. WIRE ELECTRODES.   One of the simplest methods for producing electrodes for extracellular recording is to use preinsulated wire and record from the blunt end of the wire, which has been exposed by cutting transversely with a scalpel or sharp scissors. Strumwasser (1958) implanted 80-μm stainless steel wires in the mesencephalic reticular formation of ground squirrels and recorded single-unit neuronal data. Various electrode materials have been implanted, such as nichrome (Olds, 1965; Fontani, 1981) and Pt/Ir (Palmer, 1976; Palmer et al., 1979). Another technique for obtaining a recording surface on preinsulated wire is to grind a conical tip on 25-μm tungsten wire (Kaltenbach and Gerstein, 1986).

A clever adaptation of the cut wire electrode has been described by McNaughton et al. (1983), in which two 25-μm Pt/Ir (25%) wires are twisted together and cut transversely with a sharp scissors, so that the exposed recording surfaces lie at the same level. Differential recordings are obtained from each electrode and from a remoter reference electrode. The simultaneous recordings provide useful information for improved spike-discrimination techniques. A computer-based discriminator is commercially available for use with this electrode.

3.1.3. Carbon-Fiber Microelectrodes

Another technique for fabricating extracellular microelectrodes is to use a 7–8 μm carbon fiber that has been encased in a glass micropipet for strength (Armstrong-James and Millar, 1979). These electrodes appear to have recording qualities similar to those of tungsten microelectrodes (Fox et al., 1980) and are easier to construct (Anderson and Cushman, 1981). The carbon-fiber electrode can be silver-plated to reduce the impedance and noise (Millar and Williams, 1988).

3.1.4. Printed Circuit Electrodes

The most elaborate extracellular microelectrodes are those made with printed-circuit technology. Two excellent reviews on the subject were written by Pickard (1979a,b). The advantage of this technology is that large quantities of the electrodes can be fabricated with very precise dimensions. The disadvantage of printed-circuit electrodes is the need for specialized fabrication equipment that usually is not available to most physiology laboratories.

There are two basic types of printed-circuit microelectrodes. Passive probes are those that have one or more recording sites along the shank of the electrode, as well as conductors to the top of the electrode for attaching external leads. These probes may contain one recording site (Wise et al., 1970), 24 recording sites (Kupperstein and Whittington, 1981), or up to 40 sites (Edell, 1984), to mention just a few possibilities. Active probes, on the other hand, incorporate the structure of the passive probes, but also include active electronics for signal amplification and multiplexing, to reduce the number of lead wires connected to the electrode. BeMent et al. (1986) described a 12-channel active electrode with a per-channel gain of 100, a per-channel bandwidth of 100 Hz–6 kHz, and all signals multiplexed onto a single output lead.

Both the active and passive probes show great promise, but will be useful only if they become commercially available. Currently the 24-channel passive Kupperstein electrode is commercially available, and hopefully in the near future, active probes will be marketed.

3.2. Recording Circuits and Amplifiers

3.2.1. Connections to the Electrode and the Biological Preparation

When recording with glass micropipets, if both unit potentials and slow waves or DC potentials are of interest, it is desirable to couple to the electrode and to use for a reference lead a nonpolarizable material, such as Ag/AgCl. The use of such materials will reduce the flow of DC current in the recording circuit from metal–electrolyte junction potentials to a minimum, as well as reducing noise from chemical interactions that occur with polarizable materials at the electrolyte–metal junction. Usually a small Ag/AgCl wire is used for coupling to the electrode, and a coil of larger-diameter similar wire for a reference lead. Silver wire may be chlorided by placing it in saline, and passing a DC current through the wire and a platinum or carbon electrode (silver wire positive) at a current density of 5 mA/cm^2 (Geddes et al., 1969) for 20–100 s. A technique has been described by Grubbs and Worley (1983) that produces an Ag/AgCl electrode with lower and more stable impedance. First, the silver wire is cleaned in aqua regia for 30 s, and then plated with AgCl in saline at a current density of 50 mA/cm^2 for 120 s. The electrode is then cleaned by reversing the current for 30 s.

When using metal microelectrodes where nonpolarizable coupling materials cannot be used, a blocking capacitor may be used on the input stage. (It may be necessary, when FET amplifiers are used, to provide a shunting resistance to ground of some 10^8 to 10^9 Ω so that charge buildup does not occur at the FET gate). In all cases, the input lead from the microelectrode to the input stage of the amplifier should be kept as short as possible to reduce stray capacitance and signal shunting to a minimum.

3.2.2. Amplifiers

An appropriate amplifier for extracellular, single-unit recording should have the following properties:

1. A differential input stage with a high common-mode rejection ratio. This allows recording and reference electrodes, when positioned fairly close together, to be subjected to the same unwanted signals (e.g., 60-cycle interference), which then cancel.

2. An input impedance that is at least 10× that of the highest impedance electrode to be used, and preferably 100–1000× that value. In this way, signal loss across the resistance of the electrode is minimized.

3. A leakage current at the input stage that is less than 10^{-11} amps. FET amplifiers with extremely low noise, input impedances of 10^{11}–$10^{12}\,\Omega$, and leakage currents less than 10^{-11} amps are available commercially, thus meeting these last two requirements easily.

4. Sufficiently small size (or a small input probe stage) to be positioned close to the microelectrode. This is necessary to reduce capacitance shunting and signal loss to a minimum.

5. A gain of 100–100,000×.

6. Variable bandpass filters, with lower settings of 0.01–500 Hz, and high cutoffs of 3–10 Khz. Such filters allow the recording bandpass to be restricted to the range of frequency components in the biological signal, with an attendant decrease in unwanted noise frequencies. A line frequency notch filter is also useful to reduce power-line interference. For extracellular action potentials, the frequency range of interest is from approximately 0.2 to 5 kHz.

7. An input lead that can be switched remotely (e.g., a voltage-controlled relay) out of the amplifier input circuit and into a current passing circuit so that electrode positions may be marked, or to an impedance meter so that the integrity of the insulation can be checked.

Capacity neutralization capabilities may also be desirable (cf Frank and Becker, 1964) if the electrodes are to be immersed to depths greater than 2–3 cm and if signal rise time and amplitude are variables of importance. There are a number of excellent amplifiers available commercially that meet most or all of these requirements.

3.3. Microdrives

An excellent discussion of microdrives and micromanipulators may be found in chapters by Kopac (1964) and by Frank and Becker (1964). For extracellular recording, the microdrive should allow minimal control increments of no more than 2–3 μm. Moreover, as with all microdrives for single neuron recording, mechanical backlash should be minimal. That is, when the drive passes through a particular setting in the forward and backward directions, the paths taken by the electrode tip should be as close as possible, and the tip should set at approximately the same position, whether it is advanced or retracted toward that setting. There are a number of excellent microdrives available commercially, of both the mechanical and hydraulic varieties.

3.4. Improvement of Recording Stability

A small CNS neuron may have a spike potential that is detectable over a distance of only 30 μm from its soma. To record the spike train of such a cell with an acceptable signal-to-noise ratio, the tip of the microelectrode must be positioned some 10–20 μm from the spike generating region; at closer points there is a definite possibility of cell injury. Moreover, the electrode tip must maintain that position relative to the cell (within ± 3–5 μm) if the recorded amplitude of the spike is to remain constant, thereby offering some assurance that one is indeed recording continuously from the same neuron.

Contrast these requirements, now, with the movements of the brain that are observed when the sealed pressure system around it is opened and a portion of its surface exposed to the atmosphere. Movements of the exposed surface of up to 1.0 mm in amplitude may be observed in association with each arterial pressure pulse or respiratory cycle. Clearly, such movement must be minimized if any semblance of recording stability is to be attained, or the electrode must "float" with the cortical movements so that the tip of the electrode and the cell to be recorded remain in close apposition.

There are only three basic ways of immobilizing the cortex, although in practice a combination of all three methods is often used. First, the area surrounding the exposed region can be sealed and a constant-pressure environment reinstituted; appropriate coupling devices are then used, so that the electrode can pass through this region and into the brain without pressure leakage. Second, the brain may be widely exposed, and the CSF system that bathes it drained as much as possible. Since it is by way of this fluid system that pressure pulses are communicated most effectively to the brain (particularly cerebral areas), such drainage to a certain extent "decouples" the recording site from the sources of pulsation. Finally, the sources of pulsation may be removed, for example, by vascular perfusion with a nonpulsatile pump and by artificial ventilation at a high rate and low tidal volume.

In *acute* experiments, where the animal is anesthetized and is to be sacrificed at the termination of the procedure, the following techniques may be used: To minimize movements associated with respiration, suspend the animal so that the chest can expand freely. Perform a bilateral pneuomothorax at about the second intercostal space rostral to the diaphragm, and connect the pleural cavity to the atmosphere by two small plastic tubes (3–4 mm id), which are inserted through the small openings made in the intercostal spaces. Artificially respire the animal with a low tidal volume and high rate. It is wise to monitor CO_2 levels if possible to ensure adequate ventilation.

To further restrict movement at the site of recording, use one or a combination of the following three methods:

1. Make as small an opening as possible in the skull. Then, either penetrate the dura directly with a metal microelectrode or, after making a small opening in the dura, cover the exposed area with a clear and near-liquid saline–agar gel; the gel should be boiled first, until it is clear. The electrode is then inserted through the gel after it has begun to dry and adhere to the adjacent edges of bone, and thus restore a closed pressure system. As long as the electrode is advanced no farther than the shank through the agar, a reasonably good pressure seal is maintained. If it is removed, the system must be resealed with a fresh drop of agar–saline.

2. A closed recording chamber may be attached to the skull around the defect, which can then be filled with fluid and connected to the microdrive in such a way that a closed pressure system is formed. This is essentially the method used in chronic recording experiments with an alert animal.

3. Use a radically different approach. Expose the brain around the site of electrode entry widely, and drain the CSF by inserting a small polyethylene drain tube into the cisterna magna. Cover the exposed brain area with heated mineral oil and apply a small, contoured plastic plate or "pressor foot" over the site of electrode penetration, pressing it lightly against the brain, but with sufficient pressure to dampen movement (cf Amassian, 1953; Humphrey and Corrie, 1978). Care must be taken to observe circulation in surrounding pial vessels when the plate is positioned, to ensure that blood flow is not markedly impaired. The electrode may then be introduced through a small hole in the plastic plate. In addition, surface EEG recordings may be obtained near the site of penetration by means of a Ag/AgCl ball attached to the plate, and filed flush with its bottom surface.

In the *chronic* recording situation, it is obviously technique (2) above that is employed. If the animal is alert and moving, it is wise to use a chamber that is of low mass and short height, so that its moment of inertia is small. In addition, some method of head restraint is usually also necessary in order to obtain adequate recording stability.

An alternate approach for recording from exposed pulsating cortical tissue is to allow the electrode to "float" with the cortical movements. The simplest approach is to insert manually into the cortex a microelectrode of the type described by Salcman and Bak (1976) that is tethered by an ultraflexible lead. The disadvantage of this approach is that it is difficult to adjust the depth of the microelectrode in the pulsating tissue. Burns and Robson (1960) described a technique for suspending the microelectrode from a lightweight spring. Contact is made between the microelectrode and microdrive for advancing or retracting the electrode, and then the microelectrode is released at the desired location, so that it can "float" at the end of the spring during recording.

A very elaborate floating microelectrode recording system, developed by Goldstein et al. (1975), incorporates air bearings for frictionless movement of the electrode. The instrument will follow motion along the axis of the device and produce minimal contact force on the cortical surface. The principle of the instrument is ideal for situations in which immobilization techniques cannot be applied, such as in human recordings.

It should be mentioned in conclusion that problems of recording stability always appear to be greatest when one is recording from a region near the surface of the brain, and/or near the location of a major blood vessel. Apparently, pressure introduced by the electrode shaft is sufficient to dampen pulsations partially when recordings are obtained from deep structures.

3.5. Electrode Insertion and Advancement

If possible, microelectrodes should be inserted into the brain along a path perpendicular to the dural or pial surface. This reduces the possibility of bending the tip so that it slides along the meningeal surface or enters the brain at an oblique angle. We have found, for example, that even a robust tungsten microelectrode will bend progressively into the shape of a shepherd's crook as the microdrive is advanced, if it encounters the toughened dura in a chronic monkey preparation at an angle not close to 90°.

As the advancing electrode pushes against the dura or pia, the tissue is first compressed or "dimpled," and then the electrode "pops through" to arrive suddenly at layers III to IV of the cortex as the meningeal barriers are penetrated. The extent of compression may be as much as 1.5 mm when electrodes are driven through a scarred dura mater. Moreover, once penetration occurs, the tissue does not return immediately to a decompressed state. For example, in a technical experiment conducted in our laboratory several years ago, a tungsten microelectrode was advanced through the thickened dura of a chronic monkey preparation, and advanced smoothly into the depths of the cortex until an antidromically driven PT cell was encountered. The microdrive was then withdrawn slowly over time in such a way as to maintain a recorded spike of constant amplitude, thus allowing us to track the return movements of the tissue over time. The results were amazing! A total movement of some 1.1 mm was recorded over a time-course of 50 min, with the movement–time curve declining in an exponential manner, and with a time constant of approximately 14 min. Moreover, since PT cells are all concentrated in layer V, which is 1.5–2.0 mm from the pial surface, it can be estimated that a static compression of some 0.4–0.9 mm remained even after a period of 50 min. The extent of compression observed when penetrating through only the pia mater is, of course, much less, but it may approach a magnitude of 0.2 mm.

For these reasons, it is recommended that estimates of electrode tip position that are based on measurements of the depth from first electrical contact with the pia by the microelectrode be checked histologically as often as possible, and with the aid of small marking lesions. Moreover, it is advisable, after the first signs of unit activity are seen during insertion, to withdraw the electrode rapidly until such activity signs begin to disappear. This serves to allow partial decompression of the tissue after the original meningeal dimpling. The electrode may then be advanced slowly (preferably after a waiting period of several minutes) in small, rapid increments. Tissue distortion and drag are perhaps minimal when a microdrive is employed that is driven by a small stepping motor, which advances the electrode in small and rapid steps (e.g., the microdrive unit manufactured by the Kopf Instrument Co., Tujunga, CA). Some investigators also dip the electrode in medical-grade silicon fluid just prior to insertion, in order to reduce the coefficient of friction between electrode and tissue, and thus minimize tissue drag.

It is to be emphasized that the physiological effects of tissue compression of this type on neuronal activity are not negligible. For example, we have found that, if an electrode is inserted through the pia mater in an acute preparation (reflected dura), and then is advanced slowly with no delay through the layers of the motor cortex, an average of only 2–3 antidromically driven PT cells is encountered per electrode track. However, if the electrode is first inserted through the pia until unit activity is encountered, withdrawn until it begins to disappear, and then advanced in small, rapid steps after a waiting period of 10 min, an average of 7–8 PT cells are isolated per electrode track. Thus, even without the compression caused by penetrating a scarred dura mater, tissue compression by a microelectrode may yet be sufficient to obliterate spontaneous and evoked neuronal activity for a distance around the site of penetration for periods of several minutes.

For these reasons, we recommend the practice of first inserting the electrode until it is near the superficial border of the area of interest (using also the withdrawal method described above), and then allowing several minutes to pass before further advancement of the electrode, so that the effects of tissue compression can abate.

3.6. Isolating Single Units

There are a number of techniques and several criteria that are used by experienced investigators to "isolate" single units for observation. A useful technique is that of using a peripheral and/or central (electrical) stimulus, or a repeated behavioral response in the alert animal, that the investigator suspects will evoke or be associated with activity in the cells of interest. The electrode is then advanced slowly through the area under study, while the stimulus or response is continuously repeated. The rate of electrode advance should be such that several possible responses can occur before the electrode is advanced through the potential field of a neuron of the approximate size of interest (e.g., an advancement rate of 2–5μm/s when the stimulus or response repetition rate is on the order of 1/s). A second useful technique is that of using an audiomonitor coupled to the recording amplification circuit to "listen," as the microelectrode is advanced, for patterns of voltage change that signify nearby unit activity. The apparent increase in high-frequency "noise" as a group of spontaneously active cells is approached and the faint "swishing" sound of a small group of units responding with bursts of spikes to a stimulus are both clues used by the experienced investigator to recognize neuronal activity near the microelectrode tip before it is clearly detectable on the oscilloscope screen. Once recognized from auditory cues, the activity of the cells is further isolated electrically by cautious advancement of the electrode.

3.6.1. Unit Isolation Criteria

Useful criteria are as follows: *First*, the evoked potential is probably from a single unit if it has an all-or-none amplitude (at a single recording position) with near-threshold levels of stimulation—i.e., if the amplitude is not graded as stimulus intensity is raised. This criterion is particularly valuable for separating single-unit potentials from multiunit field potentials generated by the synaptic or spike currents of more distant cells, on which the spike potential of a single unit often appears to ride. An example is shown in Fig. 15A.

A *second* criterion is that of constancy of potential amplitude and shape, *while the electrode remains at a single recording position.* This criterion must be used judiciously, however, or potentials may be rejected that are indeed from a single neuron. For example, we have already seen that the configuration of the spikes that are generated by a cell will depend on the electrode's position within the cell's potential field. Thus, for example, if the electrode is near the spike potential reversal surface and small pulsations of the brain are present, the spike potential could in fact alternate in polarity with each arterial or respiratory-induced movement of the brain. Moreover, even at other recording points, the amplitude of the spike may vary if pulsations of the brain occur, since the electrode will move toward and then away from the cell with each brain movement. Finally, during intense synaptic activity, the synaptically induced membrane conductance changes may be of sufficient magnitude to shunt partially the currents generated by cell discharge. As these conductance increases develop, each successive spike in a high-frequency burst may be lower in amplitude than the preceding one. In a recording system with a low-frequency cutoff of 100 Hz (used to reduce 60-Hz interference), the extracellular slow potential associated with the cell's intense EPSP (excitatory postsynaptic potential) may not be seen, so that only a burst of spikes of declining amplitude is recorded extracellularly. An example of this situation is shown in Fig. 15B.

One final word of caution concerning unit isolation procedures should perhaps be added for the novice. It is a great temptation, when recording single-unit activity within a CNS structure, to concentrate principally on units with spike potentials that are large, easily distinguished from background "noise" levels, and easily held for required periods of observation. In structures with a range of cell sizes, such units are almost invariably among the larger cells. Yet, anatomic data show clearly that the majority of cells within the mammalian CNS are small, with soma diameters ranging from 10–20 μm (e.g., Jones and Wise, 1977; Humphrey and Corrie, 1978; Humphrey et al., 1978). The extracellular spikes that are generated by these small cells may

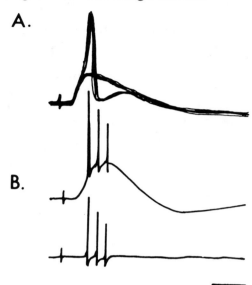

Fig. 15. Recognizing single-unit potentials. (A) An all-or-none re-sponse at threshold stimulus intensities allows a single-unit spike to be separated from background field potentials. (B) Large EPSPs and un-derlying conductance changes in a cell (intracellular potentials in upper trace) may shunt spike currents so that successive spikes in a burst are reduced in amplitude. With a high-pass filter in the recording circuit, only spikes of declining amplitude are seen extracellularly (lower trace). Hori-zontal bar: ca. 1 ms for A, 10 ms for B.

exceed an amplitude of 0.2–0.3 mV only in the immediate vicinity of the cell body; more often, when detected, their spike amplitudes are on the order of 0.05–0.1 mV (Humphrey and Corrie, 1978). Moreover, their spike potentials are detectable only over limited distances, making them difficult to "hold" uninjured by the elec-trode tip for long periods of time. Thus, the investigator must exert considerable self-discipline in order to sacrifice easily obtained, aesthetically pleasing recordings from large neurons, to sample in a more representative fashion the true neuronal populations that exist within the mammalian CNS.

3.6.2. Spike-Discrimination Techniques

Even with carefully prepared electrodes, it is often the case—particulary in the awake brain—that recordings are obtained from

2–3 U at a single electrode position. In this case, it is necessary to use electronic or computer methods to sort the recordings from each unit into separate spike trains.

The simplest method of separating single-unit spike trains is with the use of a simple *window discriminator* (*see* Fig. 16A). In such a device, the input signal is fed to two voltage comparators, whose reference inputs define the upper and lower limits of a "voltage window." Subsequent circuitry is arranged so that the device generates an output pulse only if a voltage signal that exceeds the lower limit of the window does *not* (within a following finite time period) also exceed the upper limit. By having several such windows, whose upper and lower limits are adjustable, it is possible to separate the spike trains of several simultaneously recorded units. The basic requirement for such separation on the basis of peak spike amplitudes is that the difference between successive spike heights be greater than the peak-to-peak "jitter" in the baseline recording signal produced by electrical interference and background biological noise. At least 29 articles have been published describing different methods of implementing window discriminators. Schmidt (1984a) reviewed the different methods that have been used to construct this type of discriminator.

A better method of spike separation is that of using a time voltage window discriminator that has variable voltage limits, duration, and time of operation with respect to the onset of the signal to be detected (*see* Fig. 16B). In this case the action of the discriminator circuit is triggered by a simple, low-threshold, signal detection circuit, which is thrown into operation when any spike exceeding the threshold occurs. The time voltage window (usually of a duration on the order of 20–100 μs) is then enabled at some variable time after the voltage threshold has been exceeded. If a potential occurs while the window is "open" and also falls within its voltage limits, an output pulse is generated. This method allows one to discriminate spike potentials of even identical peak amplitude, provided that, over some short interval during their time-course, they differ by the amplitude amount specified previously. A device of this type, which is also available commercially, has been described by Bak and Schmidt (1977).

A more sophisticated device that included two independent time window discriminators was described by Schmidt (1971). For a spike to be accepted, the spike potential has to pass through two successive time voltage windows.

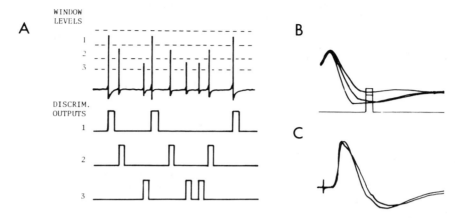

Fig. 16. Spike discrimination methods. (A) The simplest technique for sorting single-unit spike trains in a multiunit record is with a level or window detector circuit. Discrimination here is accomplished by difference in peak amplitude only. (B) A more sophisticated method involves the use of a time window discriminator. A discriminator output pulse will occur only when a voltage level occurs (and remains) within the window during a short time interval. This method allows discrimination of spikes of the same amplitude, but of different time-course. (C) The most sophisticated technique is that based on detecting differences from a stored "template" of the spike to be recognized over the entire waveform. Theoretically, this would allow even units with spikes as close in shape as those shown to be discriminated.

Proper operation of any discriminator can easily be verified by displaying the entire waveform of each accepted spike on a storage oscilloscope. Because a spike is classified only after it has occurred, the spikes must be applied to the discriminator and a delayed version of the spikes sent out to the storage oscilloscope. The storage scope is triggered from the acceptance pulse of the discriminator, so that ony the selected spikes are displayed. An instrument for accomplishing this verification technique has been described by Bak and Schmidt (1976).

Finally, the most sophisticated spike-discrimination device— and one that approaches the ideal—is one that operates on the configuration of the entire waveform, and perhaps certain of the signals that can be derived mathematically from it. This technique is accomplished by on- or off-line computer programs as described by Mishelvich (1970) and by Schmidt (1984b). Combined hardware and software discriminators are becoming commercially available for on-line discrimination.

3.7. Distinguishing Antidromically from Orthodromically Evoked Responses

For a variety of reasons, it is often necessary to be able to distinguish unit responses that are evoked antidromically, by direct stimulation of the cell's axon, from synaptically or orthodromically evoked responses. A number of criteria have been developed over the years for making such distinctions. Although none of these are completely foolproof, they will usually provide a correct decision when they are used collectively. The criteria are summarized diagrammatically in Fig. 17.

With *intracellular* recording, as shown in row 1, the two modes of activation are easily distinguished by the presence of an EPSP preceding the spike during orthodromic, but not antidromic, activation. However, with extracellular recording, the following criteria must be used.

The *first* criterion is that of *near-constant latency at threshold stimulus intensity* (Fig. 17, row 2). With such stimulation, an antidromically evoked spike will typically show a variation in latency (when the spike occurs) that is less than 20% of the spike duration. Such variation exists, of course, since even an axon's membrane potential and threshold are not constant, but vary continuously over a small range because of the "noise" inherent in many, if not all, biological processes. In contrast, a transynaptically activated cell will show a considerable variation in latency at threshold stimulus intensities, because of corresponding variability in the underlying processes (transmitter release, interaction with other postsynaptic responses, and so on); in general, the magnitude of this latency variability will increase with the number of synapses in the conduction pathway.

A *second* and related criterion is that of a *(comparatively) small decrease in latency when stimulus intensities are increased from threshold values to 2–3× threshold*. With such a change in intensity, an antidromically evoked spike typically will show a reduction in response latency of only a fraction of a millisecond. In some cases, this reduction no doubt occurs because the stimulating current

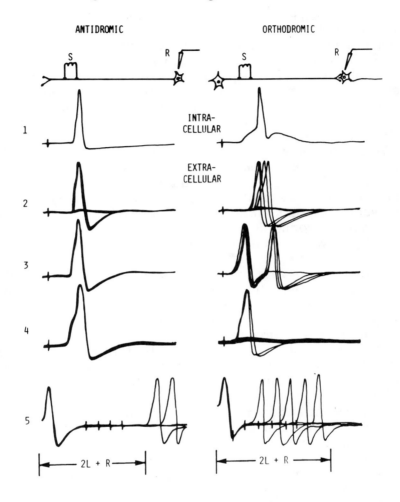

ANTIDROMIC   ORTHODROMIC

INTRA-CELLULAR

EXTRA-CELLULAR

Fig. 17. Criteria for distinguishing antidromically from orthodromically evoked spikes. Antidromically evoked spikes have the following properties: (1) Absence of EPSP preceding the spike in the intracellular record. (2) Near-constant latency at threshold stimulus intensity. (3) No marked reduction in latency at 2–3× threshold intensities, nor multiple spikes. (4) Ability to follow high stimulus-repetition rates without failure. (5) Collision between spontaneous and evoked spikes (with a "dead-time" interval equal to 2L +R). *See* text for additional details.

now spreads further along the axon, and excites it at a node of Ranvier that is nearer the recording site. With orthodromic activation, on the other hand, the decrease in latency may be on the order of several milliseconds, depending on the number of serial synapses in the transmission pathway and the extent of convergence of activated fibers onto postsynaptic cells. In addition, with increased stimulus intensities, the cell may begin to respond with multiple spikes (row 3).

A *third* criterion for antidromic activation is that of *faithful responding during high-frequency stimulation* (sometimes referred to as *frequency following*). During repetitive stimulation with a train of stimuli at pulse rates of 100–300/s, an antidromically activated cell will usually respond faithfully to each pulse in the train. In contrast, an orthodromically activated cell will respond typically only to the first few stimuli in the train, before beginning to respond intermittently (*see* Fig. 17, row 4). Often, such intermittent responding occurs with stimulation rates in excess of only 10–20 pps, depending upon the complexity of the synaptic pathway.

There are, of course, exceptions to these latter statements. For example, when antidromically activated neurons are part of a recurrent inhibitory circuit (e.g., as are PT cells in the motor cortex), they may fail to respond faithfully during high-frequency stimulation because of the surrounding inhibition generated by neighboring, antidromically activated cells. In some cases, the inhibition is not complete, but is manifest by a failure of the spike to invade the soma antidromically, so that only a small axon spike is seen following each stimulus. On the other hand, some monosynaptic pathways are extremely secure, responding faithfully to each stimulus even when delivered at rates in excess of 200 pps (e.g., the interpositorubral synapse in the monkey). For these reasons, we employ the frequency-following test with stimuli that are just suprathreshold for the unit under observation, and with stimulus trains that are at least 2 s in duration. The first measure reduces the probability of recurrent inhibition by reducing the number of antidromically activated axons; the long-duration train allows adequate time for failure of synaptic transmission resulting from transmitter depletion or other causes.

An example of a single unit that was activated both anti- and orthodromically by stimulation of the PT and nearby medial lemniscus within the brain stem is shown in Fig. 18. The responses in this figure illustrate some of the bases for criteria one and three.

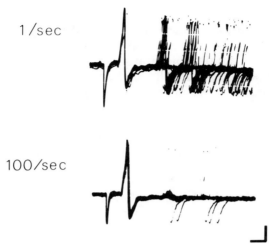

Fig. 18. Antidromically and orthodromically evoked spikes from the same PT (pyramidal tract) cell. An antidromic spike (first in record) is evoked by stimulation of the medullary PT in the monkey; later, orthodromic spikes are evoked by the same stimulating current, which spreads to the medial lemniscus. Note the marked difference in variance in latency (25–30 superimposed sweeps/record), the multiple spikes in the orthodromic response, and the failure of the orthodromic response at a stimulation frequency of 100/s.

A *fourth* criterion, and perhaps the best single criterion for concluding that a unit is activated antidromically, is the presence of a *collision between spontaneously occuring and evoked spikes* when the two are separated by an appropriate interval (cf Darian-Smith et al. 1963; Schlag, 1978). To perform the collision test, a circuit is needed that will allow both the oscilloscope sweep and, after a variable interval, the stimulating pulse that is delivered to the activating pathway to be triggered by the occurrence of a spontaneous spike at the recording site (i.e., on the part of the unit under study). The logic behind this test may be illustrated by referring to the pathway diagrams in the upper part of Fig. 17, the bottom row in the same figure, and by the following argument:

Assume, for example, that the cell is indeed activated anti-dromically by the test stimulus. Assume further that a spontaneous spike occurs at the cell soma (the presumed recording site) at time t_1. After the occurrence of this spike, a time interval L

(which is approximately equal to the latency of the cell's response to stimulation at the axonal site) will be required for it to propagate orthodromically along the axon to the stimulating electrode. During this time, any action potential set up by stimulation of the cell's axon will travel antidromically and collide with the orthodromic spike, thus failing to reach the recording site. Furthermore, after the orthodromic spike reaches (and passes) the stimulating electrode, a refractory period R must pass before the axon may again be reexcited by stimulation at that site. Thus, following the occurrence of a spontaneous spike at the cell's soma, there will be an interval

$$I = L + R \tag{13}$$

during which stimulation of the cell's axon will fail to produce a spike that reaches the (somatic) recording electrode. This interval is termed the *collision interval*. When it is measured between the time of occurrence of the spontaneous spike and delivery of the axonal stimulus, its value is given by Eq. (13). When it is measured between the time of occurrence of the spontaneous spike and the evoked spike, its value is given by

$$I = 2L + R \tag{14}$$

since the conduction time from stimulation to recording sites must be added.

Assume now, however, that the cell is activated transynaptically, as is shown in the pathway diagram on the right-hand side of Fig. 17. In this case, spontaneous and evoked spikes do not collide, and the minimum interval between them *will not correspond to the collision interval*, even though recurrent inhibition or some other process might set up a refractoriness in the cell after synchronous and spontaneous discharge by it and its nearby neighbors. Indeed, in the absence of such processes, one would expect the minimum interval between spontaneous and evoked spike in this case to approach the refractory period of the cell's membrane (e.g., as is shown in Fig. 17).

In practice, measured collision intervals are just slightly shorter than the formulae given above predict, apparently because of the way in which latencies and refractory periods are measured. The reader is referred to articles by Fuller and Schlag (1976) and Schlag (1978) for further discussion of the collision test, and for ways in which it can be applied to measure conduction time in axonal branches. In addition, papers by Towe et al. (1963) and Humphrey and Corrie (1978) may be consulted for additional discussion of the criteria for antidromic activation (*see also* Humphrey, 1968).

4. Sampling Single-Neuron Activity

The single-unit recording method is perhaps of greatest value when it is used in a systematic *population study* (cf Towe, 1973; Mountcastle et al., 1975; Humphrey et al., 1978; Georgopoulos et al., 1986). In such a study, a sensory stimulus or a behavioral response (if an alert preparation is used) is repeated under what appear to be quasi-stationary conditions, while recordings are obtained sequentially from single neurons within the neural structure or network of interest. The study typically spans several animals, and observations are collected from a sample of neurons that the investigator feels is large enough to represent the population under study.

The basic data that emerge from such a study are usually (a) a classification of cells with different response properties into a number of subsets, and (b) a description of the numbers (percentages) of cells of each type and their response properties. From these data, and those of correlated lesion and/or stimulation studies, inferences are then made about the functions of the tissue region under study, and the neuronal mechanisms by which these might be performed. Clearly, the inferences are bound to be affected by the statistics of the unit sample. For example, if, in a particular experimental paradigm with a moving animal, the cells in area X are found to fire in relation to the velocity of limb movement, then one is naturally inclined toward the interpretation that region X has something to do with limb movement, in particular its speed.

The basic population approach is used in many laboratories, and has provided much useful data. Yet it is quite clear to most investigators who use the method that its validity depends strongly on the adequacy and freedom from systematic bias of the unit-sampling procedures, and it is equally clear that there are a host of factors that can potentially introduce such bias, even when the investigator is experienced in the basic method and aware of the existence of these factors. The following rather simple example may help to illustrate how such biases can be introduced.

Let us assume, for example, that the cells in structure X can be divided into three subsets (A, B, and C), each of which processes sensory input in a different way or contributes to the control of a different parameter of movement (see Fig. 19). Let us assume further (a) that the number (N) of cells in each subset are such that $N_A < N_B < N_C$, and (b) that the average size (S) of the cells in each group is also different, such that $S_A > S_B > S_C$—in brief, a parent population in which the smallest cells are the most numerous, which is a common property of many CNS structures. Let us consider now the ways in which commonly used experimental methods might act to distort or bias the statistics of a sample of units that is observed within this population.

One obvious source of bias is the use of an anesthetic that obliterates in a selective fashion the responses of a particular subset of cells, while leaving others relatively unaffected. The fact that certain anesthetics may in even low doses effectively silence certain neuronal subsets, while leaving others relatively unaffected, is well known. Less obvious, but potentially a source of equivalent bias, is the selection of a sensory "hunting" stimulus (i.e., the stimulus employed while searching for unit responses) or a behavioral response that fails to activate a particular subset of cells in the structure of interest. Assume, for example, that type B cells fire principally in relation to inputs from velocity-sensitive receptors in a particular joint capsule, but that unit responses are examined only in relation to static limb position. Clearly, few recordings would then be obtained from units in subset B, and the conclusions concerning the functions of the parent population are biased toward those inferred from the activity of cells in subsets A and C.

A second source of potential bias is the use of a limited range of stimulus or behavioral response intensities, so that not all of the cells in structure X that might fire in relation to these variables are activated during the sampling process. This factor would not distort the *ratios* of cells of each type that are observed, but it would reduce their total number, and could lead to the (perhaps erroneous) conclusion that many of the cells within structure X must be involved in the performance of some other function.

Finally, there is the problem of variations in neuronal size (cf Towe and Harding, 1970; Humphrey et al., 1978; Humphrey and Corrie, 1978). For reasons that are outlined below, a serious sam-

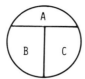

1. Parent population, with three subsets (A, B and C).

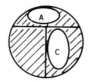

3. Limited stimulus- response intensity range activates only a portion of A and C cells.

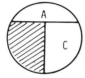

2. Anesthetic or stimulus- response selection pre- cludes detection of B cells.

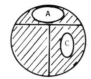

4. Size-related sampling bias results in isolation of only a few C cells.

Fig. 19. Potential effects of various experimental and physiological variables on the unit sampling process. Panel 1 depicts a parent population of neurons, with three subsets whose numerical sizes are indicated by the area associated with each letter. *See* text for further details.

pling bias and perhaps interpretive error can arise if there are subgroups of cells that differ markedly in functional properties, and also in geometric size. For example, the average size relation $S_A > S_C$ would tend to bias the sample toward an overrepresentation of A cells; i.e., their relative number with respect to B and C cells would be overestimated, as could be their functional importance.

The theoretical result of the joint operation of all of these factors is shown in Fig. 19. In this case, only two of the three subcategories of cells have been identified, and their estimated numerical ratios are the reverse of those that actually exist in the parent population. The conclusions that might be drawn from these results, both of which are wrong, are (a) that the nucleus consists mostly of unresponsive neurons (a conclusion reached by comparing the number of active cells observed/track with those expected on the basis of the packing density in the nucleus), and (b) that of the responsive neurons, the majority are of the A type.

What might be done to reduce such sources of error and/or to correct for their effects? Clearly, at our present stage of development in neurophysiological science, there are no well-tested and universally suitable remedies. However, there are some obvious measures that might be taken. First, for example, the effects of anesthetics on the population under study can be tested, when possible, by obtaining samples of smaller size from the un-anesthetized animal, provided that this can be done in a humane and acceptable fashion. Moreover, a wide range of stimuli and/or behavioral responses—covering a suitable intensity range—can be used in the initial exploratory studies, to determine if there are subsets of cells in the structure or network of interest that are active only with certain stimuli or responses. Such measures are clearly called for if an estimate of the number of responsive units in the structure studied is markedly less than the number one would expect to encounter on the basis of estimates of the average field sizes and packing densities of the cells sampled. Finally, if axonal conduction velocities can be measured, or cells in each category can be stained by microinjection and measured histologically, correction formulae can be applied to remedy the distortions in the unit sample statistics that arise from variations in cell size (*see below* and Humphrey et al., 1978).

It should be clear from these remarks that one of the areas in single-unit methodology that is currently in need of greatest research is that of further identifying possible sources of sampling error, and devising methods that can be used to correct for their effects. Until such developments emerge, conclusions about the functions of CNS structures that are based solely upon unit population studies must necessarily be accepted with caution.

4.1. How Sampling Biases Can Arise from Variations in Cell Size

Perhaps the first formal consideration of the effects of cell size upon single-unit sampling processes is that by Towe and Harding (1970), who used an empirical curve-fitting procedure to estimate the magnitude of the bias that affected samples of cat PT neurons. This paper is a classic, and should be consulted by all who are interested in this problem area. Here, we shall consider additional factors, not clearly addressed in the Towe and Harding paper, that may serve to clarify intuitively just how variations in neuronal size can lead to systematic biases in extracellular recording studies. Some of these arguments have been presented previously (Humphrey and Corrie, 1978; Humphrey et al., 1978).

There are perhaps three ways in which a systematic sampling error may arise from variations in cell size. *First,* a failure to detect the spikes of very small cells can occur when the exposed length of the microelectrode tip begins to approach some appreciable fraction of the dimensions of the steeper part of the voltage gradient that surrounds a discharging neuron. This is particularly true if the field contains both positive and negative potential areas during the peak of the action potential (e.g., as in the field of a pyramidal cell). Imagine, for example, a small neuron whose spike potential varies from an amplitude of 0.1–0.05mV over a distance of only 20–30 μm in the vicinity of the cell body. An electrode with an exposed tip length that lies within or spans this region will present an isopotential surface that can distort the cell's action currents and literally "short out" the potential variations that would normally occur along the region occupied by the exposed metal. At best, the recorded potential would be some average of that along this exposed region of metal, or on the order of only 0.04–0.05 mV with respect to ground. Yet this same electrode could easily detect the spikes of larger cells, both because they are larger to start with, and because the dimensions of their extracellular fields are considerably larger than those of the electrode tip.

A *second* source of bias is differential cell injury. Because the spikes of a small cell are detectable with acceptable signal-to-noise ratio over a comparatively small distance, an electrode must lie much closer to its soma and major dendritic trunks than is the case when recording from a large cell. As a result, there is a greater probability of injuring the small neuron before adequate data can be obtained. This factor naturally predisposes a sample toward a spuriously high representation of larger neurons.

Finally, however, even with tip dimensions that are very small and recording stability so good that one can safely record from even the smallest neuron, a sampling bias will exist in *extra*cellular recording studies simply because the spikes of large cells are detectable over greater distances than are those of small cells (*see,* for example, Fig. 7). The following example may help to illustrate how such differences in field size can introduce a bias that favors the isolation of large neurons.

Consider an experiment in which extracellular recordings are obtained across a series of transcortical electrode tracks from two functionally different classes of cells (A and B). Assume, for simplicity, that the cells *within* each class are nearly homogeneous in size and shape, and consider two hypothetical cases.

Case 1: No difference in average cell size across groups. In this case, the fields generated by the cells of each type will be roughly equivalent. Thus, if no other factor exists that favors the isolation of one cell type over the other (e.g., differences in levels of spontaneous activity, responsiveness to various stimuli, and so on), their *relative* densities within the tissue under study will be estimated accurately by the ratio $(R_{A:B})$ of the average number of each type (N_A, N_B) observed electrode track:

$$R_{AB:B} = N_A/N_B \qquad (15)$$

Case 2: Cells in one class larger than those in the other. Assume, for example, that A cells are larger than B cells, and that along each electrode track recordings are obtained from all cells of each type whose observed spikes are greater in amplitude than some minimum (and constant) voltage value, V_{min}. In this case, the spikes of the smaller *B* cells may be greater than V_{min} only if the discharging neurons lie within a particular radial distance (r_1) of the electrode track, as is shown schematically in Fig. 20. Thus, each electrode track will define the axis of a nearly cylindrical *effective recording volume* (U_{eff}) of magnitude

$$U_{eff}(B) = \pi\, r_1^2 h_1 \qquad (16)$$

where $r_1 =$ the maximum radial distance that a type B cell may lie from the electrode track and yet have its observed spike exceed V_{min} in amplitude, and $h_1 =$ the thickness of the region of cortex under study (for tracks normal to the cortical surface) or of the cortical layers that contain type B neurons.

Note now, however, that because of their larger sizes A neurons may generate spikes that exceed V_{min} even when they are located at a much greater distance from the electrode track than are detectable B cells. Thus, the effective recording volume will be significantly larger for A than for B cells, as is shown schematically in Fig. 20.

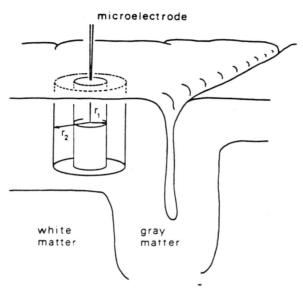

Fig. 20. Concept of effective recording volume. An electrode traversing the cerebral cortex (or any other structure) will record from all cells within a roughly cylindrical area. Since the fields of larger cells can be detected over a greater distance, this cylindrical volume will be larger when recording from large cells than when recording from small cells. For example, small cells may be detectable only when they lie within the radial distance r_1 from the electrode track, whereas larger cells may generate spikes that can be detected as long as they lie within the radial distance r_2 from the track. Thus, the volume of tissue "sampled" depends on the size of the cells recorded from.

Thus, it is clear that *the volume of tissue that a microelectrode "sees" or "samples" as it traverses a given region is not constant, but is in fact an increasing function of the size of the cells from which the recordings are obtained.* This volume is larger when recording from larger neurons and introduces a systematic bias that will lead—if uncorrected—to a spuriously high estimate of the relative densities of the larger cells. In the second case considered above, for example, the experimentally observed or biased ratio of large to small cell densities would be given by

$$R_{A:B} = N_A/N_B \qquad (17)$$

where again N_A and N_B are the average numbers of each type observed/electrode track. The *true* or unbiased ratio would be given, however, by

$$R'_{A:B} = (N_A/U_{eff}(A)/(N_B/U_{eff}(B))) \qquad (18)$$

Thus, to arrive at an unbiased estimate of the relative densities of cells of different sizes, it is necessary to divide experimentally obtained measures of their apparent densities by an estimate of their respective effective recording volumes.

With the use of

1. mathematical neuron models of the type employed by Rall (1962)
2. experimentally obtained measurements of axonal conduction velocities and
3. measurements of soma diameter distributions in populations of HRP-labeled neurons

it has been shown that the effective recording volumes for cortical pyramidal tract cells are proportional to the following quantities (Humphrey and Corrie, 1978; Humphrey et al., 1978a):

$$U_{eff} \propto v \text{ to } v^{3/2}$$

and

$$U_{eff} \propto d^2 \qquad (19)$$

where v = axonal conduction velocity, and d = transverse soma diameter. Thus, if either of these quantities are measurable from the populations under study, a correction may be made for the effects of size-related sampling bias. An example of application of this technique may be found in Humphrey and Corrie (1978) and Humphrey et al. (1978).

To what extent are such corrections necessary? Clearly, this will depend both on the nature of the cell populations under study and on the nature of the experimental questions asked. When all cells are of approximately the same size, or if functionally different groups have similar size distributions, then the effects of size-related bias should be negligible. An answer to this question will have to be formulated by each investigator in accordance with the properties of the populations under study and the information sought.

References

Amassian V. E. (1953) Evoked single cortical unit activity in the somatic sensory areas. *Electroencephalogr. Clin. Neurophysiol.* **5,** 415–438.

Amatnieck E. (1958) Measurement of bioelectric potentials with micro-electrodes and neutralized input capacity amplifiers. IRE Trans. Med. Electronics **PGME-10,** 3–14.

Anderson C. W. and Cushman M. R. (1981) A simple and rapid method for making carbon fiber microelectrodes. *J. Neurosci. Methods* **4,** 435–436.

Armstrong-James M. and Millar J. (1979) Carbon fibre microelectrodes. *J. Neurosci. Methods* **1,** 279–287.

Bak A. F. (1958) A unity gain cathode follower. *Electroencephalogr. Clin. Neurophysiol.* **10,** 745–748.

Bak A. F. (1967) Testing metal microelectrodes. *Electroencephalogr. Clin. Neurophysiol.* **22,** 186–187.

Bak M. J. and Schmidt E. M. (1976) An analog delay circuit for on-line visual confirmation of discriminated neuroelectric signals. *IEEE Trans. Biomed. Eng.* **BME-18,** 155–157.

Bak M. J. and Schmidt E. M. (1977) An improved time–amplitude window discriminator. *IEEE Trans. Biomed. Eng.* **BME-24,** 486–489.

Baldwin H. A., Frenk S., and Lettvin J. Y. (1965) Glass-coated tungsten microelectrodes. *Science* **148,** 1462–1464.

Barrett J. N. and Graubard K. (1970) Fluorescent staining of cat motoneurons in vivo with bevelled micropipettes. *Brain Res.* **18,** 565–568.

BeMent S. L., Wise K. D., Anderson D. J., Najafi K., and Drake K. L. (1986) Solid-state electrodes for multichannel multiplexed intracortical neuronal recordings. *IEEE Trans. Biomed. Eng.* **BME-33,** 230–241.

Braga P. C., Dall'oglio G., and Fraschini F. (1977) Microelectrode tip in five seconds. A new simple, rapid, inexpensive method. *Electroencephalogr. Clin. Neurophysiol.* **42,** 840–842.

Brown K. T. and Flaming P. G. (1974) Bevelling of fine micropipettes by a rapid precision method. *Science* **185,** 693–695.

Bultitude K. H. (1958) *Quart. J. Microscop. Sci.* **99,** 61.

Burns B. D. and Robson J. G. "Weightless" microelectrodes for recording extracellular unit action potentials from the central nervous system. *Nature* **186,** 246–247.

Darian-Smith I., Pillips G., and Ryan R. D. (1963) Functional organization in trigeminal main sensory and rostral spinal nuclei of the cat. *J. Physiol.* (Lond.) **168,** 129–146.

DeValois R. I. and Pease P. L. (1973) Extracellular unit recording, in *Bioelectric Recording Techniques*, Part A, (Thompson R. F. and Patterson M. M. eds.) Academic, New York, pp. 95–135.

Edell D. J. (1984) Basic design considerations for chronically implantable neural information sensors. *IEEE Solid State Sensors Conf.* 44–46.

Evarts E. V. (1968) Relation of pyramidal tract activity to force exerted during voluntary movement. *J. Neurophysiol.* **31,** 14–27.

Fatt P. (1957) Electric potentials occurring around a neuron during its antidromic activation. *J. Neurophysiol.* **20,** 27–60.

Fontani G. (1981) A technique for long term recording from single neurons in unrestrained behaving animals. *Physiol. Behav.* 26: 331–333.

Fox K., Armstrong-James M., and Millar J. (1980) The electrical characteristics of carbon fibre microelectrodes. *J. Neurosci. Methods* **3,** 37–48.

Frank, K. and Becker M. C. (1964) Microelectrodes for recording and stimulation, in *Physical Techniques in Biological Research,* vol. 5, part A (Nastuk W., ed.), Academic, New York, pp. 22–87.

Frank K. and Fuortes M. G. F. (1955) Potentials recorded from the spinal cord with microelectrodes. *J. Physiol. (Lond.)* **130,** 625–654.

Freeman J. A. (1969) A simple method of producing in quantity metal microelectrodes with desired taper and impedance. *Electroencephalogr. Clin. Neurophysiol.* **26,** 623–626.

Freeman J. A. and Nicholson C. (1975) Experimental optimization of current source-density technique for anuran cerebellum. *J. Neurophysiol.* **38,** 369–382.

Freygang W. H. and Frank K. (1959) Extracellular potentials from single spinal motoneurons. *J. Gen. Physiol.* **42,** 749–760.

Fuller J. H. and Schlag J. D. (1976) Determination of antidromic excitation by the collision test: Problems of interpretation. *Brain Res.* **112,** 283–298.

Fuortes M. G. F., Frank K., and Becker M. C. (1957) Steps in the production of motoneuron spikes. *J. Gen. Physiol.* **40,** 735–752.

Geddes L. A., Baker L. E., and Moore A. G. (1969) Optimum electrolytic chloriding of silver electrodes. *Med. Biol. Eng.* **7,** 49–56.

Georgopoulos A. P., Schwartz A. B., and Kettner R. E. (1986) Neural population coding of movement direction. *Science* **233,** 1416–1419.

Gesteland R. C., Howland B., Lettvin J. Y., and Pitts W. H. (1959) Comments on microelectrodes. *Proc. IRE* **47,** 1856–1862.

Gielen F. L. H. and Bergveld P. (1982) Comparison of electrode impedance of Pt, PtIr (10%) and Ir-AIROF electrodes used in electrophysiological experiments. *Med. Biol. Eng. Comput.* **20,** 77–83.

Goldstein S. R., Bak M. J., Oakley J. C., Schmidt E. M., and VanBuren J. M. (1975) An instrument for stable single cell recording from pulsating human cerebral cortex. *Electroencephalogr. Clin. Neurophysiol.* **39,** 667–670.

Green J. D. (1958) A simple microelectrode for recording from the central nervous system. *Nature* **182,** 962.

Grubbs D. S. and Worley D. S. (1983) New techniques for reducing the impedance of silver-silver chloride electrodes. *Med Biol. Eng. Comput.* **21,** 232–234.

Hubel D. H. (1957) Tungsten microelectrode for recording from single units. *Science* **125,** 549–550.

Humphrey D. R. (1966) Regions of the medulla oblongata mediating carotid sinus reflexes: An electrophysiological study. Ph.D. thesis, University of Washington.

Humphrey D. R. (1968) Re-analysis of the antidromic cortical response. II. On the contribution of cell discharge and PSPs to the evoked potentials. *Electroencephalogr. Clin. Neurophysiol.* **25,** 421–442.

Humphrey D. R. (1976) Neural networks and systems modeling. in *Biological Foundations of Biomedical Engineering,* (Kline J., ed.), Little, Brown and Co., Boston, pp. 639–672.

Humphrey D. R. (1979) Extracellular, single-unit recording methods, in *Electrophysiological Techniques* (Humphrey D. R., ed.), Society for Neuroscience, Bethesda, pp. 199–261.

Humphrey D. R. and Corrie W. S. (1978) Properties of the pyramidal tract neuron system within a functionally defined subregion of primate motor cortex. *J. Neurophysiol.* **41,** 216–243.

Humphrey D. R., Corrie W. S., and Rietz R. R. (1978) Properties of the pyramidal tract neuron system within the precentral wrist and hand area of primate motor cortex. *J. Physiol (Paris)* **74,** 215–226.

Jones E. G. and Wise S. P. (1977) Size, laminar and columnar distribution of efferent cells in the sensory-motor cortex of monkeys. *J. Comp. Neurol.* **175,** 391–438.

Kaltenbach J. A. and Gerstein G. L. (1986) A rapid method for production of sharp tips on preinsulated microwires. *J. Neurosci. Methods* **16,** 283–288.

Kernell, D. (1966) Input resistance, electrical excitability and size of ventral horn cells in cat spinal cord. *Science* **152,** 1637–1640.

Kopac M. J. (1964) Micromanipulators: Principles of design, operation and application, in *Physical Techniques in Biological Research,* vol. 5 (Nastuk W., ed.) Academic, New York, pp. 191–233.

Kupperstein M. and Whittington D. A. (1981) A practical 24 channel microelectrode for neural recording in vivo. *IEEE Trans. Biomed. Eng.* **BME-28,** 288–293.

Lee B. B. G. and Stean J. P. B. (1969) Micro-electrode tip position marking in nervous tissue: A new dye method. *Electroencephalogr. Clin. Neurophysiol.* **27,** 610–613.

Levick W. R. (1972) Another tungsten microelectrode. *Med. Biol. Eng.* **10,** 510–515.

Levick W. R. and Cleland B. G. (1974) Selectivity of microelectrodes in recordings from cat retinal ganglion cells. *J. Neurophysiol.* **37,** 1387–1393.

Loeb G. E., Bak M. J., Salcman M., and Schmidt E. M. (1977) Parylene as a chronically stable, reproducible microelectrode insulator. *IEEE Trans. Biomed. Eng.* **BME-24,** 121–128.

Lorente de Nó R. (1947) Action potential of the motoneurones of the hypoglossus nucleus. *J. Cell. Comp. Physiol.* 29, 207–288.

MacNichol E. F. Jr. and Svaetichin G. (1958) *Am. J. Ophthalmol.* **46,** 26.

McNaughton B. L., O'Keefe J., and Barnes C. A. (1983) The stereotrode: A new technique for simultaneous isolation of several single units in the central nervous system from multiple unit records. *J. Neurosci. Methods* **8,** 391–397.

Merrill D. G. and Ainsworth A. (1972) Glass-coated platinum-plated tungsten microelectrodes. *Med. Biol. Eng.* **10,** 662–672.

Millar J. and Williams G. V. (1988) Ultra-low noise silver-plated carbon fibre microelectrodes. *J. Neurosci. Methods* **25,** 50–62.

Mishelevich D. J. (1970) On-line real-time digital computer separation of extracellular neuroelectric signals. *IEEE Trans. Biomed. Electronics* **BME-17,** 147–150.

Mountcastle V. B., Lynch J. C., Georgopoulus A., Sakata H., and Acuna C. (1975) Posterior parietal association cortex of the monkey: Command functions for operations within extrapersonal space. *J. Neurophysiol.* **38,** 871–908.

Nastuk W. (1953) The electrical activity of the muscle cell membrane at the neuromuscular junction. *J. Cell. Comp. Physiol.* **42,** 249–272.

Nelson P. G. and Frank K. (1964) Extracellular potential fields of single spinal motoneurons. *J. Neurophysiol.* **27,** 913–927.

Olds J. (1965) Operant conditioning of single unit responses. *Proc. XXIII Int. Congr. Physiol. Union* (Tokyo) **4,** 372–380.

Palmer C. (1976) A microwire technique for long term recording of single units in the brains of unrestrained animals. *J. Physiol.* (Lond.) **263,** 99P–101P.

Palmer C., Bak M. G., Dold G. M., and Schmidt E. M. (1979) Stable simultaneous single unit recordings from groups of motor cortical neurons in the unanesthetized and unrestrained cat. *Soc. Neurosci. Abstr.* **5**, 381.

Pickard R. S. (1979a) Printed circuit microelectrodes. *Trends Neurosci.* **2**, 259–261.

Pickard R. S. (1979b) A review of printed circuit microelectrodes and their production. *J. Neurosci. Methods* **1**, 301–318.

Rall W. (1962) Electrophysiology of a dendritic neuron model. *Biophys. J.* **2**, 145–167.

Rosenthal F., Woodbury W. J., and Patton H. D. (1966) Dipole characteristics of pyramidal cell activity in cat postcruciate cortex. *J. Neurophysiol.* **29**, 612–625.

Robinson D. A. (1968) The electrical properties of metal microelectrodes. *Proc. IEEE* **56**, 1065–1071.

Salcman M. and Bak M. J. (1976) A new chronic recording intracortical microelectrode. *Med. Biol. Eng.* **14**, 42–50.

Schanne O. F., Lavallee M., Laprade R., and Gagne S. (1968) Electrical properties of glass microelectrodes. *Proc. IEEE* **56**, 1072–1082.

Schlag J. (1978) Electrophysiological mapping techniques, in *Neuroanatomical Research Techniques* (Robertson R. T., ed.), Academic, New York, pp. 385–406.

Schmidt E. M. (1971) An instrument for separation of multiple-unit neuroelectric signals. *IEEE Trans. Biomed. Eng.* **BME-18**, 155–157.

Schmidt E. M. (1984a) Instruments for separation of neuroelectric data: A review. *J. Neurosci. Methods* **12**, 1–24.

Schmidt E. M. (1984b) Computer separation of multi-unit neuroelectric data: A review. *J. Neurosci. Methods* **12**, 95–111.

Schmidt E. M., Bak M. J., and McIntosh J. S. (1976) Long-term chronic recording from cortical neurons. *Exp. Neurol.* **52**, 496–506.

Schmidt E. M., McIntosh J. S., and Bak M. J. (1988) Long-term implants of Parylene-C coated microelectrodes. *Med. & Biol. Eng. & Comput.* 26: 96–101.

Schoenfeld, R. L. (1964) Bioelectric amplifiers. In *Physical Techniques in Biological Research*. vol. V, Part A. (Nastuk W., ed.), Academic, New York, pp. 277–352.

Snodderly D, M. Jr. (1973) Extracellular single unit recording, in *Bioelectric Recording Techniques*, Part A, *Cellular Processes and Brain Potentials* (Thompson R. F. and Patterson M. M., eds.), Academic, New York, pp. 137–163.

Stone J. (1973) Sampling properties of microelectrodes assessed in cat retina. *J. Neurophysiol.* **36,** 1071–1079.

Strumwasser F. (1958) Long-term recording from single neurons in brain of unrestrained mammals. *Science* **127,** 469–470.

Suzuki H. and Azuma M. (1976) A glass-insulated "Elgiloy" microelectrode for recording unit activity in chronic monkey experiments. *Electroencephalogr. Clin. Neurophysiol.* **41,** 93–95.

Suzuki H. and Azuma M. (1987) A reliable marking technique for identification of recording and stimulating sites in the brain. *J. Electrophysiol. Tech.* **14,** 121–124.

Takahashi K. (1965) Slow and fast groups of pyramidal tract cells and their respective membrane properties. *J. Neurophysiol.* **28,** 908–924.

Tasaki K., Tsukahara Y., Ito S., Wayner M. J., Yu W. Y. (1968) A simple, direct and rapid method for filling microelectrodes. *Physiol. Behav.* **3,** 1009–1010.

Thomas R. C. and Wilson V. J. (1965) Precise localization of Renshaw cells with a new marking technique. *Nature* **206,** 211–213.

Towe A. L. (1973) Sampling single neuron activity, in *Bioelectric Recording Techniques* Part A *Cellular Processes and Brain Potentials* (Thompson R. F. and Patterson M. M., eds.), Academic, New York, pp. 79–93.

Towe A. L. and Harding G. (1970) Extracellular microelectrode sampling bias. *Exp. Neurol.* **29,** 366–381.

Towe A. L., Patton H. D., and Kennedy T. T. (1963) Properties of the pyramidal system in the cat. *Exp. Neurol.* **8,** 220–238.

Tweedle, C. D. (1978) Single-cell straining techniques, in *Neuroanatomical Research Techniques* (Robertson R. T., ed.) Academic, New York, pp. 142–174.

Wolbarsht M. L., MacNichol E. F., and Wagner H. G. (1960) Glass insulated platinum microelectrode. *Science* **132,** 1309–1310.

Wise K. D., Angell J. B., and Starr A. (1970) An integrated-circuit approach to extracellular microelectrodes. *IEEE Trans. Biomed. Eng.* **BME-17,** 238–247.

From: *Neuromethods, Vol. 15: Neurophysiological Techniques: Applications to Neural Systems* Edited by: A. A. Boulton, G. B. Baker, and C. H. Vanderwolf Copyright © 1990 The Humana Press Inc., Clifton, NJ

Techniques to Study Spinal-Cord, Peripheral Nerve, and Muscle Activity in Freely Moving Animals

Joaquín Andrés Hoffer

1. Introduction

In the past dozen years, newly developed chronic recording techniques have made possible the direct study of peripheral nerve and spinal cord function in conscious, freely moving animals. Two complementary approaches were introduced in the mid-1970s: floating microelectrodes to record the activity of single neurons, and nerve cuff electrodes to record the activity of neuronal populations. Thus far, these techniques have been largely implemented in two areas of research: the functional roles in the control of posture and movement of several kinds of peripheral neurons have been assessed by recording their activity patterns in alert, unrestrained animals, and contrasting these to the activity present during stereotyped movements in more classical decerebrate, anesthetized, or otherwise reduced preparations; and the development, plasticity, and disorders of the neuromuscular system have begun to be studied in longitudinal experiments carried out in individual animals. Important new insights on the function of the peripheral nervous system have already emerged through the use of these novel experimental approaches.

Floating microelectrodes have been implanted in cat dorsal roots (Prochazka et al., 1976) or ganglia (Loeb et al., 1977a) to record from sensory neurons, in ventral roots to record from motoneurons (Hoffer et al., 1981b, 1987a–c) and in the lateral columns of the lumbar spinal cord to record from spinocerebellar tract neurons (Cleland and Hoffer, 1986a,b; 1987). Cuff recording electrodes have been implanted on hindlimb nerves to study afferent and efferent nerve traffic during locomotion (Hoffer et al., 1974; Hoffer, 1975; Stein et al., 1975, 1977) and posture (Hoffer and

65

Sinkjaer, 1987; Sinkjaer and Hoffer, 1987b), and to monitor the evolution of activity in axotomized or regenerating nerves (Davis et al., 1978; Gordon et al., 1980; Krarup and Loeb, 1987). In combination with floating microelectrodes, nerve cuff electrodes have been used to determine the direction and velocity of axonal conduction of single neurons (Hoffer et al., 1981a, 1987a; Loeb et al., 1985a). Nerve cuff stimulating electrodes and blocking cuffs have been used to characterize the input sources of recorded neurons (Hoffer and Loeb, 1983; Loeb and Hoffer, 1985; Loeb et al., 1985b, 1987) and to study reflex responses during posture (Hoffer et al., 1983; Hoffer, Leonard et al., in press; Sinkjaer and Hoffer, 1987a and in press).

The functional significance of the natural activity patterns recorded from peripheral and spinal-cord neurons can become clear only if analyzed within the context of the ongoing movement. To this end, various implantable transducers have been developed to record electromyographic activity (EMG), force, and length of limb muscles. In addition, detailed knowledge of dynamic changes in tendinous structures, muscle fibers, and muscle spindles during normal posture and locomotion (factors of critical importance to interpret both the origin of discharge patterns of muscle receptors and motor unit force production) has recently also become available using implanted piezoelectric crystals (Hoffer, Caputi et al., in press).

This chapter provides an integrated overview, mainly based on the author's own experience, of some theoretical design considerations as well as practical details of fabrication, implantation, recording procedures, and data interpretation for eight types of implanted devices: floating microelectrodes, nerve recording, stimulating and blocking cuffs, muscle force, EMG and length transducers, and piezoelectric crystals. Two books by Lemon (1984) and Loeb and Gans (1986) have covered several of these and related topics in considerable detail, and should also be consulted.

2. Floating Microelectrodes for Recording from Single Neurons

In contrast to the brain, which is relatively immobile with respect to the skull, the spinal cord and roots can undergo considerable movement within the articulated vertebral column. For this reason, peripheral and spinal-cord neurons have been elusive systems to study during normal motor behavior.

The activity of individual neurons in the brain of head-restrained animals can be readily recorded using the "chamber" approach first introduced over 30 yr ago (Hubel, 1957; *see also* Evarts, 1968; Humphrey, 1970). A micromanipulator is attached to a sterile chamber that covers an opening through the skull, permitting the repeated advancement of a stiff metal or glass microelectrode until neurons are encountered (reviewed by Lemon, 1984). Variations on the chamber approach have also been used to record from spinal-cord neurons in sleeping cats (Glenn and Dement, 1981; Morales and Chase, 1981), in awake cats restrained in a box (Collins, 1985), and in awake monkeys (Bromberg and Fetz, 1977) or cats (Marshall et al., 1984; Glenn et al., 1988) that had several vertebral segments surgically fused and/or were rigidly fixed to an external frame to prevent displacement of the spinal cord with respect to the externally attached electrode. However, none of these chamber-based approaches has been appropriate to study the activity of peripheral or spinal-cord neurons in fully weight-bearing, unrestrained animals during the performance of normal movements.

Floating microlectrodes were first introduced to study single-neuron activity in the brains of unrestrained animals (Strumwasser, 1958; Salcman and Bak, 1973; Schmidt et al., 1976). Floating microelectrodes differ from conventional microelectrodes in their mode of external attachment. Instead of being rigidly connected to manipulanda, floating microelectrodes are only connected via a fine, compliant lead wire. The main advantage of floating microelectrodes is their positional stability during unrestrained movement. A floating electrode tip placed in close proximity to a neuron (or a few neurons) will typically stay in the same position and record from the same neuron(s) for many hours, or even several days. The recorded neuron may thus be rigorously identified and characterized, and its activity may be studied for a wide range of natural movements and experimental conditions. On the other hand, in studies where the sampling of large numbers of neurons is required, the positional stability of floating microelectrodes can be a disadvantage. Since the electrode tip cannot be repositioned after implantation and the tip tends to migrate only very slowly through the tissue, the day-to-day encountering of new neurons is typically low.

Like all implanted devices, floating microelectrodes can produce variable degrees of damage to the tissue (*see* section 8.1.). To study the normal discharge patterns of a neuron, it is essential that both the intrinsic excitability of the recorded cell and its patterns of presynaptic input remain intact. The presence of an electrode near the cell body could alter the cell membrane properties, or damage its dendritic arbor and/or presynaptic cell terminals. If so, aberrant discharge patterns could be recorded. This potential problem is avoided if the electrode is placed close to the axon, far away from the sites of synaptic integration and action potential generation. Therefore, floating microelectrodes are, in general, best suited for chronic recording from axons rather than cell bodies.

Recording from axons has other practical advantages: axon bundles or tracts are, in general, easy to locate, axons of cells of similar modality are often clustered, and axons are more densely packed than cell bodies, so that the electrode tip need not migrate far to reach another unit. A practical limitation of recording from axons is that mainly the larger myelinated axons of medium or high conduction velocity will typically produce extracellular potentials sufficiently large to be resolved with floating microlectrodes (*see* section 3.5.).

Axonal size is not, however, the sole determinant of how well a unit can be recorded. In ventral root fiber recordings, no correlation was found between the extracellular potential amplitude recorded from a unit, and its corresponding axonal conduction velocity (*see* section 3.5.), indicating that the recorded potential amplitude depends importantly on the proximity of the microelectrode tip to the fiber (in particular, perhaps, to the nearest node). For a given unit recorded over several days, it is frequently observed that the potential amplitude will gradually increase or decrease, as if the electrode tip is moving closer to or farther from the axon. Additional evidence on the importance of proximity comes from microstimulation experiments through implanted ventral root microelectrodes (*see* sections 2.3. and 5.2.).

2.1. Microelectrode Design:
Theoretical and Practical Considerations

In its simplest form, a floating microelectrode consists of a flexible, insulated fine wire, bared at the tip to reveal a recording surface. The tip of the wire must be sufficiently sharp and stiff to penetrate the tissue without bending. However, if the leadout wire is also very stiff, excessive movement of the electrode tip may damage the cells. Thus, the electrode design and the materials and dimensions of the wire and insulation must be carefully chosen, since they will affect the following mechanical properties:

The ease of insertion into the target tissue
The positional stability of the electrode during movement
The amount of tissue damage caused at insertion and during movement
The longevity of the leads and
The rate of encountering new neurons over days and weeks.

In addition, the electrode design, dimensions, and choice of materials will determine the following electrical properties:

The amplitude of extracellular potentials recorded from single axons
The background activity recorded from other neurons and
The movement artifact and other noise pickup recorded.

The floating microelectrodes originally implanted in cat dorsal roots (Prochazka et al., 1976) or dorsal root ganglia (Loeb et al., 1977a) were of very simple design. Prochazka has always used 17-μm diameter Karma wire (Ni-Cr) with enamel insulation, most recently with the insulation stripped off for the final 25 μm, and with the end cut at an angle with a surgical blade (Prochazka, 1984). This wire is quite compliant, but can still be inserted, without bending, into the fragile dorsal rootlets. Loeb et al. initially used 50-μm diameter 90% platinum (Pt)/10% iridium (Ir) wire insulated with 12 μm of Pyre Tri-ML polyimide (California Fine Wire) over-coated with 12 μm of Parylene-C (Loeb et al., 1977b; Schmidt, 1983). A recording surface was exposed by an oblique scissor cut. Since, for a given wire material, stiffness increases as the fourth power of diameter, the high stiffness of this wire facilitated inser-tion into cat dorsal root ganglia, which have a thick matrix of connective tissue. The relatively large cross-sectional area of the 50-μm wire also gave a low electrode impedance (100–200 kΩ), a desirable feature to reduce noise when recording during move-ment (*see* section 2.6). In early attempts to record from motor axons, similar 50-μm wire electrodes were inserted through the L5

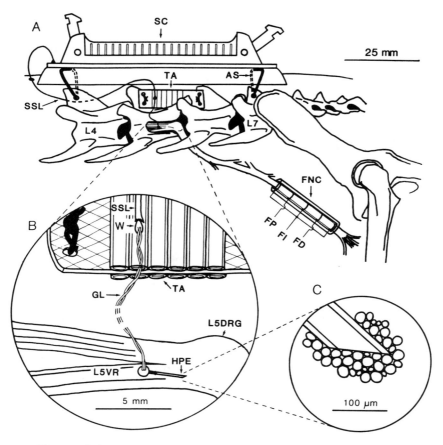

Fig. 1. Schematic diagram of implantation of devices in the left lumbar and inguinal regions of cats. The fifth ventral root (L5 VR) and dorsal root ganglion (L5 DRG) are exposed through a burr hole in the L5 vertebra. Up to 12 "hatpin" microelectrodes (HPE) are implanted in the L5 VR or L5 DRG. One HPE is shown in A and at greater magnifications in B and C. The HPEs consist of a stiff, insulated Pt/Ir wire, 2–3 mm long, microwelded to 1 or 2 strands of flexible gold leadwire, 20 mm long (GL). Each GL is microwelded to a Teflon™-coated, stainless-steel lead (SSL). Welds (W) are protected with epoxy. Each SSL is anchored inside one of 12 silicone tubes in a premade array (TA) attached to the L5 and L6 spines. Forty SSLs from hatpins and other implanted devices emerge around and are soldered to an external "backpack" or "saddle" connector (SC), firmly

dorsal root ganglion to reach the L5 ventral root (Hoffer et al., 1981b). Electrodes of this design remained stably placed when inserted through the tough dorsal root ganglion, but the excessively stiff 50-μm leads caused considerable damage when directly inserted into the fragile ventral roots.

To reduce lead wire stiffness for ventral root recordings and still retain desirable electrode tip properties, the two-piece "hatpin" microelectrode concept was adopted (Hoffer et al., 1981b, 1987a). Hatpin microelectrodes, originally designed for chronic recording from cortical neurons (Salcman and Bak, 1973), consist of a short, stiff wire electrode that is microwelded to a compliant lead wire made of a softer metal (Fig. 1B). Electrodes of this design have also been used to record from ascending and descending neurons in the lateral columns of the spinal cord (Hoffer and Cleland, 1986; Cleland and Hoffer, 1986a, 1987).

2.2. Fabrication of Floating Microelectrodes

Hatpin microelectrodes suitable for implantation in cat L5 ventral roots (Hoffer et al., 1981b, 1987a), dorsal root ganglia (Loeb et al., 1985a), or white matter in the lateral columns of the spinal cord (Cleland and Hoffer, 1986a, 1987) have usually had 1–4 mm long electrode shafts made of 25- or 37.5-μm Ir or 50-μm 80% Pt/20% Ir wire, triple-coated with enamel (Tri-ML; California Fine Wire). Tungsten can also be an appropriate (and less expensive) choice for the electrode shaft. To make a "hatpin," the stiff wire is microwelded (Black & Webster/Ewald microwelder WHD5A) to either a single 37.5-μm gold wire or two 25-μm gold wires twisted together. Since gold wire is very compliant, this design permits easy orientation and insertion of the electrode shaft into the tissue.

---

anchored by sutures (AS) to the L4 and L7 spines. A recording surface is exposed in each HPE by oblique scissors cut. Recording tip size relative to VR axons is shown in C. One other implanted device, a femoral nerve cuff (FNC) containing five circumferential electrodes within a silicone tube, is shown in A. The middle and two end electrodes are connected together to serve as common indifferent (FI). The separation between the proximal and distal recording electrodes (FP and FD) is accurately known (reprinted from Hoffer et al. 1987a, Fig. 1).

The length of the fragile gold lead wires should be limited to 10–20 mm. The other end of the gold lead is microwelded to the bared end of a Teflon™-coated, multistrand stainless-steel wire (Bergen BWR 3.48 or Cooner AS 632). To provide insulation from body fluids and add mechanical strength, each weld is covered with a small drop of epoxy (EPY 150 or equivalent; low water permeability). After thorough cleansing with more than one organic solvent (acetone, alcohols) the entire assembly is insulated either by vapor deposition of Parylene-C (Loeb et al., 1977b) or by several cycles of dipping in Epoxylite varnish followed by baking.

2.3. Surgical Implantation of Floating Microelectrodes in Ventral Roots, Dorsal Root Ganglia, or Spinal Cord

The same basic surgical approach can be used for implantation of floating microelectrodes in a single lumbar dorsal root ganglion (DRG), ventral root (VR), or spinal cord segment (SCS). An alternative surgical protocol for dorsal root microelectrode implantation was given by Prochazka (1984). For consistency, the L5 DRG, L5 VR, or L1 SCS will be considered as examples. The cat is sedated with subcutaneous Atravet (Acepromazine Maleate, 0.5 mg/kg), intubated with an infant intratracheal catheter (3.5–4.5 mm od), deeply anesthetized with Halothane gas in a 50% O_2/50% N_2O mixture, and placed prone on a heated table. Alternatively, an ip injection of Pentobarbital (30–40 mg/kg) followed by iv Pentobarbital titration (3–6 mg/kg) can be used, but recovery after several hours of surgery can be slower (*see* section 7.). Large skin fields are shaved. The L1-L7 dorsal spines are palpated and marked on the skin with indelible ink. The intended location for the backpack connector (section 2.4.) is drawn on the skin. The skin is washed down with antiseptic solution (Betadine-Providone). Through an 8-cm long midline incision centered about the segment of interest, the skin is separated from the fascia, and the fascia is opened longitudinally. The medial paraspinal muscles are bilaterally separated over the spinal segment to be implanted plus one adjoining segment, and removed. The bone is carefully scraped clean of muscle debris to reduce the chance of infection.

Using a high-speed dental drill with a No. 8-10 spherical burr, a 2 × 8-mm hole is drilled over either the VR and DRG (Fig. 1A), or over either the dorso- or ventrolateral spinal columns (further described in section 3.6.). This method reduces the amount of bleeding that can occur from the bone. For VR or DRG implants, the dura is slit open over several mm with fine microsciscors. For spinal-cord implants, however, the risk of damage from postsurgical swelling is reduced if several small slits (0.5 mm) are made in the dura, one for each microelectrode to be inserted. Surgical preparation of the site should be completed before the delicate fine-wire electrodes are brought into the surgical field.

Typically, up to six hatpin electrodes can be inserted in a single operation in a DRG, VR, or single SCS. For L5 VR or DRG implants, a prebuilt tube array consisting of 6–12 silicone tubes 0.5 mm id, 5 mm long (TA in Fig. 1A,B) is first attached with sutures to the L5 and L6 dorsal spines; for an L1 SCS implant, the tube array is attached to the L1 and L2 spines. The multistrand stainless-steel wire lead corresponding to one microelectrode is then passed through one silicone tube and anchored with silicone adhesive (Dow Corning 891), such that the remaining length of gold wire will reach the target site (Fig. 1B). Prior to its insertion into the tissue, a recording surface is exposed at the end of the microelectrode wire with an oblique scissor cut.

Using a surgical stereomicroscope at 40-fold magnification, the hatpin electrode is grasped at the epoxy ball with cupped forceps, oriented towards the target tissue, and inserted. The *in situ* impedance measured using a 1-kHz sinusoidal test signal will typically fall between 70 and 300 kΩ. The patency of the wire insulation can be verified by the absence of impedance changes as saline solution is irrigated into and suctioned out of the surgical area.

The accuracy of placement of each VR microelectrode can be immediately verified by microstimulating through it. Low levels of stimulation should evoke the progressive recruitment of single motor unit potentials recorded by EMG electrodes (previously implanted in each of the target muscles; section 4.2.–4.4.). For constant current stimuli 50 μs in duration, thresholds should fall in the 5–20 μA range (O'Donovan et al., 1983). If the level of stimulation required to evoke motor unit potentials in the target muscles is much higher than 20 μA, the tip may be brought closer to target axons by carefully moving the electrode in or out. If the threshold does not drop, the microelectrode probably should be pulled out and repositioned.

After all microelectrodes are installed, the dural openings are closed with fine monofilament suture (size 8-0) and the tissue planes are closed back in layers. The multistrand leads are passed subcutaneously to points of emergence through the skin, and are individually soldered to an external connector mounted on the cat's back (SC in Fig. 1A; *see* section 2.4.).

2.4. Connectors

In chamber-based preparations, leads often converge onto an external connector that is rigidly fixed to the skull with bolts and dental cement (e.g., Schmidt et al., 1976; Lemon, 1984). Skull connectors have also been used by Prochazka, who brought leads from 3–4 devices implanted in the lumbosacral area to a connector in the head (e.g., Prochazka et al., 1976; Lemon, 1984). However, when a larger number of devices is implanted in hindlimbs and/or lumbosacral spinal areas, it is more practical to have the leads emerge onto a nearby connector that is attached to the cat's back.

In a commonly used "backpack" or "saddle" connector design (Hoffer and Loeb, 1980, 1983; Loeb and Gans, 1986), up to 40 leads from the implanted devices emerge percutaneously in bundles, and are soldered to a 4 × 8 cm printed circuit board carrying a standard 40-pin computer ribbon plug (e.g., 3M Scotchflex 3432), built over a 1-mm thick piece of Dacron™-reinforced silicone sheet (Dow Corning 501-7). Catheters (described in sections 3.7. and 7.) to access veins or nerves can also be fitted. The connector rides outside the skin and is firmly anchored by two heavy Dacron™ sutures (size 2 or 5) passed through holes drilled in two vertebral spines (Fig. 1A). Alternatively, in experiments where the spinal cord or roots need not be surgically exposed, two sutures can be firmly anchored by simply driving a curved needle (4-cm diameter, half-circle, cutting) transversely and deep through skin and fascia, around the dorsal intervertebral ligaments. A good test is to be able to lift the cat (rather than just skin) by pulling up on the ends of each suture.

Cats usually tolerate very well these methods of anchoring a backpack connector. To reduce the chance of postsurgical infection, it may be best to make the leads emerge just outside the perimeter of the connector rather than under it, to provide air circulation for rapid scarring of the skin puncture wounds. An important precaution is to protect the connector with a cover made of a bite-proof material, e.g., aluminum. The cover should be of larger perimeter than the connector (to protect the leads at their skin emergence), and should be easily removable during recording sessions.

2.5. Amplification, Discrimination, and Recording of Single-Unit Potentials

To reduce the effects of lead capacitance that contribute to noise pickup and movement artifact (section 2.6.), it is best to current-amplify single-unit records close to the source. This function can be obtained from a 12-channel set of single-ended hybrid FET input amplifiers in a $25 \times 25 \times 3$ mm package (Bak Electronics MMRS-1P, voltage gain = 0.7) mounted on a card that plugs onto the backpack connector (section 2.4.). Other signals that arise from relatively low-impedance sources can travel without preamplification along a 1-m-long flexible ribbon cable to an overhead rack. Microelectrode signals should be filtered (1–10 kHz) and further amplified (1000–10,000-fold) prior to digitization or recording on magnetic tape (FM, 10 kHz bandpass).

Although only 1–4 microelectrodes out of 12 may usually be expected to give adequate quality records on a given day, full analysis of the identity and activity patterns of even one neuron will require the simultaneous recording of various other signals. These signals typically include several EMG channels (bandpass: 50 Hz–5 kHz), two nerve cuff channels (1–10 kHz), one or more muscle length and/or muscle fiber length channels (DC—100 Hz), one or more tendon force channels (DC—100 Hz), a time code signal (e.g., IRIG-B generated by a Datum 9300-100) used both for synchronization of simultaneous videotape recording of movements and for off-line digitization of tape-recorded signals to eliminate wow and flutter effects, treadmill speed monitor, stimulation monitor, and spoken comments.

Unitary potentials recorded by floating microelectrodes can be isolated using a threshold and window discriminator (e.g., Bak DIS-1). When more than one discriminable unit is present, it is possible to isolate independently two at a time with a dual discriminator (e.g., Bak DIS-2). Discriminable unitary potential amplitudes are typically in the range of 25–75 µV, against background activity and peak-to-peak noise of about 10 µV. Examples are shown in later sections.

2.6. Minimization of Noise Pickup and Movement Artifact

A floating microelectrode is a specialized antenna designed to pick up the clearest possible signal from a single neuron, in spite of the inevitable presence of other, often much larger sources of electrical potentials, regarded as unwanted "noise." Intrinsic sources of bioelectric noise within the animal include other neurons, nearby muscles, or the heart; extrinsic sources can include the recording equipment itself, air conditioners, power supplies, motors, fluorescent lights, or capacitive discharge associated with the animal's movement. A thorough discussion on how to reduce different types of noise present in electromyographic recordings can be found in Loeb and Gans (1986). Since microelectrodes have relatively high impedances, noise pickup can be a more severe problem for them than for most other implanted electrodes.

A major way to reduce noise problems is to reduce the tip impedance of the microelectrode. In contrast to rigid extracellular microelectrodes used in acute recordings, with tip impedances typically in the $M\Omega$ range, floating microelectrodes with tip impedance values between 100 and 200 $k\Omega$ usually have the best signal-to-noise ratios. Microelectrodes with tip impedance below 50 $k\Omega$ can rarely resolve unitary potentials much larger than background noise, given the range of axonal current sources (1–6 nA; see section 3.1.). Microelectrodes with high impedance values may record larger potentials but, because of the capacitance in lead cables, also become stronger antennae for extrinsic noise pickup.

A second important way to reduce pickup of extrinsic noise and movement artifact is to reduce lead length by placing the first stage of amplification as close as possible to the signal source, usually in the external connector plug (section 2.5.). In this way, the cable from the animal to the equipment rack is driven by the amplifier output stage, a low-impedance source. Coaxial shielding of the microelectrode lead wires inside the animal can also aid in noise rejection (e.g., Prochazka, 1984).

As with all biological recordings, marked improvement in extrinsic noise rejection can usually be obtained with careful grounding of the animal. This can be accomplished by installing a single, large surface area ground wire (for example, a 5-cm length of deinsulated, multistrand stainless-steel wire loop) subcutaneously within the leg or back of the animal.

Depending on its frequency spectrum, noise that cannot be eliminated at the source can often be reduced prior to tape recording with bandpass filtering. For mammalian myelinated axons, the bandpass of interest is 1–10 kHz, whereas electromyographic or electrocardiographic activity picked up by microelectrodes have frequency components, largely below 1 kHz, that can be filtered out. Other extrinsic noise sources, for example length transducer AC carrier signals (section 6.2.), can also be removed with bandpass filtering if the carrier frequency is set higher than 10 kHz (usually 25–35 kHz).

Some sources of noise that often appear when recording from unrestrained animals are easy to eliminate. For example, if a cat is fed from a stainless-steel bowl on a metal surface, the lapping movements can cause intermittent noise large enough to overload the amplifiers. This can be corrected if a plastic feeding dish is used. Similarly, a cat walking on a rubber treadmill within Plexiglas™ walls can generate static electricity when rubbing against the sides of the enclosure, if the ambient humidity is low. The resulting static discharge noise can be prevented if a humidifier is placed near the treadmill.

2.7. Criteria for the Identification of Recorded Neurons

Sensory or motor neurons recorded with floating microelectrodes from spinal roots or ganglia can be rigorously identified on the basis of direction of conduction and axonal conduction velocity, using the technique of spike-triggered averaging of peripheral nerve or muscle potentials recorded up- or downstream by nerve cuff electrodes or by EMG electrodes in the target muscle. These approaches are detailed in sections 3.5. and 4.4.

Spinal-cord neurons recorded from the white matter tracts in the lumbothoracic cord, in particular ventral or dorsal spinocerebellar tract (VSCT, DSCT) neurons, can often be identified by indirect methods. For example, VSCT neurons may be synaptically excited at short latency by electrical stimulation of contralateral peripheral nerves (section 3.6.) at intensities sufficient to excite group I, but few group II muscle afferents (e.g., Bloedel and Courville, 1981). In the case of DSCT neurons, their characteristic monosynaptic projection patterns can often be revealed with ipsilateral nerve stimulation. The classification of a VSCT or DSCT neuron can sometimes be further supported by demonstrating a spinal ascending projection using spike-triggered averaging (Cleland and Hoffer, 1986a; *see* section 3.9.).

Conclusive identification of presumed VSCT or DSCT neurons by antidromic activiation with electrical stimulation of the cerebellar peduncles has also been attempted in chronically implanted cats. Stimulating electrodes were stereotaxically implanted in the appropriate inferior (for DSCT; Cleland and Hoffer, unpublished) or superior cerebellar peduncle (for VSCT; Caputi and Hoffer, unpublished) using dorsolateral approaches that matched the inclination of the target tract within each peduncle. Electrodes consisted of 125-μm tungsten wire electrolytically sharpened at the tip, insulated with Epoxylite varnish, with large tip exposure (about 1 mm; tip impedance about 10 kΩ). Monopolar as well as parallel or concentric needle bipolar electrode configurations were tested. Under halothane/N_2O anesthesia, the advancing electrodes were stimulated at 1–2 Hz with 0.5-ms pulses at current levels of 10–50 μA. Optimal electrode tip locations were determined from maximal compound action potentials recorded from the lateral columns by implanted spinal-cord ENG electrodes (described in section 3.9.). Once in place, the electrodes were fixed using standard skull electrode implantation methods (e.g., Lemon, 1984).

In the above experiments, it usually was not possible to demonstrate by antidromic stimulation the identity of spinal-cord neurons that were classified as VSCT or DSCT neurons from indirect criteria (*see* section 3.9.). The stiff brainstem electrodes probably damaged some fibers, but more importantly, it was difficult to restrict the stimulation exclusively to the peduncles. Thus, the stimuli spread to fibers in other ascending or descending brainstem tracts that also projected along the lateral columns (*see* section 3.9.) before all the spinocerebellar axons could be recruited. In contrast to acute experiments, in chronic preparations it may often be difficult or impossible to use antidromic stimulation as sole criterion for identification of spinal-cord neurons.

3. Peripheral Nerve Cuff Electrodes

Nerve cuffs can be used to record, stimulate, or block conduction in peripheral nerve axons. Most aspects of construction and implantation are very similar for the various types of nerve cuffs.

This discussion will focus primarily on nerve cuff recording electrodes, because some of the design requirements are more critical and the applications more specific.

3.1. Nerve Cuff Recording Electrodes: Theoretical and Practical Considerations

Nerve cuff recording electrodes are designed to serve two purposes: first, to resolve potentials generated by nerve fibers by constraining the flow of action currents within a narrow resistive path, and second, to maximize the rejection of EMG and other signals generated by extraneural sources. The theory on how to record the activity of intact nerves chronically was developed by Marks (1965), Frank (1968), Stein and Pearson (1971), Hoffer et al. (1974), Hoffer (1975), Stein et al. (1975), Hoffer and Marks (1976), Marks and Loeb (1976), and Stein et al. (1977). A cuff electrode consists of an insulating cuff within which three or more circumferential electrodes are arranged in balanced tripolar configurations to maximize noise rejection. Two parameters, cuff inside diameter and interelectrode separation, determine the resulting neural potential shapes and amplitudes.

In analogy to the role of paraffin oil in acute recordings with "hook" electrodes, a nerve cuff, usually made of silicone rubber tubing, electrically insulates a length of nerve from surrounding tissues. Insulating the nerve causes action currents, generated by axons inside the cuff, to flow to "ground" along a long resistive pathway provided by the enclosed tissue and fluid.

3.1.1. Theoretical Considerations

Consider a nerve enclosed within an insulating cuff of diameter D and length L. A circumferential recording electrode (E_{rec}) is centrally placed. Two circumferential reference electrodes (E_{ref}), placed at the ends of the cuff and shorted together, are used for differential recording. The amplitude of extracellular potentials recorded from single axons can be calculated as follows. Assuming uniform longitudinal resistivity ρ_l for the nerve and surrounding fluid, a resistive pathway equal to two resistors in parallel separates the central electrode from ground. The total resistance (R) between the cuff midpoint and its ends is:

$$R = \frac{\rho_1 L}{\pi D^2} \tag{1}$$

When action potentials travel along a myelinated axon, a longitudinal current $i(t)$ flows at each node. Using node current values for frog and cat fibers of different diameters, Marks and Loeb (1976) calculated that, near the center of a cuff, the maximum extracellular potential V_{max} was approximately:

$$V_{max} = \frac{1}{3} i_{max} R \tag{2}$$

where i_{max} is the calculated maximum inward node current. For example, for a 64-m/s fiber within a large nerve, $i_{max} = 3.3$ nA (Marks and Loeb, 1976); assuming $\rho_1 = 1630\ \Omega$ mm (Tasaki, 1964), and using a cuff with $L = 20$ mm and $D = 2$mm, Eq. 1 gives $R = 2.5$ kΩ and Eq. 2 predicts $V_{max} = 3\ \mu V$. If a similar fiber courses within a smaller nerve branch, using a cuff with $L = 5$ mm and $D = 0.3$ mm, Eq. 1 gives $R = 27.5$ kΩ and Eq. 2 predicts $V_{max} = 33\ \mu V$.

Nerve cuff records are dominated by the activity of the largest axons in a nerve and slightly biased in favor of superficial axons with nodes near the center electrode. Potential amplitudes recorded from deep axons are attenuated by up to two- or threefold with increasing radial depth within the nerve (Marks and Loeb, 1976; Hoffer et al., 1981a).

Extracellular potentials recorded from axons by balanced tripolar nerve cuff electrodes are typically triphasic (positive, negative, positive), with the second phase of largest and the third phase of smallest amplitude. The actual shape of a recorded potential will depend on the relationship between the interelectrode distance within the cuff and the shape of the traveling extracellular potential wave. This is shown schematically in Fig. 2A. The extracellular potential wave generated by a 64 m/s axon (the negative of the intraaxonal potential; adapted from Marks and Loeb, 1976; Fig. 2) is shown traveling from left to right inside the cuff. Cusps occur at nodes, i.e., at fixed locations along the axon. Since the end electrodes are always at the same potential, a tripolar electrode set inside the cuff can be envisioned as a cord traveling from right to left along the wave. The vertical distance at mid-cord between the cord and the traveling extracellular potential wave represents the instantaneous potential difference, ΔV, between the center electrode (E_{rec}) and the reference electrodes (E_{ref}).

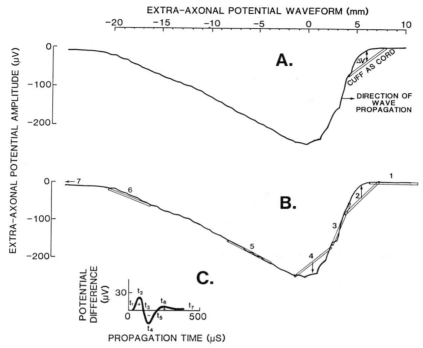

Fig. 2. (A) Schematic representation of the extraaxonal potential waveform generated by a 64 m/s fiber (adapted from Marks and Loeb, 1976), shown traveling in space from left to right. A 5 mm long, tripolar cuff electrode is represented as a cord, with its isopotential ends touching the waveform at all times. The instantaneous potential difference ΔV, recorded by the center electrode with respect to the end electrodes, is given by the vertical distance from cuff midpoint to waveform. (B) Seven positions of the cuff (as cord) are shown as the wave travels through it. (C) The development of the triphasic signal $(+, -, +)$ recorded by the tripolar cuff electrodes as the wave travels past them is shown. The times t_1-t_7 correspond to the cuff positions shown in B (modified from Hoffer, 1975, Fig. 1).

Before the wave enters the cuff, ΔV is zero (e.g., time t_1 in Fig. 2B). As the wave proceeds past one reference electrode, ΔV turns positive (e.g., time t_2 in Fig. 2B). When the peak of the wave is near the center electrode, ΔV is negative (time t_4), and as the wave exits the cuff, ΔV is positive again (time t_6). The resulting triphasic potential recorded, positive-negative-positive, is characteristic of the "center vs tied ends" recording geometry, which in effect resolves the second derivative of an action potential wave with respect to time (Stein and Pearson, 1971). The seven time points shown in Fig. 2B represent the inflexions and peaks in the extracellular potential wave.

A balanced tripolar electrode configuration is the optimal way to reduce pickup of EMG and other noise generated by current sources external to a nerve cuff (Hoffer, 1975; Stein et al., 1975, 1977). Since the resistance offered by the tissue path inside the cuff (10 kΩ in the above example) is much higher than the parallel shunt resistance in body fluids and muscles (about 500 Ω), only a fraction of EMG currents will flow through a well-sealed cuff. However, since muscles are far larger current sources than nerves, even a "small" amount of EMG pickup could badly contaminate neural recordings. Using a balanced tripolar electrode configuration (with the end electrodes tied together and symmetrically placed around the center electrode) and differential recording, potentials generated by all outside sources act as "common mode", and are rejected.

The signal amplitudes obtained in the first recordings from intact nerves using implanted cuff electrodes confirmed theoretical predictions (Eq. 2). In rabbit tenuissimus nerve (about 0.2 mm in diameter), using cuffs 0.3 mm in diameter and 5 mm long, single-fiber potentials ranged from 20–90 μV (Hoffer et al., 1974; Hoffer, 1975; Hoffer and Marks, 1976). In the much larger cat sural, femoral, or sciatic nerves, ranging from 1–3 mm in diameter, single-fiber potentials ranging from 2–10 μV were recorded (Stein et al., 1975, 1977; Hoffer et al., 1981a).

3.1.2. Practical Considerations

Nerve recording cuffs have been implanted on the sciatic, femoral, hamstring, tibial, common peroneal, superficial peroneal, medial gastrocnemius, lateral gastrocnemius-soleus, saphenous, and sural nerves in the cat hindlimb. The following discussion will focus on the femoral nerve of the cat, for which the most complete studies are available.

In large cats, the femoral nerve can be mobilized for 30–35 mm proximally to the inguinal canal, in a region where the nerve does not send out branches or receive major transverse blood vessels, and courses well away from joints. This situation is favorable for chronic implantation of a nerve recording cuff. To prevent compression neuropathy caused by postsurgical edema (Aguayo et al., 1971; Hoffer, 1975; Davis et al., 1978), the cuff inside diameter should be at least 20% larger than the diameter of the nerve. Compression neuropathy causes a reduction in axonal conduction velocity, and tends to affect most severely the largest diameter axons in a peripheral nerve (Sunderland, 1968; Gillespie and Stein, 1983). Evidence that a properly fitting, chronically implanted nerve cuff need not cause compression damage stems from the values of axonal conduction velocity measured within a femoral nerve cuff, which can reach and even exceed 120 m/s (e.g., see Fig. 6A), in agreement with α-motoneuron and primary afferent conduction velocity values typically measured in acute cat experiments (e.g., Stuart and Enoka, 1983).

3.2. Fabrication of Nerve Cuff Recording Electrodes

Nerve recording cuffs can be either fabricated in advance of implantation, or molded *in situ* by, for example, wrapping electrodes around a nerve and pouring an elastomer to obtain a conformal fit when it sets (e.g., Frank, 1968; Julien and Rossignol, 1982). Prefabricated cuffs can reduce surgical installation time and the chance of malfunction caused either by nerve compression neuropathy in case of a tight fit, or by lead crosstalk if wires touch or are improperly sealed. When prefabricated cuffs are used, it is of course necessary to be familiar with the nerve and site of implantation. It is prudent to have more than one size available, since in different cats, nerve diameters and branching patterns can vary considerably.

For the femoral nerve of adult cats, recording cuffs can be 15–30 mm long, typically made from 2.5-mm inside diameter (id) silicone rubber tubing (Extracorporeal). Originally (e.g., Davis et al., 1978; Hoffer et al., 1981a,b), cuff recording electrodes were made with 90% Pt/10 %Ir Telfon™-coated, multistrand wire (Medwire 10 Ir 9/49 T), locally deinsulated and sewn to the inside wall of the silicone cuff over most of its circumference (Fig. 3), leaving a gap for a longitudinal opening. More recently, less costly stainless-steel, Teflon™-coated flexible multistrand wire (Cooner AS 631) has been used for cuff electrodes, with similar success (e.g., Hoffer et al., 1987a).

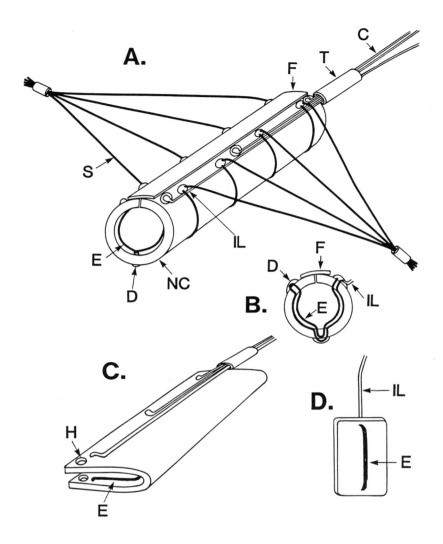

Fig. 3. (A) Schematic diagram of a tripolar nerve cuff recording electrode. The insulating nerve cuff (NC) is made of flexible silicone tubing. Three of more flexible multistrand stainless-steel wire electrodes (E) are deinsulated and sewn circumferentially to the inside wall. Their insulated leads (IL) are gathered in a short length of silicone tubing (T) and run subcutaneously as a cable (C) toward the back of the cat. A silicone sheet flap (F) adhered over the cuff opening ensures a tight seal. Several sutures (S) attached to the outside of the cuff are pulled apart to open the cuff and are individually tied to close the cuff tightly after the nerve is placed inside. (B) Diagram showing a method for attaching the

A minimum of three electrodes are placed, one carefully centered and one near each end of the cuff. The end electrodes, connected together, serve as a reference for differential recording. Measurements of axonal conduction velocity are more precise using a longer cuff (24–30 mm) with five evenly spaced electrodes configured in two tandem tripolar recording sets (Fig. 1a). The central and two end electrodes are connected together as the common indifferent against which the two active electrodes (Proximal Femoral, FP, and Distal Femoral, FD, placed 11.5–15.0 mm from each other; Figs. 1A, 5A), record differentially. The conduction velocity of individual axons can thus be estimated from the latency in the arrival times of potentials recorded at the two precisely spaced recording sites, using the technique of spike-triggered averaging (*see* section 3.5.).

The leads from the three or five electrodes are gathered within a 5–10 mm length of fine silicone tube (0.5–1 mm id) to orient them together. From the point of emergence from the fine tubing, the individual stainless-steel leads should run independently from the cuff to the backpack connector. It is not recommended to enclose the wire leads further within, for example, a long length of silicone tubing, since this can add considerably to the stiffness of the leadout cable and possibly compromise the nerve.

Sites on the outside surface of the cuff where bare wire may show must be carefully covered with small drops of silicone adhesive, to prevent the shunting of nerve signals and EMG pickup from neighboring muscles. Next, several sutures (Dacron™ or

---

electrodes (E) to the cuff wall. A 1-cm length of 125-μm tungsten wire "needle" (not shown), microwelded to the deinsulated end of each wire, is sewn through the cuff wall. The points of emergence of bare wire on the external cuff wall are covered with a drop (D) of silicone adhesive. (C) Schematic diagram of a tripolar nerve patch recording electrode. Three deinsulated flexible wire electrodes (E) are sewn to the inside wall. To retain the nerve inside the electrode, sutures are passed through holes (H) punched in the wall. (D) Schematic diagram of a spinal-cord patch recording electrode. The deinsulated electrode portion (E) of a flexible, multistrand stainless-steel wire is sewn to a 2 × 3 mm piece of silicone sheeting, 0.25 mm thick. The electrode is introduced through a small burr hole in a vertebral body, and placed either extra- or intradurally with the recording wire facing the dorso- or ventrolateral columns.

Nylon, braided, size 3-0 or 4-0, 8–10 cm in length) are placed circumferentially every 5 mm and adhered with silicone adhesive, leaving a 2-mm gap where the cuff will be slit open (Fig. 3A). The ends of the sutures are gathered, and either knotted or held together within small silicone sheeting tabs or tubing. The sutures provide two important functions: the cuff can be easily opened by pulling on the sutures and, after the nerve is inside, a good seal is ensured by knotting the sutures together.

After the silicone adhesive has set, the cuff is carefully slit open along its entire length using a sharp No. 11 scalpel blade or razor blade. To avoid damaging the electrodes, glass or metal tubing should be placed inside the lumen of the cuff. The alignment of the blade with respect to the electrodes inside the cuff should be continuously verified, preferably under a stereo dissecting microscope at low power. A rectangular piece of silicone sheeting (0.25 mm thick, 2 mm wide, and the same length as the cuff) is then placed over the cuff opening and adhered to one side to further improve the seal (Fig. 3A).

Femoral nerve cuffs can also be fitted with a catheter for infusion of lidocaine for reversible blockade of small axons in the nerve (section 3.7.).

3.2.1. Nerve Patch Recording Electrodes

Particular anatomical situations may require that the nerve be left attached to local feeder vessels or connective tissue. In such cases, a cuff can be replaced by a nerve patch electrode made of a U-shaped silicone sheet patch (Fig. 3C) that only partially wraps around the nerve. For example, it is best to only partially mobilize the saphenous nerve branch of the femoral nerve from the edge of the sartorius muscle, because the nerve is fragile and receives local blood supply. Predictably, the EMG pickup using this type of electrode is unacceptably large to carry out useful neural recordings in the moving animal. However, patch electrodes made of 0.25 mm thick silicone sheet (10 mm wide, 15–20 mm long) gave excellent records of cutaneous and joint afferents using spike-triggered averaging (Hoffer et al., 1981a; *see* section 3.5. and Fig. 5C), because such neurons can be activated in the anesthetized cat in the absence of EMG activity. A second useful application of cutaneous nerve patch electrodes is to elicit cutaneous reflexes during posture or locomotion, using low-threshold stimulation (e.g., Loeb et al., 1985b, 1987).

3.3. Surgical Implantation of Nerve Cuff Electrodes

Surgical manipulation of peripheral nerves should be carried out with great care. It is particularly important to avoid imposing rapid stretches to a nerve, since this can cause mechanical damage leading to conduction blockade, especially in the largest diameter nerve fibers (Sunderland, 1968). The best instruments for manipulating nerves are glass hooks (e.g., made by heat-sealing the end of a Pasteur pipet, pulling it to 0.5–1 mm thickness, and shaping it into a gentle hook) in combination with fine microscissors. Two instruments made of different metals should never be used simultaneously, since if they touch each other, the nerve can be accidentally stimulated and the limb may move. To separate a nerve fully from the fine surrounding fascia, it is gently lifted with a glass hook, and the connective tissue is cut well away from the nerve.

To minimize the chances of injuring the nerve, it is advisable to tunnel the cuff leads from the nerve site to the place of lead emergence near the backpack connector (section 1.5.) after the nerve has been mobilized, but before the nerve is placed within the cuff. This is done by driving a tunneling probe (at least 25 cm long, made of 4- or 5-mm (od) stainless-steel tubing with a removable bullet nose) in the distoproximal direction, initially close and parallel to the nerve. The probe must establish a cuff-cable path that will minimize torques applied on the nerve by the cable once the cuff is installed.

After the cuff electrode leads have been tunneled to the back and out through the skin, the nerve is gently lifted with one or two glass hooks, and the cuff is positioned under it. The nerve is allowed to drop into the cuff as the cuff is held open by pulling apart on its sutures. Under visual inspection to ensure a good seal, the sutures are then tied. Impedances to ground, tested with a 1-kHz test signal (Stein et al., 1978), should measure about 500–750 Ω for end electrodes and 2–5 kΩ for internal electrodes.

3.4. Recording and Processing of Nerve Cuff Signals

Because of the small amplitude of the potentials of interest, low-noise preamplifiers are highly desirable. Since the source impedance of nerve cuffs is low, it is best not to use very high input impedance amplifiers; a very good, ultra-low noise, low input impedance preamplifier (QT—5B) has been designed by Leaf Electronics in Edmonton for the specific purpose of recording neural activity with cuff electrodes. If adequate preamplifiers are not available, a step-up, impedance-matching audio transformer (Stein et al., 1975, 1977) can provide several useful functions when recording neural activity with cuff electrodes:

1. The apparent impedance of the cuff electrodes is increased, providing a better impedance match for most amplifiers.
2. Transformers provide amplification of the recorded potentials.
3. Since the noise level is increased only as the square root of the voltage gain, the signal-to-noise ratio is improved.
4. If sufficiently inexpensive, audio transformers typically act as bandpass filters in the 100–5000 Hz range, which overlaps with the range of interest for neural recordings.
5. Transformer-coupling helps to isolate the nerves electrically from the recording equipment.

Several types of audio transformers have been successfully used in nerve recording applications (e.g., Hammond 585 D or 585 F; JAF-1; Triad).

In typical applications, a total gain of 10^5–10^6 is needed to boost nerve cuff signals into the Volt range. This can be accomplished by using either a transformer (gain 10–30) or a low-noise preamplifier (gain 100) as the input stage, followed by one or two AC amplifiers of the type conventionally used for EMG recording (gain 10–1000/ stage; e.g., Bak Electronics MDA-1).

3.4.1. Cross-Correlation and Spectral Analysis

Using computational methods, it is possible to obtain separate measures of sensory and motor traffic in a mixed nerve. If neural activity is recorded by two sets of tripolar electrodes placed a distance l apart, either along the same nerve (Fig. 4A) or on a nerve trunk and one of its branches, motor fiber impulses traveling with velocity v will reach the distal electrode set at a time that is $\Delta t = l/v$ after they are recorded by the proximal set. If the signals recorded by the proximal electrode are electronically delayed an amount Δt and multiplied by the signals recorded by the distal electrode, for each motor spike traveling at velocity v, a positive output will result. In turn, sensory spikes will contribute a positive output if the signals at the distal electrode are delayed by Δt, since they conduct in the opposite direction. For delays other than Δt, positive or negative products may result, but, in the absence of correlated activity, these will average out to a small value over time. The use of spectral analysis facilitates calculation of these average products for many values of Δt. The power spectrum of each signal and the cross-spectrum of the two signals can be computed. The amplitudes of the sensory and motor peaks in the resulting cross-correlogram (Fig. 4B,C) are related to the total number of impulses recorded from all fibers that conduct at a given velocity, and to their average unitary spike amplitude (Gordon et al., 1980).

3.4.2. Patterns of Whole Nerve and Muscle Activity

An example of neural activity recorded from the tibial nerve of a cat walking on a treadmill is seen in Fig. 4D (from Gordon et al., 1980). Also shown is EMG activity generated by the long extrinsic muscles of the toes and the ankle extensor muscles, recorded by exposed wire electrodes sewn to the outside of the nerve cuff.

Two differences between neural and EMG activity are apparent. (1) Neural spikes are much smaller than muscle potentials. However, the smaller neural signals are still clearly distinguishable from the noise level of the recording system, even though recordings were made in an unscreened room with the treadmill motor nearby. (2) Action potentials recorded from nerves are much briefer and therefore contain higher frequency components that those recorded from muscles. The power spectra computed for the neural and EMG activity recorded over several steps are shown in Fig. 4E (from Gordon et al., 1980). The peak of the tibial nerve power spectrum occurs well above 1000 Hz, whereas the peak of the EMG spectrum is near 100 Hz. Neural records can be contaminated with variable amounts of EMG pickup from nearby muscles (e.g., Fig. 4B), but if the tripolar electrode configuration is balanced and the cuff is well sealed, most of the power occurs at frequencies near the neural peak. The neural spectrum (Fig. 4B) should be routinely examined in computing the cross-correlation function for each nerve (Fig. 4C), since it provides a useful way of assessing EMG contamination. If necessary, the signals recorded by the neural cuff can be further filtered to reduce the low-frequency components picked up from EMG, with a sharp high-pass analog filter (e.g., 80 dB/decade; Krohn-Hite model 3700) or a digital filter.

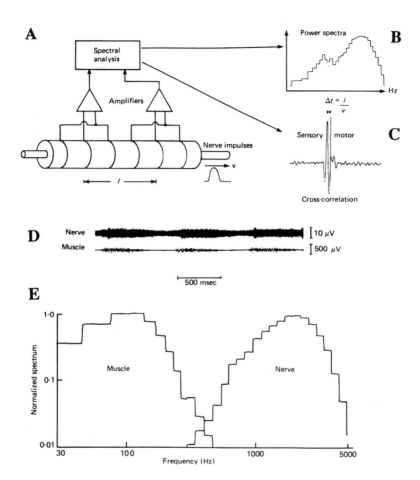

Fig. 4. (A) Cross-correlation of the neural activity recorded at two tripolar sets of electrodes on a peripheral nerve. (B) Power spectra are computed for the signals at each site. (C) The cross-correlation function is obtained from the inverse Fourier transform of the cross-spectrum. Nerve impulses traveling with velocity v between two electrodes separated by a distance l will reach the second electrode at time $\Delta t = l/v$ after they are recorded at the first electrode. If the signals recorded by the proximal electrode are delayed an amount Δt and multiplied by the signals recorded at the distal electrode, a positive output will result for each motor spike traveling at velocity v. The cross-correlation in this way measures the amount of correlated activity between the two recording sites as a

The electrodes in cuffs record impulses from all large myelinated sensory and motor fibers without too much attenuation (Marks and Loeb, 1976; Stein and Oğuztöreli, 1978; Hoffer et al., 1981a), whereas EMG electrodes are mainly sensitive to potentials from muscle fibers close to the electrodes. Neural spikes are more numerous than muscle potentials, so neural recordings often have a smoother envelope despite their small amplitude (Fig. 4D).

3.5. Estimation of Axonal Conduction Velocity of a Recorded Neuron Using the Spike-Triggered Averaging Technique

The axonal conduction velocity of a single peripheral neuron can be estimated from the difference in the time of detection of its traveling action potential wave recorded at several electrodes. For units that are recorded by floating microelectrodes and isolated using a threshold and window discriminator (e.g., Bak DIS-1), each occurrence of the discriminated spike can be used to trigger

←――

function of time delay Δt between the two signals. Motor impulses occur with a positive latency at the distal electrode, whereas sensory impulses have a negative latency, since they travel in the opposite direction. (D) Examples of neural and EMG signals recorded in a cat walking on a treadmill. Neural signals were recorded from the tibial nerve and EMG from the long extrinsic muscles of the toes and the ankle extensor muscles. The tibial nerve shows a diffuse burst in phase with the extensor EMG activity. Although the amplitude of the neural spikes is smaller than the EMG spikes, modulation in the neural signal is clearly distinguishable from the noise level. Tibial nerve spikes are much more numerous than EMG spikes in synergistic muscles, because of the large number of afferent fibers that are being recorded. (E) Nerve action potentials are much briefer and therefore contain higher frequency components than those recorded from the muscles, as can be seen from the power spectra computed for the same steps as in D. Spectra computed from the neural and EMG signals were normalized with respect to the highest peak. The units of each spectrum before normalization were $\mu V^2/Hz$. Both coordinates in E are logarithmic. The EMG peak occurs at 100–200 Hz, whereas the neural peak occurs at 2000–3000 Hz. Because of the 10-fold separation in frequency, further filtering can be used to reduce EMG pickup by the neural recording cuffs (*see* B) while preserving the neural components (adapted from Figs. 1 and 2, Gordon et al., 1980).

the sweep of a signal averager. In the case of α-motoneuron recordings in ventral roots (Hoffer et al., 1981b, 1987a), the ventral root electrode signal as well as the proximal and distal femoral cuff signals are all delayed 1–2 ms using a pretrigger buffer, in order to see the entire waveshape of the recorded VR potential. In the case of afferent recordings from the dorsal roots or ganglia (Fig. 5), a delay of 4–8 ms is needed to resolve the earlier-occurring nerve cuff potentials (Hoffer et al., 1981a; Loeb et al., 1985a). To resolve the neural waveshapes, each channel must be sampled at least every 40 μs (25 kHz). If an L5 VR or DRG axon projects through the femoral nerve cuff, correlated neural potentials will typically be resolved at fixed latencies. Usually 500 sweeps will suffice to render femoral nerve cuff potentials with signal-to-noise ratio greater than 3 (Fig. 5). The shapes and latencies of the triphasic neural cuff potentials from a given motoneuron or group I afferent are quite reproducible with repeated averaging. This method permits rapid on-line identification of recorded afferents and motoneurons. The identity of the neuron can be confirmed later by playing back from tape and reaveraging the nerve cuff data as well as the EMG data (section 4.4.).

The axonal conduction velocity is best calculated from the time delay between the occurrences of the negative peaks in the dual nerve cuff potentials recorded by the FP and FD electrodes (Figs. 5C–E). Since the negative peaks are the events of fastest change in slope, their times of occurrence can be most precisely determined. The distance between the FP and FD electrodes, which are sewn directly inside the cuff wall, can be measured within ±0.3 mm (±2–3%, if the distance between FP and FD is 10–15 mm). The fact that the cuff is initially 20% larger than the nerve does not necessarily introduce misalignment errors, because the five circumferential electrodes spaced every 5–6 mm contribute to align the nerve inside the cuff. Estimates of conduction velocity for fast-conducting fibers (about 120 m/s) usually carry a ± 5% uncertainty (Hoffer et al., 1981a, 1987a); precision is higher for slower-conducting fibers. In contrast, axonal conduction velocity estimates that are based on the conduction delay from the root to a single femoral cuff recording electrode generally carry larger errors. This is partly because axons can course tortuously through the lumbar plexus and the conduction distance may be estimated only within about ±10% (Hoffer et al., 1987a). However, an even larger source of uncertainty in root-to-nerve cuff conduction velocity measurements can arise from chronic damage locally produced in the recorded axon by the microelectrode (section 8.1.).

The single-axon potential amplitudes recorded inside cuff electrodes can be calibrated in units of current by injecting a 10-nA peak-to-peak, 3-kHz, single-cycle sinusoidal wave (e.g., generated by a Wavetek model 112 B) and averaging the recorded signal (Hoffer et al., 1981a, 1987a). This calibration method may underestimate the actual action current in nerve fibers, but it corrects for changes in tissue impedance that typically occur over weeks (Stein et al., 1978) and provides a normalization procedure for comparison of action currents estimated in different cats (Fig. 6A).

The spike-triggered averaging approach can also be used within the spinal cord to obtain the direction and velocity of conduction of spinal ascending or descending neurons chronically recorded with floating microelectrodes (section 2.3.). This requires the implantation of spinal cord patch recording electrodes, usually at a high- or mid-thoracic level, several centimeters proximal to the location of the microelectrodes (*see* section 3.9.).

3.6. Peripheral Nerve Stimulating Electrodes

The requirements for stimulating peripheral nerves are basically similar to, though not nearly as stringent as those in recording from nerves (e.g., Altman and Plonsey, 1986). Chronic stimulation essentially involves:

1. Implanting one or more electrodes near the nerve
2. Using an insulating sleeve to constrain the flow of current and
3. Minimizing mechanical damage to the nerve

If current leakage pathways are present, the only consequence may be a need for somewhat higher stimulation currents to reach threshold (in contrast to the devastating noise pickup that can disrupt recordings with leaky cuffs). A tight-sealing cuff may be required only to avoid spreading current to nearby nerve branches. Alternative methods of cuff construction (e.g., unsealed spiral cuffs; Naples et al., 1988) can also work well for stimulating nerves. In some applications, where stimulus spread and elevated current thresholds were apparently not an important problem, stimulating wire electrodes have been attached directly to nerves without the benefit of insulating cuffs (e.g., Thoma et al., 1984).

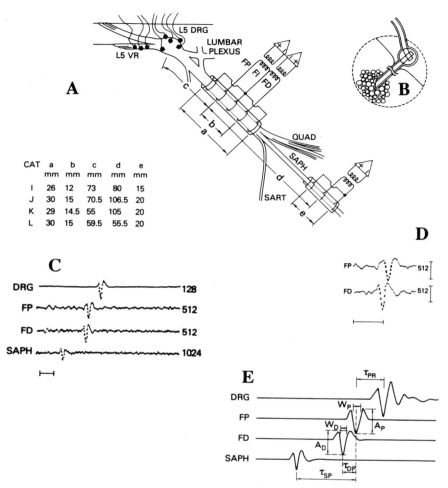

Fig. 5 (A) Method of estimation of axonal conduction velocity of anterior thigh afferent and efferent neurons, from spike-triggered, averaged femoral nerve cuff electrode records. As in Fig. 1, up to 12 microelectrodes are inserted in the L5 dorsal root ganglion (DRG) or ventral root (VR). Inset B shows dimensions of hatpin electrode tip (37–50 μm shaft) relative to DRG cells. A cuff with five circumferential electrodes is implanted on the femoral nerve, distal to the lumbar plexus. The central and two end electrodes, shorted together, serve as indifferent (FI) in two tripolar differential sets, centered about the proximal (FP) and distal (FD) recording electrodes. A U-shaped patch containing a tripolar electrode set is wrapped around the cutaneous saphenous nerve (SAPH). The separations between recording sites (b, c, and d) establish the conduction

To stimulate peripheral nerves, the active and reference electrodes can be only a few millimeters apart. Implantable nerve cuffs for stimulation can consist of a short length of silicone tubing (3–6 mm) containing two near-circumferential electrodes similar to the type used in recording cuffs. A third electrode can be added as a local ground reference, to reduce spread of stimulus artifact to other recording devices. Although Pt/Ir or other noble metal alloys may be preferable, stainless-steel wire electrodes are acceptable as long as maximum charge density limits are not exceeded (Hambrecht and Reswick, 1977; Mortimer, 1981). Tantalum/tantalum oxide capacitive electrodes have been shown to be excellent for stimulation purposes (Hambrecht, 1985).

Applications of nerve cuff or patch stimulating electrodes have included testing of reflex responses of single sensory (Loeb et al., 1985b) or motor neurons (Loeb et al., 1987), reflex effects on EMG (Duysens and Stein, 1978) or EMG, ENG, force, and length recorded from cat hindlimb muscles (Hoffer et al., 1983; Abraham et al., 1985; Hoffer, Leonard et al., in press; Sinkjaer and Hoffer, in press; *see* section 3.7.), as well as H-reflex conditioning in behaving primates (Wolpaw, 1987). Responses to electrical stimulation of

---

distances over which axonal velocity is measured. The other femoral nerve branches (QUAD and SART) supply the anterior thigh muscles. (C) Spike-triggered, averaged records obtained from a guard hair afferent fiber supplying the medial portion of the foot dorsum. The four traces correspond to the single-unit electrode (DRG), the proximal femoral (FP), distal femoral (FD), and saphenous (SAPH) nerve electrodes. All records were delayed 5 ms prior to averaging. Number of sweeps accumulated in each average are shown at right. (D) The proximal and distal femoral nerve records are reproduced in expanded scales. Consecutive points occurred every 20 μs. Vertical calibration bars indicate 1 nA, horizontal bars indicate 1 ms. (E) Parameters measured from averaged records, shown diagrammatically, are the amplitude of the proximal and distal femoral cuff potentials (A_P, A_D), their duration (W_P, W_D), and the latency from the occurrence of the negative peak in each record with respect to the proximal femoral record (τ_{SP}, τ_{DP}, τ_{PR}). Conduction distances shown in A were divided by these latencies to obtain the various estimates of conduction velocity (from Figs. 1 and 2, Hoffer et al., 1981a).

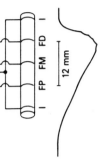

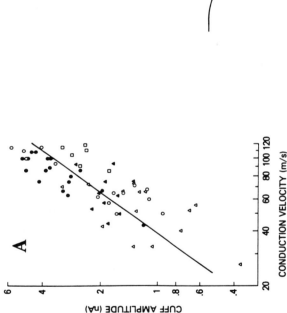

Fig. 6. (A) Relation between fiber conduction velocity (measured between proximal and distal femoral cuff electrodes) and neural potential amplitude, shown in double-logarithmic plot. Parameters of least-squares fit were: slope = 1.3 ± 0.2, intercept = −2.1 ± 0.3; n = 61. (B) Diagram of femoral cuff configuration used to measure the effect of interelectrode distance on amplitude and duration of fiber potentials. Middle contact (FM) was used either as recording electrode (with end electrodes [I] as indifferent, spanning 24 mm; FULL CUFF) or, by shorting FM to the end electrodes, FP and FD were used as recording electrodes (each tripolar set spanning 12 mm; HALF CUFF). An extracellular waveform calculated for a 64 m/s fiber (from Marks and Loeb, 1976) is shown to scale. Note that cuff dimensions were roughly comparable to fiber wavelength.

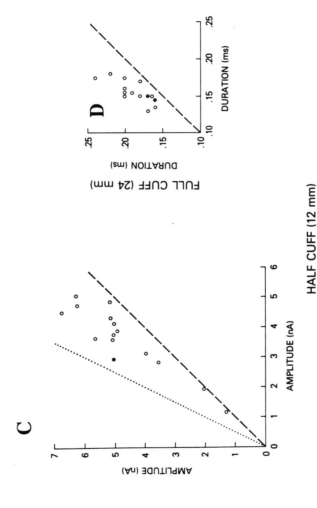

Fig. 6. (C) Unitary spike amplitudes recorded by the long tripolar set (FULL CUFF; ordinate) plotted against the average values recorded by FP and FD (HALF CUFF; abscissa). Full cuff amplitudes were larger, plotting somewhere between the 1:1 relation (dashed line) and 2:1 (dotted line). (D) Unitary spike DURATION for full-cuff vs half-cuff electrode configurations. Greater interelectrode separations rendered longer triphasic spike durations (from Figs. 5 and 7, Hoffer et al., 1981a).

low-threshold afferents via cuffs implanted in one or more peripheral nerves have provided a useful way to identify spinocerebellar tract neurons recorded with floating microelectrodes. Figure 7B (from Cleland and Hoffer, 1986a) shows an example of natural activity recorded from a VSCT neuron. Figure 7C shows that the same neuron was excited at short latency by low-intensity electrical stimulation of both the contralateral sciatic and femoral nerves through cuff electrodes. The minimum intensity of electrical stimulation of the sciatic nerve that was required to excite this VSCT neuron was $0.8 \times T_m$ (where T_m = threshold current to detect muscle EMG or twitch), showing that Group I afferents projected to the VSCT neuron. The evident variability in latency with repeated stimulation (lower traces) indicates that the response was synaptically mediated. The minimum latency of this VSCT neuron to higher intensity stimulation on the sciatic nerve was 2.7 ms, consistent with receiving monosynaptic projection. Comparison of responses of individual VSCT neurons to peripheral nerve stimulation in the awake and anesthetized cat further suggested their monosynaptic nature. The thresholds, but not minimum latencies, were increased by pentobarbital anesthesia (Cleland and Hoffer, 1986a).

3.7. Peripheral Nerve Blocking Cuffs

Blocking cuffs can be used to cause transient, reversible conduction block in a subpopulation of nerve fibers (e.g., small myelinated fusimotor axons with sparing of the larger Group I afferent fibers). Alternatively, the entire population of afferent and efferent fibers in a nerve can be blocked.

Since identified gamma fusimotor neurons innervating limb muscles have been impossible to record using floating microelectrodes in awake animals because of their small axonal size (conduction velocity = 20–50 m/s), fusimotor firing patterns have been indirectly inferred from comparisons of the normal discharge patterns of spindle afferents and the "passive" spindle response to similar limb movements in the absence of fusimotor bias (Hoffer and Loeb, 1983; Loeb and Hoffer, 1985). The method relies on the well-known increased sensitivity of peripheral nerve fibers of small diameter to sodium-channel blocking anesthetics. Infusion of a weak solution of lidocaine sodium was used to cause conduction blockade in gamma motoneurons with sparing of the much larger

Group Ia afferent fibers, as was done in acute cat experiments (Matthrews and Rushworth, 1957) and in humans (Hagbarth et al., 1970). Selective blockade of fine-caliber fibers allowed the discharge of single-spindle Ia fibers to be monitored in normal cats walking in a treadmill, through periods of progressive functional spindle deefferentation and subsequent reefferentation.

A femoral nerve recording cuff provided access to the perineural space via an implanted catheter made of silicone tubing 1.0 mm id, 2.1 mm od (Dow Corning 602-205), and about 200 mm long (Fig. 8A). The distal portion of the catheter was made of finer tubing (0.5 mm id, 1.0 mm od, and 10–30 mm long [Dow Corning 602-135]) that penetrated a hole punched through the nerve cuff wall about halfway along the length of the cuff. The catheter emerged percutaneously just lateral to the spinal column and mated onto a length of stainless-steel hypodermic tubing (1.1-mm od) bonded with epoxy to the backpack connector. This catheter access port was normally sealed with a tight-fitting silicone cap. To prevent plugging or formation of air bubbles, the catheter was flushed every 2 d with 1 mL of sodium heparin (50 U/mL) sterile solution in mammalian Ringer's.

Infusion of a 0.3% solution of sodium lidocaine in small doses over several minutes caused progressive conduction blockade of small myelinated fibers, including fusimotor neurons (Hoffer and Loeb, 1983; Loeb and Hoffer, 1985). This caused progressive changes in the discharge patterns recorded from individual Group I spindle afferents. The cat did not appear to mind the procedure, and the EMG, force, and length records were largely unchanged. The functional deefferentation of the spindles gradually reversed after flushing with mammalian saline solution (Fig. 8B).

In reflex-gain experiments that required reversible blocking of all ankle flexor afferents as well as brief electrical stimulation of all alpha motoneurons (Hoffer, Leonard et al., in press), two silicone cuffs were implanted on the common peroneal (CP) nerve of cats (Fig. 9). A nerve stimulating cuff (2.5 mm id, 5 mm long, with two stainless-steel wire electrodes sewn 3 mm apart) was placed distal to the proximolateral tendon of the lateral gastrocnemius muscle. It was used to electrically stimulate the α-motoneurons in the CP nerve to generate force in the ankle flexor muscles. A proximally placed nerve blocking cuff (4.0 mm id, 8 mm long) had snug-fitting 2.5-mm id silicone tubing rings at its ends. A 1-mm id silicone tube catheter led from the midpoint of the blocking cuff to a stainless-

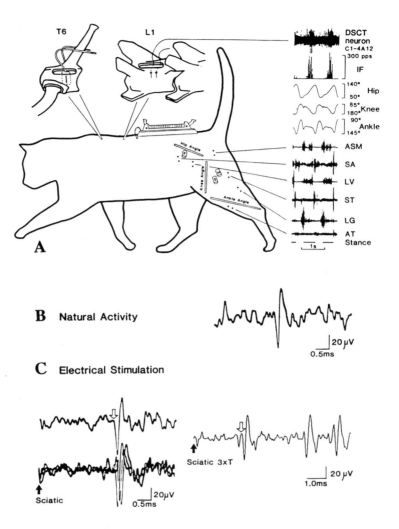

Fig. 7. (A) Diagram of chronic cat preparation to record spinal-cord neuron activity. Each cat was implanted with bipolar EMG electrodes in six hindlimb muscles, distensible length transducers across hip, knee, and ankle joints, stimulating cuff electrodes on the sciatic, femoral, and hamstring nerves, two spinal-cord patch electrodes at T6, and up to 12 floating microelectrodes in dorso- or ventrolateral columns in T13-L3 spinal segments. (B) Example of naturally occurring potentials recorded from a VSCT neuron during normal movement. (C) The same neuron was excited at short latency by low-intensity electrical stimulation of both the

steel port in the external connector, as in the experiments described above. Full-strength (2%) lidocaine sodium solution was infused to block centripetal conduction in all nerve fibers.

The effectiveness of the CP nerve conduction blockade during lidocaine infusion was assessed from records from a sciatic nerve recording cuff (10 mm long, 4 mm id with balanced tripolar stainless-steel wire electrodes) that was also implanted. The amplitude of the compound action potential elicited by stimulation of the CP nerve was monitored in the sciatic nerve.

Reflex-gain experiments were performed once the cat had fully recovered from surgery, typically 1–2 wk after implantation. While the cat walked on a treadmill, the appropriate DC offset, balance, and gain of each amplifier and bridge were established. Next, with the cat sitting or lying down, conduction in the CP nerve was blocked. An initial dose of 0.35 mL of 2% lidocaine sodium was delivered into the catheter leading to the lumen of the CP blocking cuff. The catheter volume was 0.1 mL. Over the next several minutes, the progressive diminution of the compound action potential evoked in the sciatic cuff by periodic CP nerve stimulation was monitored. The nerve was usually completely blocked after 20–30 min. If required, the initial lidocaine dose was followed with 0.05-mL boosts at 5–10 min intervals until a complete block was reached. The cat then stood on the treadmill belt or on four pedestals, and the recording session began. On an average of once per second, the left ankle joint was dorsiflexed by stimulating the α-motoneurons in the CP nerve at 2–2.5 × threshold, using either single or paired negative current pulses 0.1 ms in duration (5–10 ms between stimuli) delivered through a stimulus isolation unit (Bak BSI-2). The ankle extensor EMG responses to reproduc-

←———————————————————————————————

contralateral sciatic and femoral nerves. Top records are single traces; bottom records are several traces superimposed to show the variability in latency. Stimulation of the femoral nerve (Left, filled arrow) at 1.5 × T_m (where T_m = threshold for α-motoneuron activation) in the awake cat excited the recorded neuron at a latency of 3.4 ms (open arrow). Threshold intensity was 0.9 × T_m. Stimulation of the sciatic nerve at 3.5 × T_m (Right; threshold = 1.5 × T_m) excited the same neuron at a latency of 4.6 ms. The variability in latency shown in the lower traces indicates that the responses were synaptically mediated (from Figs. 1 and 2, Cleland and Hoffer, 1986a).

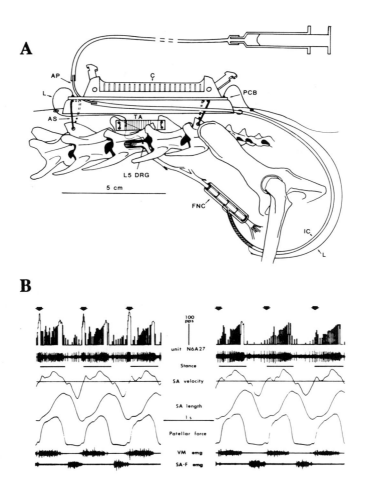

Fig. 8 (A) Schematic diagram of method for reversible blockade of anterior thigh fusimotor neurons with lidocaine infusion. A five-electrode femoral nerve cuff (FNC) had a flexible catheter that emerged percutaneously and ended in a stainless-steel access port (AP) mounted on the "backpack" connector. Other labels as in Fig. 1. A syringe was temporarily connected via a long flexible tube to the catheter access port in order to deliver dilute lidocaine to the femoral nerve while the cat was walking. (B) Example of blockade of fusimotor activity with lidocaine infusion. The left half shows normal activity recorded during three con-secutive steps from a Ia afferent (conduction velocity = 94 ± 5 m/s)

ible stretch were quantified in the normal cats. The experiments were repeated after the cats were decerebrated, in order to compare stretch reflex gain in the normal and decerebrate cats at matched background muscle activity conditions (Hoffer, Leonard et al., in press).

3.8. Applications of Nerve Cuffs to the Study of Other Systems

3.8.1. Small Limb Nerves

In normal and dystrophic mice weighing about 25 and 15 g, nerve cuff and surface EMG electrodes were chronically implanted to follow changes in the activity of the common peroneal and tibial nerves and the anterior tibial and lateral gastrocnemius muscles over several months (Milner and Hoffer, 1987). A dual neural recording cuff array was designed to fit separately around the common peroneal and tibial nerves where they branched from the sciatic nerve. The cuff array was constructed from two 7.5-mm lengths of Dow Corning medical grade silicone tubing (id 300 μm; od 640 μm) placed side by side and glued together with silicone adhesive (Dow Corning 891). A single slit was made along the length of each tube, so that it could be spread apart when inserting the nerve. One end of the joined tubes was enlarged by removing a 3.5 mm long section between the longitudinal slits and patching the resulting gap on each side of the cuff with a small rectangle of

---

supplying a spindle in the proximal part of the SA-m muscle. Traces show: instantaneous frequencygram and raw microelectrode record from afferent unit; bars indicating stance phase of gait; electronically derived velocity of SA; length of SA obtained with an implanted distensible transducer; force generated at the patellar ligament; and EMGs recorded from the VM and SA-m muscles. Arrows indicate the times of occurrence of a sharp burst at the end of the swing phase of each step. The right half of B shows activity recorded during three consecutive steps from the same afferent, 90 s after lidocaine infusion via a femoral nerve catheter. Note the disappearance of the sharp bursts at the end of the swing phase, unaccompanied by any major changes in the kinesiological parameters monitored. The normal spindle activity bursts were attributed to fusimotor drive that was transiently blocked by lidocaine influsion. (modified from Figs. 1 and 2, Hoffer and Loeb, 1983).

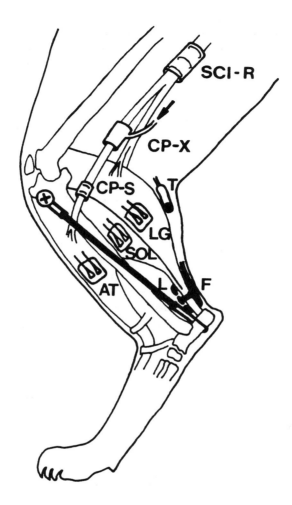

Fig. 9. Schematic diagram of devices for measurement of reflex responses, implanted in the left hindlimb of cats. Bipolar EMG electrodes were implanted in the SOL, LG, and AT muscles. Two cuffs were implanted on the common peroneal (CP) nerve: a bipolar stimulating cuff (CP-S) used to stimulate ankle flexor motoneurons to cause a brief ankle dorsiflexion, and a blocking cuff (CP-X) used to block central conduction in CP afferents by infusing lidocaine through a percutaneous silicone catheter (arrow). A tripolar recording cuff on the sciatic nerve (SCI-R) monitored compound action potentials when the CP nerve was stimu-

silicone sheet (125 μm thick). One patch was glued only along a single edge, so that it could be folded back when loading the sciatic nerve. Tripolar recording electrodes were made of single strands of 90% Pt/10%Ir wire, Teflon™-coated, 25 μm thick (Medwire).

When chronic recording devices are implanted on such small nerves and muscles, considerable care must be taken to avoid traumatizing the nerves. It is desirable to keep nerve cuffs as short as possible and electrode leads very flexible, so as not to impart torsional torques or pull the nerves away from their natural course. In some of the experiments described above, it was not possible to meet these criteria perfectly. Consequently, some nerve conduction block occurred in the days following implantation, but conduction was slowly recovered over several weeks (Milner and Hoffer, 1987). In other experiments where it was possible to use shorter cuffs with fewer leads, less trauma took place.

3.8.2. Cranial Nerves

Nerve cuff electrodes, chronically implanted in the vagus nerve, were used to record the activity of pulmonary stretch receptors in newborn lambs (Ebly et al., 1986a,b; Ebly, 1986). The design of tripolar nerve cuff recording electrodes was identical to that used in cat hindlimb nerves. For the vagus nerve of newborn lambs, 3–10 d old, 2.5-mm id silicone tubing was used. A cuff length of 15 mm was adequate to record action potentials generated by pulmonary stretch receptor afferents (conduction velocity ≈30 m/s, duration 0.5 ms; Paintal, 1953, 1966; *see also* Marks and Loeb, 1976; Hoffer et al., 1981a) and allowed implantation of two such recording cuffs plus a more distally placed, 10 mm long stimulating/ blocking cuff, along the available length of the right vagus nerve, distal to the nodose ganglion and proximal to the branch point of the recurrent laryngeal nerve. Afferent and efferent activity was computed from the two cuff records using cross-correlation methods (section 3.4.). Lidocaine was infused into the blocking cuff to eliminate afferent traffic transiently. The stimulating elec-

←——————————————————————————————

lated at the CP-S cuff. A saline-filled silicone length transducer (L) spanned either the length of SOL or (not shown) the length of LG. A force transducer (F) was placed on the tendon of either triceps surae or one of its heads. A thermistor (T) was subcutaneously implanted over the ankle extensor muscles (from Fig. 1 in Hoffer, Leonard, et al., in press).

trodes were used to demonstrate the completeness of the lidocaine blockade (*see* section 3.7.) and to test the integrity of the nerve from day to day. The vagal neurogram was found to be dominated by the rhythmic activity of pulmonary stretch receptor afferents in the quietly breathing, alert lamb. In six implanted lambs, it was possible to record vagal activity for up to 57 d. The typical reason for failure was lead breakage caused by rapid animal growth (e.g., a lamb's weight increased from 6 to 38 kg over 44 d; Ebly, 1986).

3.9. Spinal Cord ENG Electrodes

From an electrical standpoint, the bony canal surrounds the spinal cord in a manner that resembles an insulating cuff surrounding a length of peripheral nerve. Thus, in analogy to recording the electroneurogram from a peripheral nerve, the cat spinal cord electroneurogram can also be chronically recorded, if individual spinal cord patch electrodes (*see* Fig. 3D) made of fine multi-stranded stainless-steel wire (Cooner AS 631) deinsulated over several mm and sewn to a 2 × 3 mm backing piece cut from silicone sheeting (0.25 mm thick; Dow Corning) are implanted either intra- or extradurally. For extradural recording, two such electrodes are introduced through 1 × 3 mm slots drilled on opposite sides of a thoracic vertebral body (T6 to T12) and positioned against the lateral surfaces of the spinal cord. For intradural recording, the bone openings are made somewhat larger, so that a 2-mm slit can be cut in the dura on each side. After introducing each electrode, the dura is reconstructed with 8-0 nylon monofilament sutures that prevent the silicone piece from coming out. Potential amplitudes recorded by intradural electrodes are about twice as large as those recorded by similar extradural electrodes (Cleland and Hoffer, unpublished observations). However, the risk of causing damage to the cord is higher if the dura is opened.

Spinal cord patch electrodes of this design were used to determine the conduction velocity and direction of propagation of spinal ascending and descending neurons chronically recorded with floating microelectrodes (section 2.3.), using spike-triggered averaging (section 3.5.) and/or antidromic stimulation. An example of a VSCT neuron recorded at the T12 level, whose ascending projection was demonstrated by spike-triggered averaging of records from spinal cord patch electrodes implanted at the T6 level (2000 sweeps), was shown by Cleland and Hoffer (1986a; their Fig. 3).

4. EMG Electrodes

The field of chronic recording of electrical activity generated by muscles is too vast for the scope of this review because of the inherent complexity and great variety of architectural designs present in most skeletal muscles. A useful discussion of EMG electrode design, construction, and implantation procedures can be found in the book by Loeb and Gans (1986). The following discussion is specifically focused on the design of EMG electrodes suitable for identifying single motor units recorded by floating microelectrodes in ventral roots (*see* section 4.4.), and on recently introduced methods to study correlations in the patterns of activity of individual motoneurons and their target muscles during normal movement. These approaches have demonstrated that there can be distinct functional partitioning of motor units within individual muscles that are involved in the execution of different motor tasks.

4.1. EMG Recording: Theoretical and Practical Considerations

When motoneuron discharge patterns during locomotion were obtained using floating microelectrodes in the L5 ventral root (Hoffer et al., 1981b, 1987a–c; section 2.3.) it became necessary to identify also the target muscle of each recorded axon. This was done with spike-triggered averaging of records from EMG electrodes of appropriate design, implanted in each of the muscles of the anterior thigh: quadriceps (VI, VM, VL, and RF) plus sartorius (SA-a, SA-m, anterior and medial heads), the muscles innervated by the femoral nerve (Fig. 10A,B). The EMG electrodes were specifically designed to: (1) maximize sampling of motor units in each individual muscle head, and (2) minimize cross-talk from motor units in neighboring muscles. These goals tend to be mutually exclusive; on one hand, single motor unit territories may occupy a small fraction of the volume of a large muscle; on the other hand,

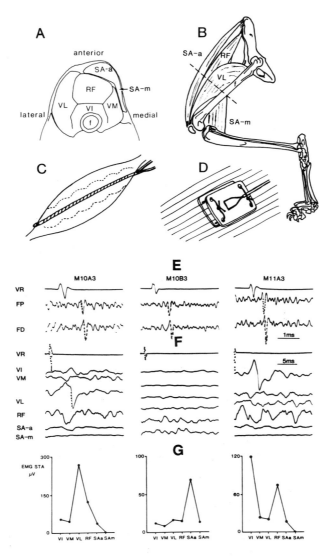

Fig. 10. (A) Cross-sectional diagram midway through the anterior
thigh of the cat, showing the femur (f) and the six muscles innervated by
the femoral nerve: vastus lateralis (VL), intermedius (VI) and medialis
(VM); rectus femoris (RF); sartorius anterior (SA-a) and medialis (SA-m).

cross-talk is in general minimized by using closely spaced electrode pairs for differential recording, which restricts the volume from which signal sources are recordable. To preserve some properties of closely spaced electrode pairs and also to match the geometry of large muscles, two special designs were used: spiral bipolar multi-contact electrodes for the fusiform heads of quadriceps (Fig. 10C) and dual patch "sandwich" electrodes for the thin, broad heads of sartorius (Fig. 10D).

←──

(B) Lateral view of hindlimb, showing the origin and insertion of anterior thigh muscles. The three vasti (only VL is shown) take origin on the femur and insert on the patella. RF and SA-a originate from the superior iliac crest and also insert on the patella. SA-m originates from the superior iliac crest and inserts on the medial edge of the tibia. Dashed line indicates the level of section represented in A. (C) Schematic representation of the location and presumed recording volume of a spiral bipolar EMG electrode implanted within the vasti or RF. The rationale behind this electrode design is detailed in the text. (D) Diagram of dual patch "sandwich" electrodes implanted across one of the portions of SA. The exposed electrodes face the muscle and are backed by silicone sheet to reduce cross-talk from other muscles. (E) Comparison of the results of spike-triggered averaging for three motoneurons recorded from the same cat on the same day. Units M10A3 and M10B3 were simultaneously recorded by the same floating ventral root microelectrode. Spike-triggered averaged records from proximal (FP) and distal (FD) femoral nerve cuff electrodes and the averaged record from the microelectrode (VR) are shown. All records were digitally delayed to show entire waveform. Sampling interval/channel: 4 μs. Total sweeps: 512. The total gain/channel was the same for all three units. (F) Spike-triggered averaged records from all six EMG electrodes and the occurrence of the VR spike are shown. Sampling interval/channel: 20 μs. For units M10A3 and M10B3, the records were digitally delayed 1 ms, and a total of 512 sweeps were accumulated; for unit M11A3, the delay was 0.5 ms, and 1,024 sweeps were accumulated. EMG vertical display gains are not the same in all cases. The background noise levels in the EMG records differed for unit M10B3, which was a flexor motoneuron; therefore, the vasti and RF were inactive while the unit was active. (G) Plots of the peak-to-peak amplitude of the EMG signature recorded from each motor unit within each muscle. Ordinates calibrated in microvolts (A–D from Fig. 2 in Hoffer et al., 1987a; E–G from Fig. 5 in Hoffer et al., 1987a).

4.2. Fabrication and Surgical Implantation of EMG Electrodes

Spiral bipolar EMG electrodes are made of two flexible, Teflon™-coated, 90%Pt/10%Ir stranded wires (Medwire 9/49T) coiled around a core of silicone tubing 0.5 mm in diameter (Dow Corning 602-135). The wires are alternatively deinsulated every 5 mm and sewn to the silicone tube to keep them from touching each other. The proximal ends of the coiled wires are soldered or microwelded to multistrand Teflon™-coated, stainless-steel leads. The coil is positioned near the core of the muscle belly (Fig. 10C) by pulling a 3-0 suture tied to the distal coil end through the muscle. At the point emergence, the suture is sewn to the tendinous sheet for stability. This device is very compliant and can follow normal changes in muscle length. The alternating recording surfaces are meant to approximate the summation of a series of closely spaced bipolar electrodes (Fig. 10C) with the objective of resolving motor unit potentials generated in any portion of the muscle, while still effectively rejecting signals from distant sources. A practical drawback of this design is that, after a few weeks, the mechanically stressed Pt/Ir wires tend to fatigue and break, most commonly near the Pt-Ir/stainless-steel junction. A more rugged alternative for this application may be to coil very fine, flexible multistrand stainless-steel wire instead of Pt/Ir wire.

Dual-patch "sandwich" electrodes consist of two square pieces of silicone sheeting, $10 \times 10 \times 0.25$ mm (Dow Corning 500-3), each with the deinsulated end of a Teflon™-coated, stranded stainless-steel wire lead sewn onto one side. The patches are positioned on opposite surfaces of the muscle with the recording electrodes facing each other (Fig. 10D) and are anchored across the muscle using 3-0 sutures. This design ensures that the electrodes cannot migrate. The volume of tissue from which activity is recorded is constrained by the insulating silicone patches, thus helping reduce crosstalk among SA-a, SA-m, and the deeper quadriceps muscle.

4.3. EMG Signal Recording and Processing

Ordinary AC-coupled differential amplifiers with variable gain from 10^2–10^4 (e.g., Bak Electronics MDA-2) are suitable for recording EMG in moving animals, given the low impedance source represented by implanted EMG electrodes (0.5–2 kΩ) and relative large amplitudes of muscle potentials (1–20 mV). To extract, with spike-triggered averaging, single motor unit potential signatures from gross EMG recordings, the frequency bandpass should include the range from 50–5000 Hz. To preserve features in the motor unit signatures that will permit the determination of muscle of origin (section 4.4.) and aid in repeated identification, higher frequencies than would normally be recorded in whole-muscle EMG studies should be included.

4.4. Determination of the Target Muscle of a Recorded Motoneuron Using Spike-Triggered Averaging

To determine the muscle of destination of a L5 VR axon that is recorded by a floating microelectrode (section 2.3.), two independent, complementary techniques have been used. First, spike-triggered averaging will generally reveal the associated muscle unit potential in EMG records obtained from the anterior thigh muscles during posture or locomotion. Averaging can be done on-line and reconfirmed off-line. Using sampling intervals of 20 μs per channel, 500–2000 sweeps typically need to be accumulated (Fig. 10E–G). Hoffer et al. (1987a) found that, for 76% of motoneurons tested, the muscle that contained the motor unit (the "target muscle" of the recorded axon) could be clearly identified by spike-triggered averaging. The reproducibility of results should always be confirmed by repeated averaging of different data epochs, since EMG electrodes in more that one muscle can sometimes resolve potentials of comparable latency, because of volume conduction (e.g., Fig. 10E–G). To identify the correct target muscle in cases of ambiguity, it is important to take into account not only the latency of the resolved potentials, but also the absolute voltage amplitude of the potentials recorded in each muscle, the presence of higher frequency components in each potential, and the possibility that a malfunctioning wire caused monopolar EMG recordings.

To identify the target muscle of a recorded motoneuron by an independent method, the variance is computed between the profile of the instantaneous frequency burst of the motoneuron and the modulations in the rectified, smoothed EMG burst profiles of each of the several synergist muscles during locomotion (procedure shown in Fig. 11). This approach was used by Hoffer et al.

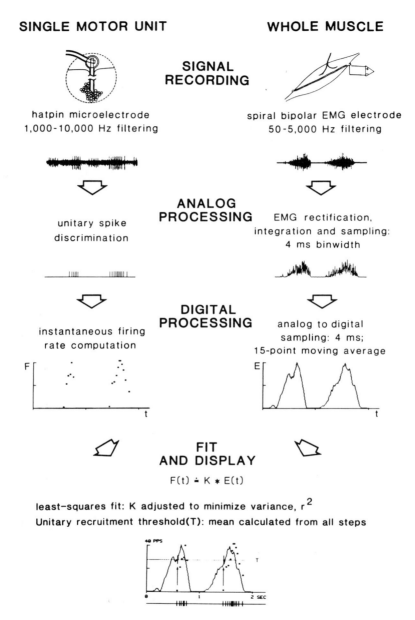

Fig. 11. Schematic diagram of the methodology used to record, process, and analyze the locomotor activity patterns of single motoneurons in relation to the EMG of their target muscles (from Fig. 1 in Hoffer et al., 1987b).

(1987b) in a study of anterior thigh muscles that demonstrated that the EMG profile of the target muscle of a motoneuron characteristically accounts for a larger fraction of the variance in that motoneuron's instantaneous frequencygram than does the EMG profile of any synergist muscle.

5. Tendon Force Transducers

The force produced at muscle tendons or ligaments in cats, sheep, and horses has been chronically recorded with implanted transducers (Barnes and Pinder, 1974; Kear and Smyth, 1975; Walmsley et al., 1978; Hoffer and Loeb, 1980; Lochner et al., 1980; Gregor et al., 1981; O'Donovan et al., 1983; Hoffer, Leonard et al., in press). The same basic approach has also been used to measure force in the human achilles tendon (Komi et al., 1984).

5.1. Fabrication and Surgical Implantation of Tendon Force Transducers

The typical approach consists of fabricating an elastic spring steel element shaped either as a letter "E" or as a "buckle," through which the intact tendon is slipped. Two similar semiconductor or resistive strain gages are bonded to the steel element in tension and in compression, to provide higher gain and temperature compensation. Insulated leadout wires, similar to those used for nerve or EMG electrodes, are soldered to the gage elements. The transducers are sealed against moisture with one or more conformal layers of insulating material (e.g., BLH Barrier "D" and/or Parylene C; viz., Loeb et al., 1977b).

The shape and orientation of the elastic steel element must closely fit the geometry and size of the tendon, and there must be no sharp edges that could tear the tendon. Prior to implantation, the tendon or ligament is carefully dissected free and the transducer is slipped on. "Buckle" transducers are kept in place with a cross-bar; "E" transducers can be fixed with retaining sutures passed through holes drilled near the ends of the arms of the "E" so the tendon cannot slip out (Fig. 12B). The leads are tunneled subcutaneously to emerge near a connector (section 2.4.). The fascial planes must be reconstructed to restore the original geometry of the muscles and tendons.

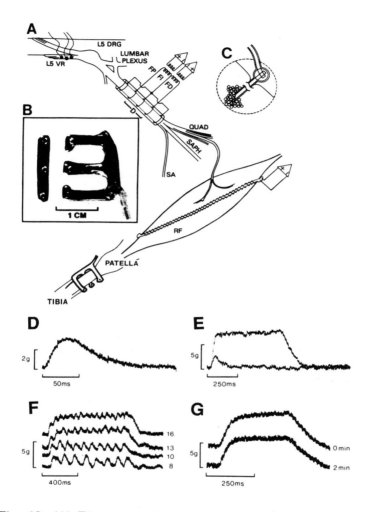

Fig. 12. (A) Diagrammatic representation of microstimulation of single motor units in intact cats using chronically implanted devices. For simplicity, only three ventral root "haptin" electrodes are shown inserted in the L5 ventral root. A femoral nerve cuff, bipolar EMG electrodes in RF, and a force transducer on the patellar ligament are shown. (B) Photograph of the implanted force transducer and retaining bar. (C) Schematic view of a "hatpin" electrode implanted in the ventral root, used for stimulating single axons. (D) Contractile characteristics of a microstimulated vastus intermedius motor unit. Each record is a stimulus-triggered average of

5.2. Tendon Force Signal Recording and Calibration

A simple DC bridge with two test arms is required (Walmsley et al., 1978; Hoffer and Loeb, 1980). Chronically obtained force records can be quite linear over the physiological range. An active low-pass filter with 100-Hz cutoff may be placed at the output to remove high-frequency noise, if present. Since small variations in leg temperature during locomotion can cause drift in the DC level, it is useful to unload the joints of interest briefly to provide a "zero-force" check every few minutes.

Static and/or dynamic calibration of an implanted force transducer is done in a final acute experiment, in which the tendon is left attached to a bone chip, tendons from other muscles are cut, and an external transducer is attached in series with the implanted transducer. Static and/or dynamic forces can be generated in the decerebrated animal by reflex stimulation, or in the anesthetized animal by electrical stimulation of the muscle or its nerve. Static calibration can also be done by pulling the passive muscle with a motor or by hanging weights.

In chronic applications, it is important to be aware that tendons remodel quickly after a tendon transducer is implanted. As is the case with any implanted device, tendon transducers become ensheathed in connective tissue within a few days of implantation. Over the course of 2–3 mo, it appears that the strain is increasingly borne by the newly formed tissue, because implanted force transducers, even though still in place, tend to register a continuously decreasing fraction of the actual force (Hoffer and Loeb,

---

the patellar force recorded with the implanted force transducer. Unpotentiated twitch, 256 sweeps, digitally smoothed. (E) Single twitch (unpotentiated) and tetanus (100 Hz), 32 sweeps, digitally smoothed. (F) "Sag" test showing four unfused tetani and different stimulation frequencies (Hz) indicated at the end of each record (32 sweeps each). (G) Fatigue test. The unit was stimulated at 40 Hz for 330 ms at a repetition rate of 1 Hz, and averages (32 sweeps) were performed initially (0 min) and 2 min later (2 min). This unit did not display sag in an unfused tetanus and did not fatigue during the 2 min of stimulation, suggesting that it was a type S motor unit according to the criteria adopted for other cat hindlimb muscles (Burke et al., 1973) (from Figs. 1 and 4 in O'Donovan et al., 1983).

unpublished observation). It is thus advisable to calibrate tendon transducers within a few days of recording important data.

5.2.1. Single Motor Unit Forces Measured in Chronically Implanted Cats

If signal-averaging techniques are used, the resolution of an implanted force transducer can be sufficient to obtain single motor unit twitch and tetanic force information, as well as to perform "sag" and fatigue tests (Burke et al., 1973). With the cat under general anesthesia to ensure that the background force is unchanged, single motoneurons are microstimulated through implanted VR microelectrodes (O'Donovan et al., 1983). Examples of resolved motor unit forces are shown in Fig. 12.

5.2.2. Spike-Triggered Microstimulation

On occasion, it is possible to microstimulate in isolation the same motoneuron that was recorded during behavior. In such case, the physiological type and contractile properties of a recorded motor unit may be determined. However, since there are other axons in the proximity of the microelectrode, it is essential to be able to show that the recorded and the stimulated units are one and the same. To this end, a definitive test called spike-triggered microstimulation was devised by O'Donovan et al. (1983). An example is shown in Fig. 13. The test consists of microstimulating the unit a short, variable delay after the occurrence of a natural spike during voluntary activity. If the delay is long enough, two near-identical motor unit signatures should be recorded by EMG electrodes in the target muscle. If the delay is sufficiently short, the stimulus will fall within the refractory period of the unit and a stimulus-evoked spike will not occur, proving that the recorded and stimulated unit are one and the same.

6. Muscle and Tendon Length Transducers

6.1. Length Measurements: Theoretical and Practical Considerations

The origin-to-insertion length of several cat hindlimb muscles has been measured with distensible transducers (section 6.2.). However, measuring the "length" of a skeletal muscle or its tendon

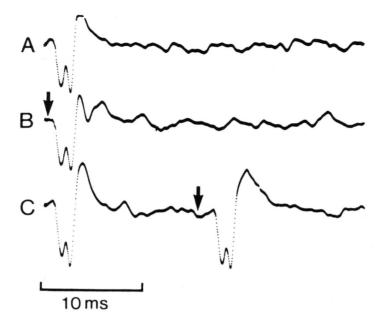

Fig. 13. Verification of the identity of a recorded and microstimulated RF motoneuron using spike-triggered microstimulation. Each record is the averaged EMG recorded from the RF muscle during treadmill locomotion, triggered on-line by the occurrence of discriminated ventral root spikes. The initial EMG response in each case is the unitary EMG recorded from the muscle fibers innervated by the axon whose spike was recorded. The averager was triggered by a pulse derived from the spike discriminator, so each trace starts 0.5 ms after the onset of the ventral root spike. A shows the spike-triggered average without subsequent stimulation. In B and C, the spike also triggered an ultrafast relay that switched the recording electrode from the input of the VR amplifier to the output of a stimulator. The stimulator was triggered after one of two different delays following the natural spike, at a voltage set to be approximately 2 × threshold for the unit suspected to be the recorded unit. In C, the record with the longer stimulus delay (15 ms) is displayed, and it can be seen that microstimulation recruits a unit that closely resembles the form and amplitude of the naturally evoked EMG. Proof of the identity of the microstimulated unit with that of the naturally occurring spike is shown in B; the stimulus delay (0.3 ms; 0.8 ms after VR spike onset) was sufficiently short to fall within the refractory period of the unit and resulted in a failure to evoke the microstimulated electromyogram. All records are displayed at the same gain (from Fig. 3, O'Donovan et al., 1983).

117

can be anything but simple. Just to define "muscle length" or "tendon length" is often difficult, since few skeletal muscles have the simple fusiform shape and architecture so often depicted in textbooks. Instead of consisting of parallel or unipinnate fibers inserted in single short tendons of origin and insertion, most muscles have complex shapes; act across more than one joint; may either originate from bone or have distributed (or multiple) tendons of origin and/or insertion; and may have complex, interdigitated fiber arrangements, often forming more than one anatomical compartment. In addition, for virtually all skeletal muscles, independently of the muscle length, the muscle fibers are quite short (typically 1–4 cm long). This means that, within the muscle belly, the muscle fibers are arranged in complex series and parallel combinations, usually involving long, compliant tendinous strands or sheets (e.g., Otten, 1988).

In spite of such complex, varied geometrical and mechanical arrangements of muscle fibers, it is generally assumed that "muscle length" is a critical parameter that the nervous system somehow monitors. It is also understood that the muscle spindles are stretch receptor organs whose afferent output reflects complex interactions between two time-dependent inputs: muscle length and centrally generated fusimotor drive (e.g., Hulliger, 1984). In analyzing spindle afferent discharge during normal movements, it has been assumed that the changes in muscle length that are measured in the behaving animal are also directly imposed onto the muscle spindles (e.g., Prochazka, 1981; Prochazka et al., 1985; Loeb et al., 1985a; Loeb and Hoffer, 1985; Hulliger et al., 1987; *see* section 3.7.).

However, in active muscles, a variable fraction of muscle stretch is taken up by the elasticity of tendons (e.g., Cavagna, 1977; Alexander and Bennet-Clarke, 1977). Thus, only a complexly distorted version of the muscle movement will be registered by the muscle fibers and spindles (e.g., Rack and Westbury, 1984; Hoffer, Caputi et al., in press). Further, fiber pinnation angles also change in active muscles (Caputi, Hoffer, and Pose, in preparation), leading to conformational changes of the muscle belly that affect total muscle length and muscle fiber length differently.

Since muscle spindles are typically arranged in parallel with extrafusal muscle fibers, it is necessary to measure muscle fiber length, rather than whole muscle length, to understand the mechanical input to spindles during normal movement. Muscle fiber length has recently been measured in freely moving cats using a technique of pulsed ultrasound (Hoffer, Caputi et al., in press; section 6.4.). It may also be essential to take into account muscle fiber length and pinnation angle changes to investigate the dynamic force production properties of single motor units in relation to their discharge rates during normal movement (sections 2.3., 4.4., 5.2.).

6.2. Fabrication and Surgical Implantation of Distensible Length Transducers

The origin-to-insertion length of a variety of cat hindlimb muscles has been measured with distensible transducers filled with either mercury (Prochazka et al., 1974) or hypertonic saline solution (Loeb et al., 1980; Prochazka, 1984). Full details of construction are found in Loeb and Gans (1986). Briefly, a thin-walled, compliant silicone rubber tube, typically 5–10 cm long and 0.5–1.0 mm id, is filled with a column of conducting fluid. A U-shaped electrode made of a 3-mm deinsulated length of multistrand stainless-steel wire (e.g., Bergen Wire or Cooner AS 631) is introduced at each end and placed in contact with the fluid. The point where the wire insulation ends is sealed beforehand with silicone adhesive to prevent later fluid loss by capillary action between wire and insulation. An air-bubble-free column of fluid is sealed in place with silicone adhesive, and a heavy suture (Dacron™ size 2) is tied around each end of the tube. The ends of the sutures are left long and are used to implant the transducer in parallel with the muscle.

For detailed studies of posture or locomotion, the anatomical layout of each muscle must be carefully matched when implanting length transducers. For example, the origin-to-insertion length of the cat medial gastrocnemius (MG) and/or soleus (SOL) muscles should be separately measured with length transducers. Even though these two ankle extensor muscles are considered to be close synergists, they have very different mechanical actions about the knee because of their different origins at the femur (MG) and fibula (SOL). For MG, the distal suture of the transducer is passed through a hole drilled through the calcaneum near the MG tendon insertion. It is best to attach the proximal suture through a hole drilled through the sesamoid bone found within the tendon of origin of MG (Hoffer, Caputi et al., in press), rather than to a bone screw placed in the femur, because large systematic errors in MG length change estimation during locomotion can be introduced by small errors in the placement of a bone screw, given the variable MG torque arm as the knee joint angle changes (*see* Goslow et al., 1973). For SOL, the distal suture is also attached to the calcaneum. Since the SOL muscle originates from the fibula over a 3–5 cm long region, it is impossible to approximate the origin of SOL as a single point; only a "representative" length for the SOL muscle can be obtained. Because the fibula is fragile and difficult to reach, it is safer to tie the proximal suture to a bone screw placed on the tibia, 1–2 cm below the knee (Fig. 9; Hoffer, Leonard et al., in press).

6.3. Measurement of Whole Muscle Length with Distensible Length Transducers

The end-to-end resistance R of the fluid column is proportional to its length L and inversely proportional to its cross-sectional area A. Since the fluid volume ($V = A \cdot L$) is constant, R varies simply as L^2. If DC (for mercury) or AC (for saline) current is passed between the electrodes, the resulting voltage signal varies as the square of the length of the fluid column.

Saline-filled transducers are driven with an AC bridge amplifier (e.g., Bak Electronics ABI-1), typically at a frequency of 25–35 kHz (chosen to be outside the bandpass of interest for neuromuscular signals). Low-pass filtering (time constant = 5 ms) of the modulated signal gives a DC output proportional to muscle length. An absolute calibration of length transducer records for specific steps of interest can be obtained *a posteriori* from bone length and joint angle measurements made from simultaneous videotape or film records, using the cosine law to calculate muscle length, as in Goslow et al. (1973). Saline-filled length transducer signals tend to drift with small temperature changes in the leg, making it necessary to recalibrate individual records, sometimes even for data segments that were obtained a few minutes apart. To reduce DC drift, it is useful to implant two length transducers near each other; the second transducer, left slack, is used as an external reference arm in the AC Bridge (Loeb and Weytjens, personal communication).

6.4. Fabrication and Surgical Implantation of Piezoelectric Transducers

Muscle fiber length, aponeurotic sheet length, and fiber pinnation angle can be measured in freely moving animals using an ultrasound transit-time technique. The essence of this approach is the careful implantation of pairs of small piezoelectric crystals near the origin and the insertion of identified groups of muscle fibers, most readily in a unipinnate muscle. The distance between the crystals is measured from the transit time of pulsed ultrasound bursts that are emitted by one crystal and received by the other. This method was originally developed for cardiovascular research three decades ago (viz., Rushmer et al., 1956) and has also been applied to the study of diaphragm movements (reviewed by Newman et al., 1984) and, most recently, to skeletal muscles in moving limbs (Hoffer, Caputi et al., in press).

Cylindrical crystals, 1.5 mm in diameter and 1.5 mm in length, having a natural frequency of 5 MHz (CY5-2; custom fabricated by Triton Technology), fitted with Teflon™-coated, multistrand stainless-steel leads (Cooner AS 631) and a small piece of Dacron™ cloth adhered with epoxy to the outer surface, give excellent results when chronically implanted in cats (Hoffer, Caputi et al., in press). Disk crystals, tried in preliminary acute (Griffiths, 1987) and chronic experiments (Griffiths and Hoffer, 1987), tend to be extremely sensitive to small changes in their relative alignment, an undesirable feature when attempting to measure fiber length in the presence of changing pinnation angles during normal activity in, e.g., the MG muscle of the cat.

Installation of the crystals requires good surgical access to both ends of defined groups of muscle fibers. Thus far, the following approach has been used in the MG and SOL muscles in the cat. After both the deep and medial surfaces of the muscle belly are surgically exposed, the intended position for the deep crystal of each pair is marked with a grain of Methylene blue. The course of superficial tendinous fibers is used as reference for orientation and placement of the crystals. The placement of the corresponding superficial crystal in each pair is determined by electrical microstimulation at the marked point, using a concentric needle electrode (od = 0.5 mm) and stimulating at 2 Hz using 40–70 μA × 0.2-ms pulses. Each stimulus causes a tiny dimple on the opposite surface, indicating the origin of the extrafusal fibers that are

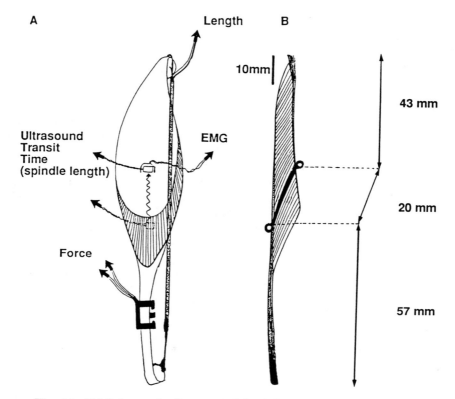

Fig. 14. (A) Schematic diagram of the left MG muscle, dorsomedial view, showing an implanted pair of piezoelectric crystals, nearby EMG electrodes, force transducer on the MG tendon, and distensible saline-filled length transducer spanning from the sesamoid bone in the tendon of origin to the calcaneum. (B) Diagram of the MG muscle in longitudinal cross-section, showing typical dimensions and orientation of its muscle and tendon fibers. The crystals recorded the length of muscle fibers and spindles in the highlighted region (from Hoffer, Caputi, et al., in press, Fig. 1).

being stimulated near their distal end. A second grain of Methylene blue is placed at the dimple. A piezoelectric crystal is then positioned directly over each marked spot, such that the cylinder axis is perpendicular to the plane determined by the long axis of the muscle and the axis of the fibers to be measured (Fig. 14). The Dacron™ cloth is sutured to the fascia with size 5-0 sutures.

Over the next 7–10 d (after implant), the crystals are progressively encapsulated by proliferating connective tissue (Hoffer, Caputi et al., in press). This encapsulation process is essential for obtaining strong signals and accurate records with piezoelectric crystals. The connective tissue replaces trapped air that absorbs ultrasound, and also adheres the crystal to the muscle surface. The location of each crystal can be accurately confirmed postmortem from the imprint left on the muscle surface. Furthermore, if the shape of the imprint exactly matches the crystal rather than appearing like a "groove," or as an extended area with unclear borders, this provides important confirmation that the crystal was intimately attached and did not systematically move with respect to the muscle during activity. For this reason, even when carrying out acute experiments with piezoelectric crystals, it is strongly recommended that crystals be preimplanted 7–10 d prior to taking data, since without the bonding process provided by connective tissue proliferation, it is difficult to ensure that the crystals do not systematically move with respect to the muscle surface, and the signal strength will also improve as trapped air is replaced.

6.5. Measurement of Tendon Length, Muscle Fiber Length, and Pinnation Angle

The measurement of distance between pairs of crystals is readily made with a commercially available instrument (Sonomicrometer 120; Triton Technology). This instrument "pings" one of the crystals 1543 times/s with a brief, high-voltage signal that causes the crystal to vibrate at its resonant frequency of 5 MHz. The crystal emits a brief burst of ultrasound that travels in all directions and is detected by the companion crystal some time later, causing it to oscillate and generate a voltage burst that can be recorded. The transit time of the burst wavefront is proportional to the distance between crystals, and inversely proportional to the speed of transmission of ultrasound in tissue at 37°C (assumed to be 1580 m/s; *see below*).

Figure 15 shows representative data from one step taken by a cat, of MG muscle fiber/muscle spindle length measured with pulsed ultrasound, whole MG muscle length measured with a saline-filled distensible transducer, locally recorded MG EMG, and MG tendon force. Systematically through the step cycle, major discrepancies between the length of the whole MG muscle and the length of its muscle fibers and spindles are apparent. The departures are largest during the "yield" phase (since the muscle stretches about 2 mm when it is suddenly loaded by the weight of the cat, but the fibers and spindles do not stretch [horizontal bar in Fig. 15A; phase II in Fig. 15B]) and as the foot is lifted from the treadmill (when the MG muscle shortens rapidly in the absence of EMG activity or load, but the fibers and spindles are largely impervious to that movement [phase III in Fig. 15B]). The implication is that compliance in tendinous structures and conformational changes in the muscle belly are responsible for the major differences in muscle length and muscle fiber/spindle length that are seen (Hoffer, Caputi et al., in press).

In recent experiments (Caputi, Hoffer and Pose, in preparation), 12 crystals were implanted on the surface of the cat MG muscle, allowing the movement of up to four groups of muscle fibers in different regions of the muscle to be monitored simultaneously, along with the movement taking place in tendon and aponeurotic sheets. By simultaneously measuring fiber length, aponeurotic sheet length, and the length of the third side of the triangle made up by the measured fiber and sheet segments, it was possible to calculate the change in the angle of fiber pinnation during active movements. Fibers (and spindles) in various proximodistal locations of the MG muscle were found to undergo systematically different length and pinnation angle changes during locomotion and postural tasks. This finding stresses the importance of knowing the location of a muscle spindle within a muscle in order to assess its mechanical input and the functional origin of its discharge pattern. Similarly, the location of a motor unit's territory will have a bearing on its dynamic force production properties for a given firing pattern.

6.5.1. Estimation of Accuracy of Muscle Fiber Length Measurement with Piezoelectric Crystals

An increase in longitudinal velocity of transmission of sound of about 1.5% has been reported for electrically activated, isometric frog muscle (Tamura et al., 1982; Hatta et al., 1988), but no change was seen in isometric cat MG muscle fibers (Caputi, Hoffer and Pose, in preparation). The Sonomicrometer is internally calibrated from 0–120 mm in 1-mm steps. The main source of measurement uncertainity can be a false trigger on other than the first wavefront

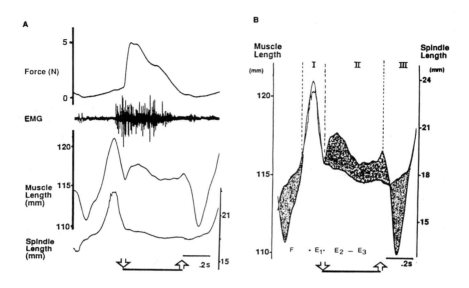

Fig. 15. (A) Signals recorded from a cat walking on a level treadmill at about 0.5 m/s, during one representative step. From top, traces are: FORCE recorded from the MG tendon; EMG recorded by bipolar electrodes sewn near the superficial MG crystals; origin-to-insertion MG MUSCLE LENGTH recorded with a saline-filled transducer; and LENGTH OF MUSCLE FIBERS AND SPINDLES in the central region of MG recorded by two piezoelectric crystals. Horizontal bar indicates weight-bearing period for the implanted hindlimb. Arrows indicate paw touchdown and liftoff. (B) Direct comparison of muscle length and muscle fiber/spindle length records obtained during the same step. Traces corresponding to the length of the MG muscle and the length of muscle spindles are superimposed to reveal three periods (I, II, III) of dissimilar relationship. The phases of the Philippson (1905) step cycle (F = flexion; E^1, E^2, E^3, extension) are also shown. Note that whole muscle and muscle fiber/spindle length are very similar in period I, when the muscle is unloaded, but the fibers and spindles do not yield as the muscle does in period II, and the fibers and spindles do not shorten with the muscle in period III, after the load is released. (from Hoffer, Caputi, et al., in press, Figs. 2 and 3).

in the received burst. This tends to happen either when signal strength declines (at relatively long fiber lengths) or when signal strength increases markedly (at short lengths). Using 5-MHz crystals, a false trigger that skips one wavelength will cause an absolute error in length measurement of 0.33 mm. In typical recordings, these false triggers are easy to detect and are also rare enough that they do not seriously distort the shape of the recorded signal (Hoffer, Caputi et al., in press). The uncertainty in measurement of changes in fiber length is generally better than ± 0.33 mm.

7. Selection, Training, and Care of Implanted Animals

The cat is the animal of choice for recording during normal posture and locomotion because, since the pioneering work of Sherrington, Eccles, and others (viz., Creed et al., 1932), most of what is known about the cellular properties and synaptic connectivity of afferent, efferent, and spinal neurons, as well as motor unit properties, has been learned from cat experiments. In addition to their well-described spinal cord anatomy and physiology, cats can be readily trained to perform complex motor tasks as varied as, e.g., dynamic force matching (Ghez and Vicario, 1978) or ladder walking (Amos et al., 1987).

For chronic experiments, cats should be carefully selected on the basis of physiotype and personality. For surgery, large-boned, lean male cats are preferable; for successful training, alert, friendly cats are required. By using food rewards and affection, cats can be trained to walk, trot, or gallop on a Plexiglas™-enclosed motorized treadmill at level, uphill (+10%), or downhill (–10%) grades, at a range of speeds from about 0.2 to over 2.5 m/s. Cats can also be trained to stand on four pedestals (Macpherson et al., 1987) and produce desired force levels with one hindlimb (Sinkjaer and Hoffer, 1987a). Against matched force backgrounds, reflex responses can be tested by perturbing the position of the implanted hindlimb with a servo-controlled motor configured to rotate the pedestal about the axis of the ankle joint. Usually 3–6 wk are needed to condition a cat to walk at moderate speeds (0.3–0.5 m/s) for up to 30 min/d, and to train it fully to perform a range of locomotor and postural tasks.

The night before surgery, and for at least the following 3 d, broad-spectrum antibiotics should be administered subcutaneously. After surgery, the cat should receive subcutaneous doses of a sedative (e.g., Acepromazine Maleate, 0.5 mg/kg) and an analgesic (morphine sulfate, 0.1 mg/kg) every 8 h for at least 24 h, or longer if it shows signs of pain or discomfort. Starting 2–3 d after surgery, the cat should be exercised on a treadmill for several minutes at slow speeds. Recordings can usually be carried out starting on the second postsurgical week, after the cat is willing to bear full weight again with the implanted hindlimb and has regained full strength and endurance.

7.1. Implanted Venous Catheter

A useful procedure for the long-term maintenance of chronically implanted cats is to implant a catheter leading into an external jugular vein from a port in the backpack connector. In the same manner as catheters used for lidocaine infusion into nerve blocking cuffs (section 3.7.), venous catheters can be made of silicone tubing (1.0-mm id, 2.1-mm od [Dow Corning 602-205]). To prevent kinking, the catheter is preformed into a U-shaped loop of ~1-cm diameter by placing the two ends of a 50-cm length of tubing into a 5-mm length of ~3-mm id silicone tubing and preserving this shape with silicone adhesive. One end of the catheter, 5 cm long beyond the loop, is cut diagonally to facilitate insertion into the distal portion of an external jugular vein. After insertion, a 3-0 suture is used to retain the catheter inside the distal portion of the vein, and a second suture is used to tie the loop to the proximal, ligated portion of the vein, thus ensuring proper alignment of the catheter. The long end of the catheter is tunneled subcutaneously to the back, emerges near the backpack, and is connected onto a length of stainless-steel hypodermic tubing (1.1 mm od) bonded with epoxy to the backpack connector. As with nerve-blocking cuff catheters, the access port is kept sealed with a tight-fitting silicone cap and, to prevent plugging and formation of air bubbles, is flushed every 2 d with 1 mL of sodium heparin sterile solution (50 U/mL).

An implanted venous catheter can serve four useful functions:

1. Fluids (e.g., 30 mL of 5% Dextrose solution) can be administered during or after surgery to replenish blood volume or to nourish the cat until it eats again.
2. Antibiotics (e.g., Chloramphenicol, 30 mg/kg) can be administered by iv route if needed.

3. Short-acting anesthetics (e.g., Thiopental) can be delivered for immediate sedation, e.g., to explore sensory fields of recorded units.

4. Systemic pharmacological effects on reflex gain or
nerve cell discharge patterns can be studied (e.g.,
Dantrolene, 2-5 mg/kg; used to alter excitation–
contraction coupling).

8. Limitations of Chronic Recording Techniques

The chronic recording techniques described here offer unique
opportunities to study natural activity patterns and functional
involvement of identified sensory, motor, or spinal tract neurons,
as well as the patterns of use of many muscles during the performance of voluntary or reflex movements in intact, conscious animals (Loeb, 1987). Some of these techniques may also have
application in the restoration of lost function in disabled humans
(section 9.). It is important, therefore, to know that implanted
electrodes or transducers may sometimes cause chronic damage or
alter the normal function of the system under study. Some studies
of altered function are reviewed below.

8.1. Assessment of Chronic Damage Caused by Implanted Devices

8.1.1. Discrepancies Between Axonal Conduction Velocity Measured from Root to Cuff and Within Cuff

Axonal conduction velocity measurements can provide a
sensitive assay of axonal integrity (e.g., Gillespie and Stein, 1983).
This criterion has been used to determine the extent of damage
caused by chronically implanted microelectrodes. For example, for
25 motoneurons recorded by Hoffer et al. (1987a–c) using floating
microelectrodes in L5 ventral roots, the conduction velocity was
independently measured in two regions of the axon: between the
ventral root microelectrode and the proximal femoral nerve cuff
recording electrode (VR-FP; see Fig. 16A), and between the proximal and distal femoral cuff recording electrodes (FP-FD). For
some motoneurons, it was found that the two estimations differed
by more than could be attibuted to measurement uncertainties
alone.

Invariably, units with a large discrepancy in the two conduction velocity estimations turned out to also have VR potentials of peculiar shape and/or prolonged duration (Fig. 16C,D). It was recognized that some chronically implanted VR microelectrodes could have damaged fibers locally and affected action potential propagation along the root. Of this sample of motoneurons, 32% shared the following characteristics:

1. Triphasic VR action potentials (+, −, +) of <0.6-ms duration (measured from first to last zero crossing, arrows in Fig. 16B)
2. Clearly resolved triphasic (+, −, +) action currents of brief duration in the FP and FD records
3. Comparable conduction velocity values (differing by not more than 20%) when measured from VR to FP and from FP to FD.

Units fulfilling these three criteria were considered to be functionally undamaged by the presence of the microelectrodes.

In contrast, for 44% of the units in this sample, the discrepancy between conduction velocities exceeded 20%, reaching 60% in one case. An example is shown in Fig. 16C (unit L2A33). The conduction velocity calculated from VR to FP was generally lower than within the femoral nerve cuff. For every one of these units, the duration of the VR action potential exceeded 0.6 ms (arrows in Fig. 16C). The VR spike was usually polyphasic (of reproducible shape with repeated averaging). The shape and prolonged duration of the VR potential, and the slow propagation from VR to FP (but not from FP to FD), suggested that the axons of motoneurons in this category had been damaged locally by the implanted VR microelectrodes.

Figure 16E compares, for 25 motoneurons, the discrepancy between conduction velocity values measured from root to cuff and those measured within the cuff (VR→FP/FP→FD; ordinate) with respect to the duration of the VR action potential (abscissa). The eight "uninjured" units in the first category (enclosed within the dashed box) all had VR action potential duration of <0.6 ms. Six units (24%) also had conduction velocity estimations within the ±20% range, even though their VR potential duration exceeded 0.6 ms. The VR axons of this third category of motoneurons appeared to be less severely damaged by the microelectrodes.

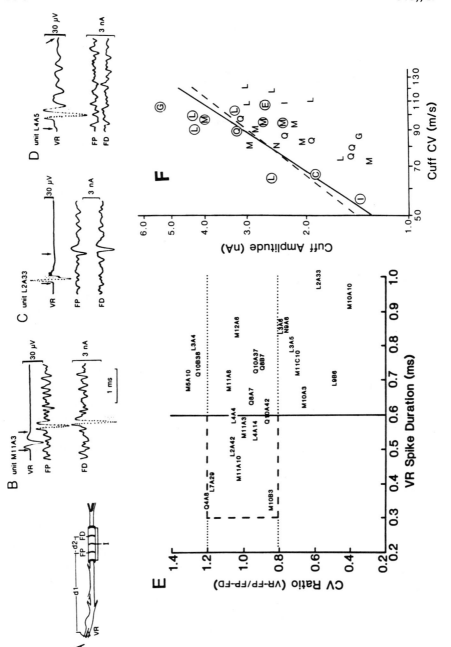

Fig. 16. (A) Diagram of the recording configuration used for spike-triggered averaging of neural signals. (B–D) Examples of spike-triggered averaged records obtained from three representative motoneurons. Signals recorded by the VR, FP, and FD electrodes are shown. All signals were digitally delayed 0.5 ms prior to averaging. The VR record was calibrated in µV and the cuff electrode records in nA. (B) Example of axon that did not appear injured by the presence of the VR microelectrodes. The VR potential was simple triphasic $(+, -, +)$, of average amplitude (30 µV), and its duration (shown by arrows) was <0.6 ms. The FP and FD records showed neural potentials well-resolved from noise, triphasic $(+, -, +)$, and at brief latencies from the VR spike. (C) Example of axon that was probably injured by the VR microelectrodes. Its VR spike was multiphasic, of larger-than-average amplitude (128 µV), and of duration considerably >0.6 ms (arrows). The FP and FD potentials were poorly resolved from noise, and the latency from the FP to the FD potential. (D) Example of axon that appeared to have suffered severe damage. It almost always fired closely spaced triplets of 65-µV amplitude; the second and third components appear washed out in the averaged record as a result of time jitter. Further details in text. (E) Summary for 25 motoneurons. The name of each unit represents its location in the plot. The ordinate shows the ratio of CV values measured in two segments of the axon, d1 and d2 (see A). In uniformly conducting axons, the ratio would be 1 (1 ± 0.2, accounting for measurement errors). See text for interpretation of data distribution within dotted and dashed areas. (F) Relation between axonal CV (measured between FP and FD within the femoral nerve cuff) and amplitude of the action currents recorded by FP and FD; double-logarithmic plot. Letters represent the cats from which the 30 motoneurons shown in this plot were recorded. The dashed line reproduces the best fit obtained for a population of 55 afferent fibers recorded in the same cats (see Fig. 6A). Twelve motoneurons deemed "undamaged" by the VR electrodes (circled data) were fitted by a line (solid) that agreed closely with the dashed line obtained for afferents. The other 18 motoneurons (uncircled data) had shown signs of damage in the VR. They tended to yield smaller averaged action currents (reproduced from Figs. 3 and 4, Hoffer et al., 1987a).

131

A fourth category consisted of axons suspected of having suffered extreme injury by a microelectrode, exemplified by unit L4A5 (Fig. 16D). Since unit L4A5 was active during the stance phase of locomotion, it probably was a motoneuron that had innervated an anterior thigh muscle. However, no correlated cuff potentials appeared with spike-triggered averaging. It was assumed that this axon was either severed by a microelectrode, or damaged sufficiently to block conduction. Interestingly, although unit L4A5 seemed to generate typical motoneuron discharge profiles during locomotion, it usually fired closely spaced triplets of action potentials with interspike intervals of ≈ 4 ms, suggesting that two additional action potentials were being generated ectopically in the cut axon (Wall and Gutnick, 1974). Repeated trials resulted in different averaged waveforms for this unit, probably because of jitter in the timing of the second and third spikes in the triplets. Only about six axons that fired this kind of aberrant pattern were encountered by Hoffer et al. (1987a–c), out of a sample of 164 ventral root axons.

8.1.2. Relation Between Amplitude of Cuff Action Current and Axonal Conduction Velocity

In the above experiments, the amplitude of the recorded extracellular action currents for 30 motoneurons, extracted by spike-triggered averaging from the femoral nerve cuff electrode records, was positively correlated with the axonal conduction velocity (Fig. 16F). A similar trend was found for afferent neurons recorded from the L5 dorsal root ganglion in the same cats (Fig. 6A), well fitted by a straight line of slope = 1.3 and intercept = –2.1. This line is reproduced, dashed, in Fig. 16F. For 12 motoneurons deemed "uninjured" by the criteria of Fig. 16E, a comparable line fit was obtained (solid line; slope = 1.5, intercept = –2.4). In contrast, 18 motoneurons deemed "injured" tended to plot below the lines. The action currents recorded with spike-triggered averaging from "injured" axons tended to be smaller, as a result of jitter in conduction along the ventral root. This finding is consistent with the view that the site of damage was in the ventral root, not in the peripheral nerve within the cuff.

These observations, taken together, indicate that a chronically implanted microelectrode can cause local damage to nerve fibers, although the damage is often minor and need not alter the normal firing patterns of the neuron. These data also suggest that axonal conduction velocity estimates should be made on the basis of latency measurements along the peripheral axon, so as to avoid potentially spurious values caused by local injury to the ventral root, and also to benefit from the higher precision of intracuff measurements (section 3.5.).

8.2. Expected Functional Longevity of Implanted Devices

Cat preparations typically work well for 1–2 mo after implantation. After this time, most implanted devices (except nerve cuffs; *see below*) tend to malfunction as a result of breakage, migration, or progressive remodeling of tissues. The expected lifetime and specific reasons for breakdown for the different implanted devices can be summarized as follows:

Single-unit floating microelectrodes can be expected to survive for 2–5 wk. The usual reason for failure is breakage of the fine lead wire. In electrodes that last more than 3 wk, a secondary reason for failure can be a progressive electrode encapsulation by fibrous tissue, which tends to move nearby neurons 10–30 μm away from the electrode tip. Evidence for this process comes from histological studies (Schmidt et al., 1976), from the progressively smaller unitary action potentials that tend to be recorded over time, and from the progressively larger currents that are needed to stimulate units over time (Hoffer et al., unpublished observations).

Implanted EMG electrodes often last many weeks without major change in their performance. The most fragile can be the spiral bipolar electrodes, or any electrodes that require the use of Pt Ir wire rather than stainless steel. With multistrand stainless-steel wire EMG electrodes, the cause of malfunction is often not breakage, but rather a slow migration from the original location that can lead to altogether erroneous recordings from other muscles.

Nerve recording and stimulating cuff electrodes are by far the most robust of all the implantable devices considered in this study. If appropriate precautions are taken in the design (section 3.1.) and surgical implantation (section 3.3.) of nerve cuffs, and if the lead-out cable is routed so that it cannot impose tugs or torques on the nerve, the long-term prognosis of a nerve preparation is excellent. This is because, as connective tissue grows inside and around the nerve cuff, the mechanical coupling of the cuff to the nerve becomes more and more stable, and as a bonus, the impedance of the electrode increases (Stein et al., 1978). As a result, recorded signals tend to improve over a period of weeks, and the likelihood of mechanical damage to the nerve diminishes with time. Ample evidence for the long-term safety and invariant performance of stimulating cuff electrodes is available from the clinical literature; chronic electrical stimulation of human nerves was first attempted over 100 yr ago and has been successfully performed on phrenic or peroneal nerves for over 20 yr (Hambrecht and Reswick, 1977; Glenn and Phelps, 1985; McNeal and Bowman, 1985). The few differences between nerve stimulating and recording cuff electrodes need not affect much the expected longevity of recording cuff electrodes. In cat regeneration studies, it was possible to record from individual nerves for 1 yr (Gordon et al., 1980).

Tendon force transducers and distensible length transducers, as well as any implanted device that must rely on mechanical deformation for its function, cannot be expected to last indefinitely. The usual reasons for malfunction are either mechanical fatigue leading to breakage, impedance changes resulting from fluid leakage and/or corrosion, or migration from the original site of implantation because of the presence of continuous forces acting on the device and the tissue. An alternative cause for failure of tendon force transducers is encapsulation by new tendinous fibers that eventually take up the load (section 5.2.). Tendon force and distensible length transducers can usually be expected to perform well for 1–2 mo. Signals recorded with implanted piezoelectric crystals improve markedly over the first 1–2 wk and remain stable for a least 1 mo after implantation. Their useful lifetime has not been yet determined.

9. Clinical Applications of Chronic Recording Techniques

At least two types of severely disabling disorders may warrant considering the use of implanted devices for the control of prostheses: high-level limb amputation (particularly bilateral) and stroke or spinal-cord injuries.

An experimental model of nerve amputation, ligation of peripheral nerves in cats (Davis et al., 1978), has shown that the proximal stumps of severed motor nerve fibers may remain viable indefinitely. Furthermore, cat motoneurons chronically disconnected from their target muscles continue to be activated in the appropriate patterns characteristic of locomotion (Gordon et al.,

1980). Thus, in amputees, the stumps of peripheral nerves that originally projected to the missing limb musculature could be used as sources of output signals to control prosthetic limbs. After axotomy, the proximal stumps of peripheral axons are known to shrink and produce smaller extracellular potentials (Davis et al., 1978; Hoffer et al., 1979; Gillespie and Stein, 1983), but they can regain their size after reinnervation (Davis et al., 1978). Thus, signals generated from amputated motor nerves could be augmented by grafting the nerve to a purposely denervated portion of a proximal "donor" muscle, and recording the resulting nerve (or muscle) signal (Hoffer and Loeb, 1980). In turn, sensory information from transducers in the prosthesis could be relayed back to sensory nerve fibers in amputated nerves, using electrical stimulation (Stein et al., 1980a,b).

In stroke or spinal-cord injury patients, the peripheral sensorimotor system usually remains viable below the lesion, but disconnected from the central nervous system. The challenge is to reestablish some measure of the two-way traffic that normally allows motor centers to monitor sensory inputs and to control movements. Partial restoration of upper and lower limb function can be achieved with functional electrical stimulation (FES) of paralyzed muscles (Mortimer, 1981). Safe and efficient parameters for muscle or nerve stimulation have largely been determined (e.g., Mortimer, 1981; Hambrecht, 1985; Grandjean and Mortimer, 1986; Sweeney and Mortimer, 1986). Contemporary FES systems, however, use open-loop control, insensitive to changes in limb position, load, or fatigue (Cybulski et al., 1984; Crago et al., 1980, 1986). Since human glabrous skin mechanoreceptors provide detailed information about contact force and impending slippage that is normally used in precision grip (Johansson and Vallbo, 1979; Johansson and Westling, 1987), closed-loop control of FES of paralyzed muscles may be achieved using skin contact force feedback information provided by nerve cuff recording electrodes implanted on cutaneous nerves (Hoffer and Sinkjaer, 1986; Hoffer and Li, 1988). Implementation will require a totally implanted telemetry system for transmitting sensory information recorded from nerves, combined with an implanted telemetered stimulation system for FES (e.g., Buckett et al., 1985). Closed-loop control systems based on feedback from implanted nerve cuff electrodes should provide reliable long-term performance and be widely accepted by users, for practical as well as cosmetic reasons. Advanced versions may incorporate multichannel recording and stimulation technology based on, for example, miniature micro-electrode arrays implanted in nerves or roots (e.g., Weissman and Schwartz, 1981; Edell, 1986), once their long-term reliability is proven, and may include other types of sensors, like Hall effect goniometers to measure joint position (Troyk et al., 1986), in addition to contact force sensors.

Acknowledgments

I gratefully acknowledge the numerous past and present collaborators and colleagues who contributed in various ways to the development of the chronic recording techniques described here. In chronological order of our association, they are: W. B. Marks, K. Frank, W. Z. Rymer, F. T. Hambrecht, E. M. Schmidt, R. B. Stein, D. Charles, L. A. Davis, T. Gordon, T. E. Milner, G. E. Loeb, M. J. Bak, M. J. O'Donovan, C. A. Pratt, N. Sugano, A. Prochazka, C. L. Cleland, R. I. Griffiths, T. Sinkjaer, A. A. Caputi, I. E. Pose and J. L. F. Weytjens.

I am also grateful to the organizations that provide grant support for my current research: the Muscular Dystrophy Association of Canada, the Medical Research Council of Canada, the Rick Hansen Man in Motion Legacy Fund of Canada, and the Spinal Cord Research Foundation of the USA.

References

Abraham L. D., Marks W. B., and Loeb G. E. (1985) The distal hindlimb musculature of the cat. Cutaneous reflexes during locomotion. *Exp. Brain Res.* **58**, 594–603.

Aguayo A., Nair C. P. V., and Midley R. (1971) Experimental progressive neuropathy in the rabbit. *Arch. Neurol.* **24**, 358–364.

Alexander R. McN. and Bennet-Clarke H. C. (1977) Storage of elastic strain energy in muscle and other tissues. *Nature* **265**, 114–117.

Altman K. V., and Plonsey R. (1986) A two-part model for determining the electromagnetic and physiologic behavior of cuff electrode nerve stimulators. *IEEE Trans. Biomed. Eng.* **33**, 285–293.

Amos A., Armstrong D. M., and Marple-Horvat D. E. (1987) A ladder paradigm for studying skilled and adaptive locomotion in the cat. *J. Neurosci. Methods* **20,** 323–340.

Barnes G. R. G. and Pinder, D. N. (1974) In vivo tendon and bone strain measurement and correlation. *J. Biomech.* **7,** 35–42.

Bloedel J. R. and Courville J. (1981) Cerebellar afferent systems, in *Handbook of Physiology, Vol. II: Motor Control* (Brooks V. B., ed.), Am. Physiol. Soc., Bethesda, Maryland, pp. 735–830.

Bromberg M. B. and Fetz E. E. (1977) Responses of single units in cervical spinal cord of alert monkeys. *Exp. Neurol.* **55,** 469–482.

Buckett J. R., Braswell S. D., Peckham P. H., Thorpe G. B., and Keith M. W. (1985) A portable functional neuromuscular stimulation system. *IEEE 7th Annual Conf in Med. Biol. Soc.,* 314–317.

Burke R. E., Levine D. N., Tsairis P., and Zajac F. E. (1973) Physiological types and histochemical profiles in motor units of the cat gastrocnemius. *J. Physiol.* **234,** 723–748.

Cavagna G. A. (1977) Storage and utilization of elastic energy in skeletal muscle. *Exerc. Sport Sci. Rev.* **5,** 89–129.

Cleland C. L. and Hoffer J. A. (1986a) Activity patterns of spinocerebellar neurons during normal locomotion, in *Neurobiology of Vertebrate Locomotion* (Grillner S., Stein P. S. G., Stuart D. G., Forssberg H., and Herman R., eds), Macmillan, London, pp. 705–723.

Cleland C. L. and Hoffer J. A. (1986b) Chronic recordings from neurons in the spinal cord of freely moving cats: cutaneous spinocerebellar neurons. *Neurosci. Lett. [Suppl.]* **26,** S364.

Cleland C. L. and Hoffer J. A. (1987) Activity of ventral spinocerebellar tract neurons chronically recorded in the spinal cord of awake, freely moving cats, in *Motor Control* (Gantchev G. N., Dimitrov B., and Gatev P., eds.), Plenum, New York, pp. 155–158.

Collins J. G. (1985) A technique for chronic extracellular recording of neuronal activity in the dorsal horn of the lumbar spinal cord in drug free, physiologically intact, cats. *J. Neurosci. Methods* **12,** 277–287.

Creed R. S., Denny-Brown D., Eccles J. C., Liddell E. G. T., and Sherrington C. S. (1932; reprinted 1972) *Reflex Activity of the Spinal Cord* (Clarendon Press, Oxford).

Crago P. E., Mortimer J. T., and Peckham P. H. (1980) Closed-loop control of force during electrical stimulation of muscle. *IEEE Trans. Biomed. Eng.* **27,** 306–312.

Crago P. E., Chizeck H. J., Neuman M. R., and Hambrecht F. T. (1986) Sensors for use with functional neuromuscular stimulation. *IEEE Trans. Biomed. Eng.* **33,** 256–268.

Cybulski G. R., Penn R. D., and Jaeger T. J. (1984) Lower extremity functional neuromuscular stimulation in cases of spinal cord injury. *Neurosurgery* **15**, 132–146.

Davis L. A., Gordon T., Hoffer J. A., Jhamandas J., and Stein R. B. (1978) Compound action potentials recorded from mammalian peripheral nerves following ligation or resuturing. *J. Physiol.* **285**, 543–559.

Duysens J. and Stein R. B. (1978) Reflexes induced by nerve stimulation in walking cats with implanted cuff electrodes. *Exp. Brain Res.* **32**, 213–224.

Ebly E. M. (1986) "Chronic recordings of pulmonary stretch receptor activity in neonatal lambs." M. Sc. thesis, University of Calgary, Calgary, Alberta, Canada.

Ebly E. M., Cleland C. L., Hoffer J. A., and Maloney J. E. (1986a) Chronic recordings of pulmonary stretch receptor activity during development in the neonatal lamb. *Soc. Neurosci. Abstr.* **12**, 303.

Ebly E. M., Hoffer J. A., and Maloney J. E. (1986b) Chronic recordings of pulmonary afferent activity from the vagus nerve in naturally breathing lambs. *Can. J. Physiol. Pharmacol.* **64**, Aix.

Edell, D. J. (1986) A peripheral nerve information transducer for amputees: long-term multichannel recordings from rabbit peripheral nerves. *IEEE Trans. Biomed. Eng.* **33**, 203–214.

Evarts E. V. (1968) A technique for recording activity of subcortical neurons in moving animals. *Electroencephalogr. Clin. Neurophysiol.* **24**, 83–86.

Frank K. (1968) Some approaches to the technical problem of chronic excitation of peripheral nerves. *Ann. Otol., Rhinol. and Laryngol.* **77**, 761–772.

Ghez C. and Vicario D. (1978) The control of rapid limb movement in the cat. I. Response latency. *Exp. Brain Res.* **33**, 173–189.

Gillespie M. J., and Stein R. B. (1983) The relationship between axon diameter, myelin thickness and conduction velocity during atrophy of mammalian peripheral nerves. *Brain Res.* **259**, 41–56.

Glenn, L. L., and Dement, W. (1981) Membrane potential and input resistance of cat spinal motoneurons in wakefulness and sleep. *Behav. Brain Res.* **2**, 231–236.

Glenn L. L., Whitney J. F., Rewitzer J. S., Salamone J. A., and Mariash S. A. (1988) Method for stable intracellular recordings of spinal alpha-motoneurons during treadmill walking in awake, intact cats. *Brain Res.* **439**, 396–401.

Glenn W. W. L. and Phelps M. L. (1985) Diaphragm pacing by electrical stimulation of the phrenic nerve. *Neurosurgery* **17**, 974–984.

Gordon T., Hoffer J. A., Jhamandas J., and Stein R. B. (1980) Long-term effects of axotomy on neural activity during cat locomotion. *J. Physiol.* **303,** 243–263.

Goslow G. E., Reinking R. M., and Stuart D. G. (1973) The cat step cycle: hind limb joint angles and muscle lengths during unrestrained locomotion. *J. Morphol.* **141,** 1–42.

Grandjean P. A., and Mortimer J. T. (1986) Recruitment properties of monopolar and bipolar epimysial electrodes. *Ann. Biomed. Eng.* **14,** 53–66.

Gregor R. J., Hager C. L., and Roy R. R. (1981) *In vivo* muscle forces during unrestrained locomotion. *J. Biomech.* **14,** 489.

Griffiths R. I. (1987) Ultrasound transit time gives direct measurement of muscle fiber length in vivo. *J. Neurosci. Methods* **21,** 159–165.

Griffiths R. I. and Hoffer J. A. (1987) Muscle fibers *shorten* when the whole muscle is being stretched in the "yield phase" of the freely walking cat. *Soc. Neurosci. Abstr.* **13,** 1214.

Hagbarth K. A., Hongell A., and Wallin G. (1970) The effect of gamma fibre block on afferent muscle nerve activity during voluntary contractions. *Acta Physiol. Scand.* **79,** 27–28.

Hambrecht F. T., (1985) Control of neural prostheses, in: *Electromyography and Evoked Potentials* (Struppler A., and Weindl A., eds.), Springer, Berlin, pp. 64–67.

Hambrecht F. T. and Reswick J. B. (eds.) (1977) *Functional Electrical Stimulation: Applications in Neural Prostheses. Biomed. Engng. and Instrum. Ser. 3,* Marcel Dekker, New York.

Hatta I., Sugi H., and Tamura Y. (1988) Stiffness changes in frog skeletal muscle during contraction recorded using ultrasonic waves. *J. Physiol.* **403,** 193–209.

Hoffer J. A. (1975) *Long-term Peripheral Nerve Activity during Behaviour in the Rabbit: The Control of Locomotion,* Publ. No. 76-8530, University Microfilms, Ann Arbor, Michigan.

Hoffer J. A. and Cleland C. L. (1986) Alternative approaches to recording activity of spinal cord neurons in behaving animals. *J. Neurosci. Methods* **17,** 198–199.

Hoffer J. A. and Li T. (1988) Real-time processing of cutaneous nerve activity to obtain contact force information. *Soc. Neurosci. Abstr.* **13,** 64.

Hoffer J. A. and Loeb G. E. (1980) Implantable electrical and mechanical interfaces with nerve and muscle. *Ann. Biomed. Eng.* **8,** 351–360.

Hoffer J. A. and Loeb G. E. (1983) A technique for reversible fusimotor blockade during chronic recording from spindle afferents in walking cats. *Exp. Brain. Res.* **Suppl. 7,** 272–279.

Hoffer J. A. and Marks W. B. (1976) Long term peripheral nerve activity during behavior in the rabbit. *Adv. Behav. Biol.* **18,** 767–768.

Hoffer J. A. and Sinkjaer, T. (1986) A natural "force sensor" suitable for closed-loop control of functional neuromuscular stimulation. *Proc. 2nd. Vienna Int'l Workshop on Functional Electrostimulation,* pp. 47–50.

Hoffer J. A. and Sinkjaer T. (1987) Decerebration causes increased spindle sensitivity in triceps surae muscles of standing cats. *Neuroscience* **22,** S659.

Hoffer J. A., Leonard T. R., and Spence N. S. (1983) A method for measuring muscle stiffness in unrestrained cats. *Soc. Neurosci. Abstr.* **9,** 470.

Hoffer J. A., Loeb G. E., and Pratt C. A. (1981a) Single unit conduction velocities from averaged nerve cuff electrode records in freely moving cats. *J. Neurosci. Methods* **4,** 211–225.

Hoffer J. A., Marks W. B., and Rymer W. Z. (1974) Nerve fiber activity during normal movements. *Abstr. Soc. Neurosci.,* p. 258.

Hoffer J. A., Stein R. B. and Gordon T. (1979) Differential atrophy of sensory and motor fibers following section of cat peripheral nerves. *Brain Res.* **178,** 347–361.

Hoffer J. A., Caputi A. A., Pose I. E. and Griffiths R. I. Roles of muscle activity and load on the relationship between muscle spindle length and whole muscle length in the freely walking cat. *Prog. Brain Res.,* in press.

Hoffer J. A., Leonard T. R., Cleland C. L., and Sinkjaer T. Segmental reflex action in normal and decerebrate cats. *J. Neurophysiol.,* in press.

Hoffer J. A., Loeb G. E., Marks W. B., O'Donovan M. J., Pratt C. A., and Sugano N. (1987a) Cat hindlimb motoneurons during locomotion. I. Destination, axonal conduction velocity and recruitment threshold. *J. Neurophysiol.* **57,** 510–529.

Hoffer J. A., Sugano N., Loeb G. E., Marks W. B., O'Donovan M. J., and Pratt C. A. (1987b) Cat hindlimb motoneurons during locomotion. II. Normal activity patterns. *J. Neurophysiol.* **57,** 530–553.

Hoffer J. A., Loeb G. E., Sugano N., Marks W. B., O'Donovan M. J., and Pratt C. A. (1987c) Cat hindlimb motoneurons during locomotion. III. Functional segregation in sartorius. *J. Neurophysiol.* **57,** 554–562.

Hoffer J. A., O'Donovan M. J., Pratt C. A., and Loeb G. E. (1981b) Discharge patterns of hindlimb motoneurons during normal cat locomotion. *Science* **213,** 466–468.

Hubel D. H. (1957) Tungsten microelectrode for recording from single units. *Science* **125,** 549–550.

Hulliger M. (1984) The mammalian muscle spindle and its central action. *Rev. Physiol. Biochem. Pharmacol.* **101,** 1–110.

Hulliger M., Horber F., Medved A., and Prochazka A. (1987) An experimental simulation method for iterative and interactive reconstruction of unknown (fusimotor) inputs contribution to known (spindle afferent) responses. *J. Neurosci. Methods* **21,** 225–238.

Humphrey D. R. (1970) A chronically implantable multiple microelectrode system with independent control of electrode positions. *Electroencephalogr. Clin. Neurophysiol.* **29,** 616–620.

Johansson R. and Vallbo A. (1979) Tactile sensibility in the human hand: relative and absolute densities of four types of mechanosensitive units in glabrous skin. *J. Physiol.* **286,** 283–300.

Johansson R. and Westling G. (1987) Signals in tactile afferents from the fingers eliciting adaptive motor responses during precision grip. *Exp. Brain Res.* **66,** 141–154.

Julien C. and Rossignol S. (1982) Electroneurographic recordings with polymer cuff electrodes in paralyzed cats. *J. Neurosci. Methods* **5,** 267–272.

Kear M. and Smyth R. N. (1975) A method for recording tendon strain in sheep during locomotion. *Acta Orthop. Scand.* **46,** 896–905.

Krarup C. and Loeb G. E. (1987) Multielectrode nerve cuffs reveal growth and maturation rates of group-identified regenerating axons. *Muscle Nerve* **10,** 189–191.

Komi P. V., Jarvinen M., and Salonen M. (1984) In vivo measurements of achilles tendon force in man. *Med. Sci. Sports Exerc.* **16,** 165.

Lemon R., (1984) *Methods for Neuronal Recording in Conscious Animals. IBRO Handbook Series: Methods in the Neurosciences,* Vol. 4. (Wiley, Chichester).

Lochner F. K., Milne D. W., Mills E. J. and Groom J. J. (1980) In vivo and in vitro measurement of tendon strain in the horse. *Am. J. Vet. Res.* **41,** 1929–1937.

Loeb G. E. (1987) Hard lessons in motor control from the mammalian spinal cord. *Trends Neurosci.* **10,** 108–113.

Loeb G. E. and Gans C. (1986) *Electromyography for Experimentalists,* Univ. Chicago Press, Chicago.

Loeb, G. E. and Hoffer, J. A. (1985) Activity of spindle afferents from cat anterior thigh muscles. II. Effects of fusimotor blockade. *J. Neurophysiol.* **54,** 565–577.

Loeb G. E., Bak M. J., Duysens J. (1977a) Long-term unit recording from somatosensory neurons in the spinal ganglia of the freely walking cat. *Science* **197,** 1192–1194.

Loeb G. E., Bak M. J., Salcman M., and Schmidt E. M. (1977b) Parylene as a chronically stable, reproducible microelectrode insulator. *IEEE Trans. Biomed. Eng.* **24,** 121–128.

Loeb, G. E., Hoffer, J. A. and Pratt, C. A. (1985a) Activity of spindle afferents from cat anterior thigh muscles. I. Identification and patterns during normal locomotion. *J. Neurophysiol.* **54**, 549–564.

Loeb, G. E., Hoffer, J. A. and Marks, W. B. (1985b) Activity of spindle aferents from cat anterior thigh muscles. III. Effects of external stimuli. *J. Neurophysiol.* **54**, 578–591.

Loeb G. E., Marks W. B., and Hoffer J. A. (1987) Cat hindlimb motoneurons during locomotion. IV. Participation in cutaneous reflexes. *J. Neurophysiol.* **57**, 563–573.

Loeb G. E., Walmsley B., and Duysens J. (1980) Obtaining proprioceptive information from natural limbs: implantable transducers vs. somatosensory neuron recordings, in: *Physical Sensors for Biomedical Applications. Proc. of Workshop on Solid State Physical Sensors for Biomedical Application,* (Neuman M. R. ed.) Boca Raton, Florida, CRC, 1980, p. 135–149.

McNeal D. R. and Bowman B. R. (1985) Selective activation of muscles using peripheral nerve electrodes. *Med. Biol. Eng. Comput.* **23**, 249–253.

Macpherson J. M., Lywood D. W., and van Eyken A. (1987) A system for the analysis of posture and stance in quadrupeds. *J. Neurosci. Methods* **20**, 73–82.

Marks W. B. (1965) Some methods for simultaneous multiunit recording. *Proc. Symp. on Informat. Processing in Sight Sensory Systems,* (Nye P. W. ed.), Caltech, Pasadena, California, pp. 200–206.

Marks W. B. and Loeb G. E. (1976) Action currents, internodal potentials and extracellular records of myelinated mammalian nerve fibers derived from node potentials. *Biophys. J.* **16**, 655–668.

Marshall K. W., Tatton W. G., and Bruce I. C. (1984) A technique for recording from single neurons in the spinal cord of the awake rat. *J. Neurosci. Methods* **10**, 249–257.

Matthews P. B. C. and Rushworth G. (1957) The relative sensitivity of muscle nerve fibres to procaine. *J. Physiol.* **135**, 263–269.

Milner, T. E. and Hoffer, J. A. (1987) Long-term peripheral nerve and muscle recordings from normal and dystrophic mice. *J. Neurosci. Methods* **19**, 37–45.

Morales F. R. and Chase M. H. (1981) Postsynaptic control of lumbar motoneuron excitability during active sleep in the chronic cat. *Brain Res.* **225**, 279–295.

Mortimer J. T. (1981) Motor Prostheses, in *Handbook of Physiology, The Nervous System II: Motor Control* (Brooks V. B., ed.) Am. Physiol. Soc., Bethesda, Maryland, pp. 155–187.

Naples G. G., Mortimer J. T., Scheiner A. and Sweeney J. D. (1988) A spiral nerve cuff electrode for peripheral nerve stimulation. *IEEE Trans. Biomed. Eng.* **35**, 905–916.

Newman S., Road J., Bellemare F., Clozel J. P., Lavigne C. M., Grassino A. (1984) Respiratory muscle length measured by sonomicrometry. *J. Appl. Physiol.* **56**, 753–764.

O'Donovan M. J., Hoffer J. A., and Loeb G. E. (1983) Physiological characterization of motor unit properties in intact cats. *J. Neurosci. Methods* **7**, 137–149.

Otten E. (1988) Concepts and models of functional architecture in skeletal muscle. *Exerc. Sport Sci. Rev.* **16**, 89–137.

Paintal A. S. (1953) The conduction velocities of respiratory and cardiovascular afferent fibres in the vagus nerve. *J. Physiol.* **121**, 341–359.

Paintal A. S. (1966) The influence of diameter of medullated nerve fibres of cats on the rising and falling phases of the spike and its recovery. *J. Physiol.* **184**, 791–811.

Philippson M. (1905) L'autonomie et la centralisation dans le système nerveux des animaux. *Trav. Lab. Physiol. Inst. Solvay, Bruxelles* **7**, 1–208.

Prochazka A. (1981) Muscle spindle function during normal movement. *Int. Rev. Physiol. Neurophysiol.* **IV**, 47–90.

Prochazka A. (1984) Chronic techniques for studying neurophysiology of movement in cats, in *Methods for Neuronal Recording in Conscious Animals. IBRO Handbook Series: Methods in the Neurosciences*, vol. 4, (Wiley, Chichester) pp. 113–128.

Prochazka A., Westerman R., and Ziccone S. (1976) Discharges of single hindlimb afferents in the freely moving cat. *J. Neurophysiol.* **39**, 1090–1104.

Prochazka A., Hulliger M., Zangger P., and Appenteng K. (1985) "Fusimotor set": new evidence for alpha-independent control of gamma-motoneurons during movement in the awake cat. *Brain Res.* **339**, 136–140.

Prochazka A., Tate K., Westerman R., and Ziccone S. (1974) Remote monitoring of muscle length and EMG in unrestrained cats. *Electroencephalogr. Clin. Neurophysiol.* **37**, 649–653.

Rack P. M. H. and Westbury D. R. (1984) Elastic properties of the cat soleus tendon and their functional importance. *J. Physiol.* **347**, 479–495.

Rushmer R. F., Franklin D., and Ellis R. (1956) Left ventricular dimensions recorded by sonocardiometry. *Circ. Res.* **4**, 684–688.

Salcman M. and Bak M. J. (1973) Design, fabrication and in vivo behavior of chronic recording intracortical electodes. *IEEE Trans. Biomed. Eng.* **20**, 253–260.

Schmidt E. M. (1983) Parylene as an electrode insulator: a review. *J. Electrophysiol. Tech.* **10**, 19–29.

Schmidt E. M., Bak M. J., and McIntosh J. S. (1976) Long-term chronic recording from cortical neurons. *Exp. Neurol.* **52**, 496–506.

Sinkjaer T. and Hoffer J. A. (1987a) A computer-controlled system to perturb the ankle joint of freely standing cats trained to maintain a given force. *J. Neurosci. Methods* **21**, 311–320.

Sinkjaer T. and Hoffer J. A. (1987b) Blocking antagonist nerve reduces the amplitude of the short-latency stretch reflex response in triceps surae muscles of cats. *Soc. Neurosci. Abstr.* **13**, 717.

Sinkjaer T. and Hoffer J. A. Factors determining segmental reflex action in normal and decerebrate cats. *J. Neurophysiol.*, in press.

Stein R. B. and Oğuztöreli M. N. (1978) The radial decline of nerve impulses in a restricted cylindrical extracellular space. *Biol. Cybern.* **28**, 159–165.

Stein R. B. and Pearson K. G. (1971) Predicted amplitude and form of extracellularly recorded action potentials from unmyelinated nerve fibers. *J. Theor. Biol.* **32**, 539.

Stein R. B., Charles D., Davis L., Jhamandas J., Mannard A., and Nichols T. R. (1975) Principles underlying new methods for chronic neural recording. *Can. J. Neurol. Sci.* **2**, 235–244.

Stein R. B., Charles D., Gordon T., Hoffer J. A., and Jhamandas J. (1978) Impedance properties of metal electrodes for chronic recording from mammalian nerves. *IEEE Trans.* **25** 532–537.

Stein R. B., Nichols T. R., Jhamandas J., Davis L. A. and Charles D. (1977) Stable long-term recordings from cat peripheral nerves. *Brain Res.* **128**, 21–38.

Stein R. B., Charles D., Hoffer J. A., Arsenault J., Davis L. A., Moorman S., and Moss B. (1980a) New approaches to controlling powered arm prostheses, particularly by high-level amputees. *Bull. Prosth. Res.* **17**, 51–62.

Stein R. B., Gordon T., Hoffer J. A., Davis L. A., and Charles D. (1980b) Long-term recordings from cat peripheral nerves during degeneration and regeneration: Implications for human nerve repair and prosthetics, in *Nerve Repair: Its Clinical and Experimental Basis* (Jewett D. L. and McCarroll H. R., eds.), C. V. Mosby, St. Louis, pp. 166–176.

Strumwasser F. (1958) Longterm recording from single neurons in the brains of unrestrained animals. *Science* **127**, 468–470.

Stuart D. G. and Enoka R. M. (1983) Motoneurons, motor units and the size principle, in *The Clinical Neurosciences* (Rosenberg R. N., ed), Churchill Livingstone, New York, pp. 471–517.

Sunderland S. (1968) *Nerves and Nerve Injuries*. Livingstone, London.

Sweeney J. D. and Mortimer J. T. (1986) An asymmetric two electrode cuff for generation of unidirectionally propagated action potentials. *IEEE Trans. Biomed. Eng.* **33**, 541–549.

Tamura Y., Hatta I., Matsuda T., Sugi H., and Tsuchiya T. (1982) Changes in muscle stiffness during contraction recorded using ultrasonic waves. *Nature* **299**, 631–633.

Tasaki I. (1964) A new measurement of action currents developed by single nodes of Ranvier. *J. Neurophysiol.* **27**, 1199–1210.

Thoma H., Frey M., Stöhr H., Gruber H., and Holle J. (1984) Epineural electrode implantation for electrically induced mobilization of paraplegics. *Artif. Organs* **8**, 384.

Troyk P. R., Jaeger R. J., Haklin M., Poyezdala J., and Bajzek T. (1986) Design and implementation of an implantable goniometer. *IEEE Trans. Biomed. Eng.* **33**, 215–221.

Wall P. D. and Gutnick M. (1974) Ongoing activity in peripheral nerves: the physiology and pharmacology of impulses originating from a neuroma. *Exp. Neurol.* **43**, 580–593.

Walmsley B., Hodgson J. A., and Burke R. E. (1978) Forces produced by soleus and medial gastrocnemius muscles during locomotion in freely moving cats. *J. Neurophysiol.* **41**, 1203–1216.

Weissman A. and Schwartz E. (1981) A flexible high density multichannel electrode array for long-term chronic implantation. *Brain Res. Bull.* **6**, 543–546.

Wolpaw J. R. (1987) Operant conditioning of primate spinal reflexes: the H-reflex. *J. Neurophysiol.* **57**, 443–459.

From: *Neuromethods, Vol. 15: Neurophysiological Techniques: Applications to Neural Systems* Edited by: A. A. Boulton, G. B. Baker, and C. H. Vanderwolf Copyright © 1990 The Humana Press Inc., Clifton, NJ

Human Evoked Potentials

Eric Halgren

1. Introduction

1.1. Organization and Scope of This Review

After the current section, the history (1.2.) of evoked potentials (EPs—for abbreviations, *see* the end of this chapter) is briefly presented, followed by a discussion of how EPs can be broken down into components (1.3.). General methodology (2.) is then presented, covering recording techniques (2.1.), including electrodes and their placement (2.1.1.), reference electrodes (2.1.2.), EEG amplifying, filtering, and digitizing (2.1.3.), and recording artifacts (2.1.4.). The discussion of methodology then turns to analysis techniques (2.2.), from averaging and peak detection (2.2.1.), and alternative analysis methods (2.2.2.), to factor analysis (2.2.3.), spectral analysis (2.2.4.), and topographical display (2.2.5.). Increasing use is being made of methods of generator localization (2.3.), from scalp EPs (2.3.1.), from evoked magnetic fields (2.3.2.), and from depth recordings and brain lesions (2.3.3.).

The different categories of EPs are then individually presented, beginning with those evoked by sensory stimuli (3.). Auditory EPs (3.1.) are divided according to their poststimulus latency into brainstem (3.1.1.), middle latency (3.1.2.), and long latency auditory EPs (3.1.3.). Somatosensory EPs (3.2.) are then discussed, including the methods (3.2.1.) used to record them, and their components and probable generators (3.2.2.), followed by the same information for visual EPs (3.3). In the next section, movement EPs (4.) are presented, from methods (4.1), components (4.2.), and topography (4.3.), to generators of the P1/N2/P2/P3 (4.4.) and RP, NS' (4.5.), and the cognitive correlates of the RP (4.6.).

Cognitive EPs (5.) are then discussed, beginning with the methods used to evoke them and their current division into components (5.1.). The cognitive correlates of the N4 (5.2.) and P3 (5.3.) are presented, followed by a critical discussion of the generation of the P3 (5.4.) and N4 (5.5.). Next is presented the Contingent Negative Variation (5.6), beginning with the methods used to record this potential and its division into components (5.6.1.), and concluding with its probable brain generators (5.6.2.). The section on cognitive EPs concludes with a discussion of their interpretation (5.7.). In the final section (6.), the actual and potential uses of EPs in general are presented.

Several comprehensive chapters and books describing EP collection and analysis are already available (Desmedt, 1977a; Goff, 1974; Harmony, 1984; Picton, 1987; Picton et al., 1984; Picton and Hink, 1974). Some concentrate on methodology appropriate for clinical studies (Spehlmann, 1985). Standards for clinical practice (American EEG Society, 1984) and publication criteria for experimental studies (Donchin et al., 1977) have been developed. Other chapters and books focus on sophisticated mathematical analysis techniques (Aunon et al., 1981; Gevins, 1984; Gevins and Aminoff, 1987; Gevins and Cutillo, 1987; Gevins and Remond, 1987; Lopes da Silva et al., 1986; Nunez, 1981; Glaser and Ruchkin, 1979; John et al., 1978; and Tukey, 1978) and are especially appropriate for the scientist whose research focuses on EPs *per se*. The general problem of EEG and evoked-potential generation from synaptic activity and propagation to the scalp has been reviewed by Goff et al. (1978), Wood (1982, 1987), Nunez (1981), Gloor (1985), Lopes da Silva and van Rotterdam (1982), Vaughan (1974), Woodbury (1960), Speckmann and Caspers (1979), Lagerlund and Sharbrough (1989), and Schlag (1973). This chapter is intended for the scientist whose focus is on brain operations and who wishes to use EPs as reliable and sensitive tools.

1.2. History

Studies of the human electroencephalogram (EEG) evoked in relation to sensory, motor, and cognitive events (i.e., evoked potentials, or EPs) have long been hampered by a lack of knowledge of their neural substrate. The ongoing EEG ultimately reflects extracellular currents generated by the brain's 10^{13} synapses, of which .1% might be active at any given moment. These 10^9 current flows all contribute, to some extent, to the potential difference recorded between any two scalp locations. The key to EP methodology is thus the extraction from the EEG of the activity of some identifiable group of brain synapses and the relation of this activity to sensation, movement, and cognition.

EPs were first recorded in animals over 100 years ago (Caton, 1875; *see* Brazier, 1984). However, they were not recorded from the human scalp until 1939 (Davis, 1939). In 1950, Dawson presented the first averaged EPs, obtained using a rotator feeding the voltages obtained at different delays into a series of capacitors. This mechanical averaging device was replaced within the decade by digital computers (Clark, 1958; Remond, 1956), which became commercially available in the 1960s, leading to an explosion of EP research that has not yet abated (*see*, for example, recent symposia edited by Desmedt, 1977a, 1979; Owens and Davis, 1985; Cracco and Bodis-Wollner, 1986; Karrer et al., 1984; Johnson et al., 1987). Averaging is necessary because visual inspection of the EEG recorded during multiple trials of seemingly identical tasks reveals no apparent consistency. However, if the EEG is averaged across 20 or more trials, then regular waveforms (EPs) are observed. Each EP is a plot of the average voltages observed at a series of points in time after trial onset. The EP is thus generated by those synapses that are activated regularly within a particular latency range after trial onset and that happen to be oriented such that their current flows summate and propagate to the scalp (Fig. 1). These criteria may be fulfilled by as few as 1% of the synapses active at any given moment (Mitzdorf, 1985; Elul, 1972).

1.3. Components

After averaging, the second most important methodological advance was the division of the EP into "components"— reproducible positive or negative peaks, or sustained potentials, with more-or-less characteristic topography, latency, polarity, amplitude, behavioral correlates, and relations to other components. Ultimately, one would like to define a component unambiguously, in terms of a specific brain generator. In fact, the identification of components has permitted EP research to advance in the absence of any definitive knowledge of their specific neural substrates. Thus, for example, an EP study may identify a component through its topography, polarity, and latency, and then proceed to better define its behavioral characteristics by observing its changes across various task conditions.

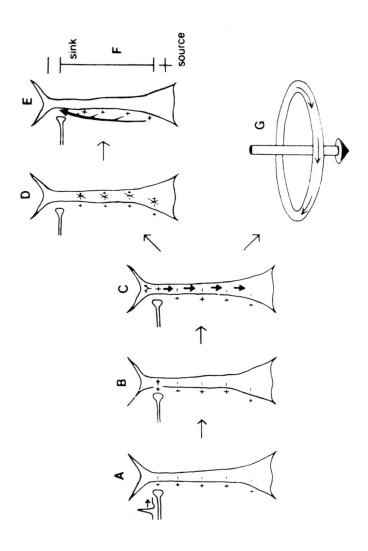

Fig. 1. A simplified schematic diagram of the sequence of events leading from synaptic activation (A) to electrical (F) and magnetic (G) fields that can be recorded at a distance. By definition, current will flow between two points in a conductive medium at different electrical potentials. In the brain, synaptic activity opens conductive pathways between points at different potentials inside *vs* outside of the neuron (A). Suppose that the activated synapse is excitatory. Then the transmembrane current will be carried by positive ions entering the cell (B). Once inside the cell, the positive ions will flow from the subsynaptic area down gradients of concentration and charge (C) into the rest of the neuron. If the synapse is located on the distal part of the apical dendrite, then the current flow into the proximal apical shaft and soma will be greater than that in the opposite direction, because the resistance to such flow is less. This flow of positive ions will tend to neutralize the negative ions on the inside of the somadendritic membrane (D). Extracellularly, the positive ions that enter the cell are replaced by ions flowing toward the synaptic regions through extracellular space (E). This flow will preferentially include those ions released by the neutralization of the negative ions on the inner surface of the neuronal membrane (D) (from Halgren et al., 1986).

By relying on a convergence of criteria for component identification, the risk of circularity is somewhat decreased. It must be emphasized that several criteria must be considered together for reliable identification. For example, both the N4 and the slow wave *(see below)* are negative, have a diffuse/frontal distribution, and can peak in the 400–500 ms range. The N4 is evoked only by complex meaningful stimuli (words, faces, and so forth), whereas the slow wave is evoked by either simple or complex stimuli, if they are responded to individually. Thus, if the evoking stimuli are simple, the negativity should be a slow wave. If the stimuli are complex, the N4 and slow wave are still differentiable, because the N4 precedes a broad positivity ("P3"), whereas the slow wave follows it. In such tasks, the N4 may peak at approximately 450 ms, and the slow wave will peak much later (approximately 800 ms), following the P3. Even where multiple criteria are followed, it is still clearly possible that what is called the same component in different tasks will turn out to be generated by distinct regions in those tasks. Conversely, what are thought to be different components may actually have the same generators (Fig. 2). These ambiguities have resulted in many controversies that, in most cases, require depth recordings for their resolution. Again, the possession of multiple criteria for component identification has permitted depth recordings to be interpreted in terms of scalp EP components, even though polarity and topography are irrelevant in depth recordings. In addition, multiple criteria are essential for the establishment of homologous EP components across species, where topographical, temporal, and behavioral correspondences are problematic. It should be clear that the ultimate criterion for the identity of an EP component is synaptic: two components are identical if and only if they are generated by the same synapses. Similarly, the two EP components belong to the same "family" if and only if they are generated by the same "family" of synapses. That is, EP components in the same family may be generated by synapses at the same level of information processing, but operate on different material, and therefore at different anatomical loci. For example, the geniculostriate synapses activated by left vs right hemifield stimulation evoke EP components identical except in topography. These might be considered "identical twins." At a more abstract level, attention to tones vs flashes or contextual integration of spoken vs written words results in EP components with differing topographies, but similar task correlates, latencies, waveforms,

Task A
(anterior topography)

Task B
(posterior topography)

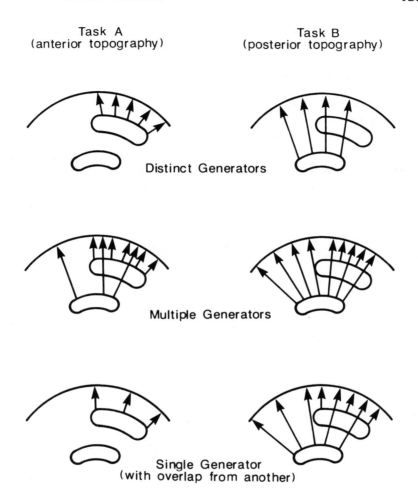

Distinct Generators

Multiple Generators

Single Generator
(with overlap from another)

Fig. 2. Possible explanations for observed differences in the scalp topography of an EP component across tasks. The more anterior topography in Task A than in Task B could indeed be caused by distinct generators with overlapping scalp projections (top), but could also be caused by differential activation of the same two generators in the two tasks (middle), or by a single generator with differential overlap from another component with a different peak latency (bottom).

and so forth (*see* Ritter et al. 1983; Pritchard et al. in press for further discussion).

To summarize, the application of the multiple criteria of polarity, topography, latency, sequence, and task correlates provides a methodology for distinguishing and classifying EP components in the absence of comprehensive recordings of brain synaptic activity. Conversely, when the activity of individual synaptic systems is monitored, these criteria allow individual EP components to be linked to their neural substrate. The promise of EP research, as yet unfulfilled, is that psychological models of cognition will be linked to biological models of the brain through EP components, which are at the same time identified with both elementary psychological processes and emergent but analyzable biological processes. Uniting the psychological and biological models is necessary to make the psychological models testable and precise, and the biological models functional.

2. Methodology

2.1. Recordings

2.1.1. Electrodes and Placement

Electrodes to record from the scalp may be either needles or shallow cups. The needles penetrate the skin and thus pose some risk of infection, especially if they are reused, and may also be painful if a small cutaneous nerve branch is injured during insertion. For these reasons, needle electrodes are falling into increasing disfavor. Cup (or disk) electrodes are usually gold, silver, or tin and often have a hole in the cup's center through which conducting gel can be applied. Cup electrodes can be attached to the scalp by applying collodion to the edge of the cup and drying with an airstream. After recording, the collodion is removed with acetone. Alternatively, a conductive paste may be applied under and just around the cup, and a gauze pad pressed over it. This method is easier, but shorter-lived and more prone to mechanical artifacts than collodion. Specialized clip electrodes are available for recording from the ear lobes. EKG-type electrodes may be used for recording from nonhairy skin away from the scalp. The quality of the contact between the electrode and the skin is determined by measuring the impedance between two electrodes. This should be

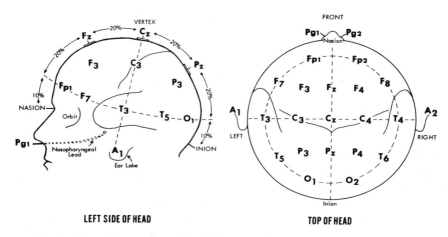

LEFT SIDE OF HEAD   **TOP OF HEAD**

Fig. 3. The International 10-20 System. Electrode placement is based on proportional spacing of electrodes from bony skull landmarks (nasion, inion, and preauricular points). The electrode positions relative to the Sylvian and central sulci are accurate to within ± 1 cm (Jasper, 1958). (Figure courtesy of Grass Instruments Co.)

between 1 and 5 Kohm/cm^2. It is reduced to this level by first removing waxy skin oils with alcohol or acetone, and then mildly abrading the skin before applying the electrode.

Electrode placement is determined by the experimental question. In most experiments, all that is required is to unambiguously identify and measure an EP component, and this can be done with one or two electrodes. At the other extreme, a detailed topography over the entire scalp may require about 100 electrodes, given the smallest likely cortical generators and how they are spread by the intervening skull and scalp. One method for selecting the optimal sites to sample, given an initial high density map, has been described by Lux et al. (1978). In any case, electrode sites are nearly always in the International 10-20 system (Fig. 3: Harner and Sannit, 1974; Jasper, 1958). When another site is chosen, as is occasionally necessary to optimize the recording of a particular component (cf American EEG Society, 1984), its location is usually described in reference to the 10-20 system. Measuring the skull locations for the 19 sites of the 10-20 system, plus supplementary sites if needed, is quite time-consuming. A much quicker (but still accurate and reproducible) method uses a system of modified cup electrodes in a flexible nylon mesh helmet (something like a bathing cap) held on by elastic straps (Blom and Anneveldt, 1982).

The standard 10-20 system sites yield relatively poor samples of activity from the basal temporal and frontal lobes. In fact, when electrodes are inserted through the nose onto the nasopharynx to record below the temporal pole, fairly large inverted potentials corresponding to the N1–P2–N2–P3 slow wave (SW) are recorded relative to a noncephalic reference (Perrault and Picton, 1984a,b). Nasopharyngeal electrodes can be uncomfortable or even painful. Clinical studies often use fine, twisted wires inserted below the sphenoidal wings to record from the basal temporal and frontal lobes (King et al., 1986; Sperling and Engel, 1985, 1986). In the absence of nasopharyngeal or sphenoidal electrodes, some indication of basal frontotemporal activity has been obtained with surface electrodes over the zygomatic process (Sindrup et al., 1981) or between the ear and eye (Sperling and Engel, 1985).

2.1.2. Reference Electrodes

EP recordings are always of voltage differences between two points. Thus, except when the data is postprocessed to estimate transskull current *(see below)*, the choice of the reference electrode can be of critical importance. Except for very early sensory EPs, a noncephalic reference can safely be assumed to be effectively inactive. Most commonly, such references use linked chest and back electrodes with a potentiometer circuit to balance out the fields generated by the heart (Lehtonen and Koivikko, 1971; Stephenson and Gibbs, 1951). Similar results are obtained with a continuous conducting neck ring (Nunez, 1981) or four neck electrodes connected by dual potentiometers (Woods, personal communication). However, these noncephalic references are prone to contamination by EMG, EKG, and movement artifacts; therefore, a nose, earlobe, or mastoid reference is often used. In order to obviate the laterality of the earlobe or mastoid, the left and right sites are often linked. However, this could alter significantly the EP field over the scalp by providing a low-resistance path, and so should be avoided when the lateralized EP scalp topography in the region of the temporal lobe is of interest. The choice of using a cephalic reference is justified when previous studies have demonstrated the relative absence of activity in the chosen reference site when recorded against a noncephalic reference. A possible strategy, if enough recording channels and time are available, would be to simultaneously record the scalp sites against a low-noise cephalic reference, and the cephalic reference site against a noncephalic reference, in order to determine whether it is indeed inactive.

Many authors have used an "average reference," that is, have analyzed the difference between voltage recorded at a given site and the average voltage of all recorded sites (e.g., Osselton, 1965; Kavanagh et al., 1978; Scherg, 1984; Lehmann and Skrandies, 1984; Walter et al., 1984). Although the average reference is theoretically justified if the entire head's electrical field is equally sampled (Bertrand et al., 1985), in practice this does not occur, because the bottom of the brain is not accessible to recording electrodes.

2.1.3. Amplifying, Filtering, and Digitizing

The EEG signal must be amplified about 20,000-fold, filtered, and digitized before averaging. Amplifiers need to have low noise, high input impedance, and a good common-mode rejection ratio to eliminate artifactual activity common to both input leads (e.g., line noise). Safety considerations are of paramount importance. Equipment leakage currents and grounding should be checked periodically by a competent biomedical engineer (Seaba, 1980). Every recording session should include a calibration signal for amplitude and phase applied to all channels.

The power of each EP component is concentrated in a particular frequency band. Since EP components are roughly sinusoidal, the frequency of interest can be estimated by taking the inverse of twice the duration of the EP component. The signal-to-noise ratio of the recording can then be improved by filtering out other frequencies with a "band-pass" filter, which is composed of a "high-pass" filter and a "low-pass" filter. A low-pass filter is also necessary in order to prevent "aliasing" or "folding" artifacts in digitization. Aliasing occurs when the digitization rate (i.e., the number of times/s that the analog-to-digital converter [ADC] samples each channel) is less than twice the highest frequency present in the input analog signal. Aliasing results in spurious signals appearing in the ADC output as harmonics of the difference between the high-frequency signal and the digitization rate. These spurious signals are difficult to distinguish from the EP component of interest.

Filters are characterized by their cutoff frequency, slope, and phase-shift. The cutoff frequency and slope are usually expressed in decibels (dB), equal to 20 × the logarithm to base 10 of the gain (for example, a gain of 1000 is equal to 60 dB). The cutoff or "corner" frequency is the point at which the gain is 3 dB down. A simple RC filter (composed of one resistor and one capacitor) has a slope equal to 6 dB/octave. That is, the signal decreases by 50% with every doubling of frequency (if it is a low-pass filter) or halving of frequency (if it is a high-pass filter). The ability of a filter to pass low-frequency signals is often characterized by its "time constant," that is, the time necessary for a step increase entering the filter to reach 63% of its maximum at the output. Phase-shift refers to the amount of delay induced by the filter on different frequencies of the signal. The phase-shift is maximal near the cutoff frequency and, all other things being equal, is larger for filters with steeper slopes.

Analog filters are generally constructed from operational amplifiers, connected to each other and to ground with resistors and capacitors in feedback circuits. The parameters of these circuits control their gain and their phase vs frequency curves. Parameters can be chosen so that the filter belongs to one of various "families" of filters, each designed to optimize different filter characteristics. Butterworth filters provide a maximally steep slope, but introduce a great deal of phase-shift. Bessel filters offer a much more constant phase-lag across frequencies (Doyle and Hyde, 1981).

Filtering can also be performed after the waveform has been digitized (Picton et al., 1984). Such "digital filters" can operate either in the time domain, by adding or subtracting to each point proportions of the values of the adjacent points, or in the frequency domain, by performing a fast Fourier transform, removing unwanted frequencies, and reconstructing the waveform (Childers and Durling, 1975). Digital filters are superior to analog filters in that they are absolutely stable and can be constructed so as to introduce no phase-shift. Digital filters are very easy to modify (by changing parameters in a computer program), and thus can be repeatedly modified and applied to the stored waveform until the optimal filtering configuration is found. Finally, since the average of filtered waveforms is mathematically equal to their filtered average, digital filtering need be done only once, on the averaged waveform. Given these advantages of digital filtering, it is probably best to use the minimal analog filter necessary to prevent aliasing, followed by digital filtering tailored to the application.

Analog-to-digital conversion, or digitization, is the translation of a continuous analog voltage at a particular instant in time into an integer, which is stored in the computer. The number of bits in this number determines the accuracy of the ADC. Suppose that the input range of a 3-bit ADC is ± 4 V. Then the ADC will divide the signal into 8 ($= 2^3$) equal steps of 1.0 V ($= 8$ V/2^3) each. For example, this ADC may assign 000 to a −4.0 V input signal, 100 to 0.0 V, and 110 to 2.0 V. However, because of the limited accuracy of this ADC, it would also assign 110 to 2.1 V, 2.2 V, and even 2.99 V. This results in a "digitization noise" being added to the signal (*see* Picton et al., 1984). This noise has a standard deviation equal to about 0.29 × the digitization step (0.29 V in our example). Its importance depends upon the digitization accuracy as well as upon how well the amplifier gain is adjusted so that the EEG fills up the entire input range of the ADC. Suppose that the EEG is amplified so that ± 3.5 × its standard deviation saturates the ADC input. Then digitization would increase the noise by a factor of $[(2^{b-1}+1)/2^{b-1}]$ for an ADC with b bits. This results in a 0.8% increase in noise for an 8-bit ADC, which could be counteracted by increasing the number of trials by 2%. Beyond 8 bits, increased ADC accuracy can still be useful, as it permits signals to be digitized with less concern that the amplifier output be carefully matched to the ADC input range.

2.1.4. Artifacts

EP components can be as small as 0.25 μV, and are recorded from fairly-high-impedance probes temporarily attached to the body (which is full of extracerebral electrical generators, such as eyes, tongue, skin, muscles, heart) within an environment (and with equipment) saturated by line, transient, and other voltages generated by power sources many magnitudes stronger than anything biological. EP recording thus requires a meticulous attention to detail in order to obtain a clean signal, clear of artifacts. The most pernicious artifacts are those that can be time-locked to the sensory stimulus or to the movement, and thus are not relatively attenuated by the averaging process.

Stimuli that are to be counted silently, or words that might be subvocalized, can produce tongue movements, resulting in artifacts of up to 100 μV (Klass and Bickford, 1960). Subjects need to be instructed not to subvocalize and must be observed during data collection. Various stimuli, especially loud sounds, can evoke EMG artifacts in the 8–80 ms latency range (Bickford, 1972). These are predominately caused by the inion, temporalis, frontalis, and post-auricular reflexes (Picton and Hink, 1974).

Electrodermal responses are typically evoked with a latency of about .5–1 s after an arousing stimulus and last for 1–5 s (Picton and Hillyard, 1972). They can be eliminated by filtering unless the contingent negative variation or other slow potentials are of interest, in which case the skin needs to be short-circuited by "drilling" until the interelectrode impedance is less than 1 Kohm/cm^2. The recording of slow potentials also requires that the electrodes be nonpolarizable and balanced by using Ag/AgCl electrodes maintained in the electrolyte between recording sessions.

Electrodes themselves can be the source of mechanical artifacts if they are loose, resulting in movement or intermittent breaks in continuity. A constant current can develop between two electrodes connected to the same amplifier if they are constructed of dissimilar metals. Common-mode rejection of line (60 cycle), EKG, and other artifacts will also be degraded if the two inputs to an amplifier have substantially different impedances. Line artifacts and intermittently drifting signals may result from absent or high-impedance grounding, or from "ground loops." Line noise can also be greatly reduced by presenting one-half of the trials on opposite phases of the power cycle. For example (assuming 60-Hz power), in a series of tones, the interstimulus interval might be x in one half of the trials, and $x + 8.33$ ms in the other half (Picton and Hink, 1974).

Stimulus artifacts can be difficult to eliminate, especially from somatosensory stimuli. The stimulator should be shielded and grounded, and anything attached to the patient should be optically isolated in order to prevent ground loops. Some of the artifact may also be averaged out if the polarity of the stimulus is inverted on alternate trials.

Another common problem in EP recording is eye movements. A large standing potential (the Electroretinogram: ERG) is generated across the retina. When the eyeball and eyelids are stationary, the ERG propagates passively across the scalp, but is constant and therefore presents no problems for EP recordings. When the eyeball moves in its socket, a large transient field propagates across the scalp. Eye blinks also cause large artifacts, partly through accompanying involuntary eye movements, and partly through conduction of the corneal potential through the eyelid (Hillyard and Galambos, 1970; Matsuo et al., 1975; Picton, 1987). Eye movements and blinks have a latency of at least 250 ms after stimulus onset, hence are only a serious problem for the movement EPs and for the later cognitive EPs. Since the eye blink may occur at a fairly constant latency after the stimulus, and is larger than the cognitive or movement EP, the eye-blink artifact can pose a very significant problem. In these cases it is essential to monitor for eye movements and either to eliminate contaminated trials from averages or to subtract the EOG (electro-oculogram) contamination from the EEG (Barlow and Remond, 1981; Gasser et al., 1986; Semlitsch et al., 1986; Elbert et al., 1985). The latter approach is especially welcome in cognitive tasks with brain-damaged subjects, when most of the trials may be contaminated by EOG.

Eye movements may be monitored by recording the EOG between electrodes around the eyes. EOG electrodes and recording techniques are essentially identical to those used for EEG. If only eye blinks are of concern, or if a purely midsaggital EEG montage is used, then monitoring vertical eye movements (for example, by recording the EOG between electrodes on the tip of the nose and in the middle of the forehead) is adequate. In studies where the lateralized topography of EP components is of primary interest, then electrode placement that is sensitive to lateral eye movements (for example, at the outer canthus) is important. The absolute position of the eyes is reflected in the absolute dc levels of EOG recordings. In practice, it is difficult or impossible to distinguish artifactual dc drift (caused by skin potentials or electrode polarization) from small nonsaccadic eye movements. Furthermore, the EOG is always contaminated to some degree by potentials generated by the underlying frontal cortex. Therefore, in some special circumstances (for example, if the task involves lateralized presentation of visual stimuli), techniques other than the EOG may be used to monitor eye movements.

2.2. Analysis

2.2.1. Averaging and Peak Detection

"Averaging" consists of adding together all of the voltage values collected at each particular peristimulus latency and dividing by the number of trials, resulting in a plot of the average voltage at the sampled peristimulus time points. The simplest model assumes that each trial consists of an EP, with constant amplitude and latency, superimposed upon noise uncorrelated with the EP and randomly varying from trial to trial. Averaging thus results in no change in the signal, whereas the noise amplitude decreases proportionally to the square root of the number of trials. Consequently, a signal that is one-tenth of the noise level in the raw signal will be ten times larger than the noise if 10,000 trials are averaged. One assumption of the standard averaging methodology is that the signal is constant in amplitude and latency across trials. The signal-to-noise ratio can be improved by adjusting the individual trials so that the components of interest have the same apparent latency before averaging (Woody, 1967; McGillem et al., 1985) or by selecting trials that appear to have strong signals (Gevins et al., 1986). These techniques work iteratively. That is, an initial constant-latency average of all trials is used as a template for latency adjustment or trial selection in the next stage. This results in an "improved" average, which serves as a template for the following stage, and so forth. The cycle is continued until the average no longer changes with iteration. Thus, inherent in these techniques is the assumption that the true signal resembles the initial average.

Despite the most strenuous efforts to eliminate artifacts from the collected data, some trials with large artifacts are likely to slip through, and may significantly distort the average if they are time-locked to the stimulus and occur on a significant proportion of the trials. Thus, it is wise to include in the averaging program an artifact-rejection routine that checks to see if a trial exceeds some amplitude criterion and, if so, either rejects the trial from the average, or limits the voltage in the offending region so that it cannot make a large contribution to the ultimate average (Picton and Hink, 1974).

In the standard analysis scheme, the average waveforms are plotted and the EP components are measured and entered into analysis of variance (ANOVA) to test the experiment's hypotheses. EPs may be plotted as in electroencephalography, with negative up (that is, with an upward deflection representing a situation in which amplifier input one is more negative than input two). Alternatively, EPs are sometimes plotted with positive up, as is standard in other fields of electrophysiology and in physics. Since no standard exists for EPs, it is essential that the polarity always be indicated in published traces.

EP peaks are usually identified visually, on the basis of latency, polarity, topography, sequence, and task correlates (Kramer, 1985). Peaks can also be identified by computer algorithms, which are more definitely objective, but also more prone to stupid errors than is the human eye. Especially for broad EP components, it is often more accurate to measure the average EP amplitude in a latency window, rather than the EP amplitude at one fixed point.

When an EP component is superimposed on another component or components, it may be necessary to acquire EPs in two situations, one of which evokes the component in question, and the other of which does not, subtract the latter from the former, and thus obtain the desired activity free of contaminants. This of course assumes that only the components of interest change between conditions, an assumption that can be partially tested by comparing the topography of the EP components in the "difference waveform" to that of the putatively unchanging EP components.

As in any scientific experiment, some indication of the reliability of the measurements is in order. Cognitive EP studies often display the "grand average" EP across all subjects in the study, and then describe the ANOVA based on peak measures from an individual subject's waveforms. An indication of variability can be derived by comparing the "flatness" of the grand average EP in the prestimulus period with the size of the EP components, and from the F-ratios in the ANOVA. However, in clinical studies each individual may be unique, and some indication of variability within a subject is useful. This indication may be visible, by superimposing replicate averages or by adding and subtracting alternate trials to obtain an estimate of the noise in the absence of a stimulus (Schimmel, 1967). Quantitative descriptors of the signal-to-noise ratio are reviewed by Picton et al. (1984).

The entire process from recording through filtering, digitization, averaging, plotting, and measuring, to analyzing can be performed by commercially available dedicated EP systems, or alternatively, by general-purpose microcomputers with appropriate peripherals: physiological amplifiers, ADC, and display devices. Compared to the dedicated averagers, the general-purpose microcomputers are much less expensive as well as more flexible and powerful (e.g., capable of collecting and analyzing more channels, points, and task conditions), but are less convenient and require more time and expertise to set up and operate.

2.2.2. Alternative Analysis Methods

In addition to ambiguities in component identification, the standard method of EP analysis—EEG averaging across trials followed by amplitude/latency measures of visually identified peaks—has been criticized for its assumption that behavior/brain response is constant across many trials, for its subjectivity, and for its disposal of the vast majority of the experimental data (Gevins, 1984; Gevins and Cutillo, 1987; John et al., 1978; Tukey, 1978). This has led to the development of many alternative analysis methods. Almost without exception, these methods have received little acceptance by the experimental investigators of EPs. This is partly because these techniques require mathematical sophistication and computational resources seldom available to the neurophysiologist or experimental psychologist. More importantly, the physiological basis for averaged EPs in post synaptic potentials (PSPs) has been well-established by a series of rigorous experiments over the past 40 years (Purpura, 1959; Elul, 1972; Mitzdorf, 1985; Schlag, 1973). In contrast, the novel mathematical measures seldom have a neural basis that is hypothesized, much less established.

Finally, an investigator who chooses to dispense with component amplitude/latency measures in favor of a different mathematically derived measure, has to a large degree cut himself or herself off from the society of scientists. The work might not be replicated or extended. It will lack the benefit of hundreds of other studies making the same measure in relation to various tasks, behavioral and neurological states, from various brain structures, and so forth. Thus, it will be difficult to be sure that the relevant experimental variables were adequately controlled, or to relate the work either to its neural basis or to cognition. Since the only possible justification for studying such an ambiguous measure as EPs is their potential for connecting the neural and the cognitive realms in humans, this is indeed a very serious problem.

Ultimately, the reason that investigators have, in general, not adopted complicated mathematical techniques for EP analysis is because they have not needed to—for all its deficiencies, the standard averaged EP component measurement methodology has proved to be extremely fruitful. Bearing these factors in mind, several advanced mathematical techniques still have considerable promise for better localization of cortical regions generating EPs and for extracting their temporal interrelationships. These techniques have long existed, but are now emerging as multichannel recordings and powerful computing come within the reach of all laboratories.

2.2.3. Factor Analysis

Principal Components Analysis (PCA) (Donchin and Heffley, 1978; Glaser and Ruchkin, 1979) provides orthogonal components of the variation of the averaged ERP waveforms across different subjects, conditions, and sites. PCA is commonly implemented using the BMDP statistical package (BMDP4M). The covariance matrix is calculated for latency X latency across different depth electrode sites, patients, and tasks. PCA has also been applied in the spatial domain, where the covariance matrix is one of electrode sites rather than latencies (Skrandies and Lehmann, 1982). Eigenvectors and eigenfactors are converted to PCA factors by varimax rotation. Varimax replaces eigenfactors with another orthogonal set, which contains more components close to zero (and others far from zero) than do the eigenfactors. Because of the autocorrelation structure of evoked potential data, the effect is to promote factor loadings whose activity is relatively localized in latency. ANOVA can be performed on PCA factor scores to test if the waveforms vary across patients, locations, or tasks. Because the PCA factors represent orthogonal components of the covariance, a separate ANOVA may be performed for each factor.

Recently, Wood and McCarthy (1984) reported simulation experiments suggesting that serious problems may exist in the application of PCA to ERP data. Using the same steps as outlined above, they found that the rotated principal components did not necessarily correspond to the original prototypes. In an extensive analysis of one situation in which this correspondence in fact appeared to be very good, a relatively small (8–10%) misallocation of the variance between overlapping components could result in a type I error rate (in the ANOVAs on principal component scores) as high as 81%. Further simulations are needed before the generality of this problem, its sensitivity to treatment effect and number of observations, and potential means of amelioration can be evaluated with any certainty. In the meantime, the possibility must always be entertained that a significant effect assigned to a given PCA component may not actually be caused by the underlying ERP component that the PCA component appears to measure. McCarthy and Wood (1985) have also called attention to the possible misinterpretation of location X condition interactions in ANOVA when waveforms are not properly normalized (*see also* Figure 2).

2.2.4. Spectral Analysis

Simple averaging will not detect event-related EEG activity with fairly constant frequency and latency, but without a fixed phase-relation to the stimulus. Such activity is predicted by Freeman's models of neuronal population dynamics (Freeman, 1975, 1978). One way to measure this activity is to apply the fast Fourier transform (FFT) to the digitized EEG from successive intervals of each trial. These epochs need to be padded on each side with the points from adjacent epochs forced to zero with a cosine function before calculation of FFT in order to minimize the addition of specious frequencies from the epochs' boundaries. Spectral intensity in each of several frequency bands at each poststimulus latency are then averaged across all trials (the "Bartlett Estimator" [Glaser and Ruchkin, 1979]). The width of the frequency bands is limited to the inverse of the duration of the analysis epochs. An analysis that yields a continuous time–frequency function, the Wigner distribution, has recently been introduced by Morgan and Gevins (1986).

2.2.5. Topography

These newly popular techniques often involve topographical mapping of the EP potential distribution over the scalp (recently reviewed by Lehmann and Skrandies [1984] and Picton et al. [1984], and the subject of a book edited by Duffy [1986]). A page of paper has two dimensions; the brain has three, and with time, four. Typically, isopotential lines in a two-dimensional projection of the scalp are mapped at an instant of time, for example, at the peak of an EP component. Alternatively, one may plot the potentials recorded in a line of electrodes across the entire EP epoch (Remond, 1962). Particularly revealing of cognitive EP components are isopotential plots of EPs recorded in a midsaggital line (*see* Fig. 3—F_{pz}, F_z, C_z, P_z, O_z) (e.g., Renault and Lesevre, 1978). Spatiotemporal plots of EPs recorded from multiple contacts along the shafts of single depth probes in the human cortex have been used effectively to visualize overlapping generators of early auditory (Liegious-Chauvel et al. in preparation) and somatosensory (Chauvel and Badier, in preparation) EPs. Much insight can be gained by examining such maps of potential distribution, but it must be remembered that in itself this is a technique for data *display* only, not for *analysis*. Equivalent dipole localization, estimation of trans-skull currents, and spatial factor analysis are methods for extracting numbers to test the hypotheses suggested by visual inspection of topographical displays.

The possibility that spontaneous EEG and/or EPs represent intrinsic cortical oscillators linked by cortico-cortical fibers has been discussed by Nunez (1981) and Thatcher et al. (1986). In a series of elegant studies, with extreme care for elimination of behavioral or recording artifacts, Gevins et al. (1983, 1984, 1985, 1989) have studied the intercorrelations between Laplacian-transformed EPs recorded at different scalp sites, in different latency windows (defined by EP component peaks), and across different tasks. They have also found that these intercorrelations are maximal at delays that are consistent for site pairs, tasks, and latencies. This technique is promising, but animal studies are needed before it can be used to draw inferences regarding the sequential communication of underlying cortical areas.

2.3. Generator Localization

2.3.1. From Scalp EPs

The final common pathway for information processing in the brain is the flow of current across neuronal membranes. These current-flows volume conduct to the scalp, where they result in differences in electrical potential: the EEG and EPs. These current-flows at the same time give rise to magnetic fields: the magnetoencephalogram (MEG) and evoked fields. The electrical and magnetic fields from different, simultaneously active sources add algebraically. This results in cancellation if the current-flows are asynchronous, as is nearly always the case with action potentials. Current-flows also cancel if they are radially symmetrical, as is the case with intracellular currents in stellate cells, or with most extracellular currents in a freely conducting medium (which the brain approximates). Summation thus usually results from the more-or-less synchronous activation of synapses on the apical dendrites of pyramidal cells in cortical structures. Increased membrane conductance at one end of the apical dendrite produces a polarized current-flow within that dendrite, which in turn produces a polarized extracellular current. Because these dendrites are aligned in parallel, and the synapses from a given pathway tend to lie in the same cortical layer, the current-flows will summate (Fig. 1). Clearly, only extracellular currents can volume conduct to the scalp to produce the EEG. Although extracellular currents also generate magnetic fields, theoretical considerations (their lack of alignment and low current density) suggest that the MEG is generated by *intracellular* currents. This interpretation has been supported by experimental observations *(see below)*. At a reasonable distance, the magnetic and electric fields generated by apical dendrites in a cortical region resemble closely those fields that would be generated by a single current dipole with appropriate orientation and strength in the center of the cortical region. This is termed the "equivalent dipole" and is used to characterize the generator.

Estimation of the intracerebral generators responsible for an observed scalp EP topography is termed the "Inverse Problem." Especially for primary visual potentials, this technique has yielded results consistent with those demonstrated by intracranial recordings in animals (e.g., Thickbroom et al., 1985a). The Inverse Problem is solved by first estimating the number, location, direction, and magnitude of the equivalent intracerebral generating dipoles. The resulting scalp topography is calculated ("Forward Problem"). From the differences between the calculated and the observed scalp topography, a better set of dipole parameters is estimated, and its propagation to the scalp is calculated. These steps continue in a cyclic fashion until a convergence criterion has been attained, or the allowed number of iterations is exceeded (e.g., Darcey 1979). Within practical limits, the initial dipole estimate does not affect the ultimate solution, but does affect how many iterations are necessary before it is found.

This method assumes that the intracerebral generator may be represented as a combination of dipoles; this assumption is supported by considerations based on physical laws (at relatively large distances from a multipole generator, the dipole term will predominate [Nunez, 1981; Wood, 1982]) and by physiological calculations of current-flows in sheets of pyramidal cells similar to the hippocampus (Freeman, 1975; Vaughan, 1974). It should be noted that a significant error in localization occurs with large sheets of pyramidal cells parallel to the head's surface (Goff et al., 1978; Nunez, 1981). Such sheets appear as a single dipole located at a much deeper level (Ary et al., 1981b).

In the limiting case, a closed sphere of cortically arranged neurons with radially symmetrical processes produces no outside potential (Lorente de Nó, 1947). The potential inside a punctured sphere may be very large, and it does not necessarily invert polarity within the cortical layer (Klee and Rall, 1977). This might be an important consideration in interpreting the lack of cortical polarity inversion sometimes observed with cognitive potentials, especially the CNV. It must be emphasized again that in laminar structures, it is the second spatial derivative of the voltage that is proportional to transmembrane current-flows (Mitzdorf, 1985; Nunez, 1981). Thus, in intracranial recordings, it is variable and steep voltage gradients that point to local generation, not polarity inversion *per se.*

Experimental observations as well as theoretical calculations indicate that the low-conductance skull significantly attenuates and smears the appearance of brain potentials at the scalp (Ary et al., 1981b; Hosek et al., 1978; Nunez, 1981). However, solution of the Inverse Problem takes about 50 times longer if the head is modeled as three concentric spheres of differing conductivity than if it is modelled as a single homogenous sphere. Since the skull effects are systematic, dipole parameters from a single-sphere model can be adjusted (made shallower and stronger) according to published tables (Ary et al., 1981b; Schneider, 1974). Provided that skull thickness is accurately estimated (by measuring skulls using magnetic resonance imaging [MRI] or computed tomography [CT]), the error in equivalent dipole localization between the three-sphere model and the corrected one-sphere model is probably less than that from other sources of error (Ary et al., 1981a).

In normal subjects, two symmetrical dipoles may often be assumed. By forcing the dipole locations and directions to be mirror images of each other across the midsaggital plane, the number of parameters to estimate is reduced from 12 (3 location, 2 direction, and 1 magnitude for each dipole) to 7 (defining the location and direction of one dipole determines those of the other dipole, whereas magnitude remains independent). Confidence limits for dipole location are estimated based on the variability of the EP measures from which they are calculated (Ary et al., 1981a; Marquardt, 1964).

Of course, in many tasks, many dipoles will be active in a spatially and temporally overlapping fashion. If one is willing to assume that these dipoles result from activation of relatively small superficial cortical regions, then it is possible to transform EPs to more directly reflect the topography of these regions (Srebro, 1985b). This Laplacian transform is estimated at a given site by subtracting proportions of the EPs from adjacent sites, resulting in an approximation of the second spatial derivative of the potential field (Nunez, 1981; Hjorth, 1976; MacKay, 1983, 1984, Koles et al., 1989). The Laplacian transform acts as a spatial filter with a characteristic frequency dependent on electrode spacing and on the polynomial used to combine voltages from different sites. For example, Srebro (1985a) found on theoretical grounds, and confirmed by experimental observation, that optimal localization of cortical areas .6–3.1 cm in diameter was obtained with a simple Laplacian transform of an electrode array with 2.5-cm spacing. An extension of these methods to the three-concentric sphere model is discussed by Nunez (1987).

2.3.2. From Evoked Magnetic Fields

The apparent generation of MEG by *intracellular* current flows gives it several advantages over EEG for localizing brain activation (Hari and Ilmoniemi, 1986; Williamson and Kaufman, 1981). Using noninvasive MEG measures, calculations of the equivalent dipole are fairly simple (given certain a priori assumptions—*see below*), because they do not need to take into account the influence of the reference electrode (MEG has none) or of the skull and intervening tissue (because these do not affect intracellular currents). Theoretical considerations (Cuffin, 1986) as well as actual measurements using artificial dipoles in a gel-filled skull (Barth et al., 1986) confirm the applicability of these simplifications and indicate that with current MEG instruments, a resolution of about 3 mm is reasonable. Furthermore, in actual physiological situations (tonotopic mapping of the auditory cortex), generators separated by as little as 2 mm and involving as few as 50,000 neurons have been distinguished (Panter et al., 1988).

One significant disadvantage of MEG compared to EEG has been its relatively low signal-to-noise ratio (S:N). The actual magnetic signals generated by the brain are very small: about one-billionth the size of the earth's magnetic field (that which a hand compass detects). Measurement of the MEG thus requires SQUIDs: superconducting quantum interference devices. These are maintained at a temperature near absolute zero in order to induce superconduction and to reduce noise. Commonly, SQUIDs are used in a "second-order gradiometer" configuration to detect the *gradient* in the magnetic field near the scalp, rather than its absolute value. Since the earth's field is essentially constant over short distances, it is effectively eliminated from recordings. Other artifacts, generated by electrical currents or by moving ferromagnetic objects, are also reduced in comparison to the brain's field. Even so, however, many common events, such as a polygraph pen moving in the next room or an elevator moving in the same building, are often sufficiently large to completely obscure physiological signals.

An effective technological solution to this challenge is to use a magnetically shielded room. The exact amount of increase in S:N made possible by these rooms depends upon many interacting factors, but a net increase of 10-fold is not unreasonable. This has especially great practical consequences for detecting cognitive evoked magnetic fields. Since S:N increases according to the square root of the number of events in averaged MEG, a 10-fold S:N increase owing to magnetic shielding results in a 100-fold decrease in the number of events needed to obtain a signal of equivalent quality. For the most part, previous MEG studies have been limited to primary sensory and motor cortices (Brenner et al., 1975; Kaufman and Williamson, 1986), because only they are reliably activated by the thousands of stimulus repetitions at high rates necessary to map fields at low S:N. Trials in cognitive tasks require the patient's active attention and participation and cannot occur rapidly; hence, the number of trials is limited by habituation and fatigue. The amount of information gathered by the MEG is limited not only by the S:N of its measurements, but by the number of locations simultaneously sampled. The magnetic field at a minimum of about 21 points must be mapped to get an initial idea of its intracerebral generator. Thus, a second technical advance of great importance in acquiring cognitive evoked magnetic fields has been the development of multisensor instruments. Current instruments have up to 14 channels, and a 100-sensor machine should be available within the decade. The "high" temperature superconductors now being developed may find their application to MEG in this context beginning in another 5 years. Because of thermal noise considerations, room-temperature SQUIDs will not be used for MEG. However, decreased operating expense and increased sensor packing may be achieved using liquid nitrogen as the coolant, rather than the currently used liquid helium.

In essence, extracranial magnetic field distribution measurements are useful because they provide the basis for calculations of the likely location of brain generators. Various calculation methods have been used, differing in their *a priori* assumptions, physical model, and integration of ancillary data. In the simplest model, the source is assumed to be a single dipole, lying in a homogenous medium parallel to (i.e., tangential to) the surface of an infinite flat plane (Williamson and Kaufman, 1981). A line is drawn between the points of maximal entry and exit of the magnetic field. The dipole then lies directly beneath the midpoint of this line, at a depth equal to the length of the line divided by the square root of two, and pointing in a direction perpendicular to the line. As we noted above, this model is not so far-fetched, given that a relatively small sheet of cortical neurons produces at a distance a field very similar to that of an "equivalent dipole." Furthermore, inhomogeneties of the head (especially the skull) seem to have little effect on the MEG (Grynszpan and Geselowitz, 1973), and for dipoles near the surface, a plane (or in a similar, slightly more complicated model, a sphere) may provide an adequate approximation for some purposes. However, this model suffers from several problems. First, localization is based entirely on only two points in the extracranial field, and thus has an undesirable sensitivity to inaccuracies in their localization resulting from measurement errors. Methods that find the best fit to all measurements are more stable and accurate. Second, the assumption of a single generating dipole is often inaccurate (Nunez, 1986; Okada, 1982). For example, many cognitive potentials result from the simultaneous activation of more than one cortical generator, together with the hippocampus. Third, the head is not a plane, or even a sphere. This fact must especially be taken into account in interpreting fields over the frontal lobe or at the base of the temporal lobe, where significant deviations from the ideal geometric forms occur. Finally, although the assumption that the dipole is tangential is no problem from a theoretical point of view, it is unfortunate for localizing brain activity. The magnetic field generated by a radial dipole makes no contribution to the extracranial field, because it is perpendicular to the direction of current flow, and thus is "underneath" the cranial surface (Hari and Lounasmaa, 1989). Although this simplifies the interpretation of MEG fields, it also means that activity in many cortical regions (for example, at the crowns of all exterior cortical gyri) cannot be detected with MEG.

   One possible solution to these challenges is to conduct source localization within more realistic and comprehensive models (He et al., 1987; Heringa et al., 1982; Meifs et al., 1987). Such models require a discrete integral equation or finite difference element method, but can model generator and head geometries as actually measured by MRI in the individual under study.

In summary, the MEG has advantages over the EEG for localizing intracerebral generators, in that it is unaffected by over-lying tissue, has no reference electrode, may have a somewhat tighter field, and has fewer degrees of freedom because magnetic fields generated by radial dipoles will not be apparent at the scalp. Conversely, EEG is much less expensive (allowing more sites to be simultaneously sampled), has a better S:N, can detect radial as well as tangential dipoles, is less sensitive to artifacts, and relates to a much larger experimental literature, which aids in interpretation of results. Both MEG and EEG have difficulties in distinguishing between alternative generator geometries that would result in similar extracranial magnetic or electrical fields, and both are in-sensitive to certain geometries. Thus, by using MEG and EEG in combination, it is possible to constrain potential EP generators with greater precision than would be possible using either tech-nique in isolation (cf Cohen and Cuffin, 1983; Wood et al., 1985).

2.3.3. From Depth Recordings and Brain Lesions in Humans

Identification of the neural generator(s) of a scalp EP com-ponent is necessary and sufficient to link the pathological and cognitive correlates of the component to actual brain biology. The topographic EEG and MEG techniques described above are very useful and in some cases can suggest likely candidates for in-tracranial EP generators. However, depth recordings in humans and scalp recordings after brain lesions are usually necessary to confirm hypothesized generators, and are always necessary to identify coactivated structures that do not propagate to the scalp (Figs. 4 and 5). Chronic depth recordings are performed in humans in order to localize the origin of medically uncontrolled seizures prior to surgical treatment (Bancaud, 1975). The first of several steps in identifying the neural generator of such seizures is to record from various intracerebral sites during task conditions that are known to evoke the scalp component. If a depth potential larger than the simultaneous scalp component is found, then the psychological identity of the depth and the scalp components must be confirmed across multiple task conditions. If this criterion is fulfilled, then a variety of physiological and lesion evidence can help to establish whether or not the depth component is locally generated in the vicinity of the recording electrode. If so, then the

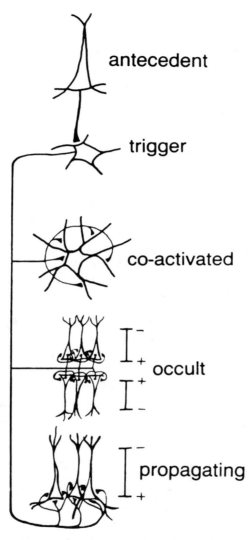

Fig. 4. Terminology used here to discuss evoked potential (EP) generators; different modes of participation by different brain regions during an EP. Projections from one or many *antecedent* structures activate a critical *trigger* structure, which projects widely, to: (1) *coactivate* neurons with synaptic currents that do not summate into an EP; (2) generate EPs that cancel and therefore remain *occult;* or (3) generate EPs that actually *propagate* to the scalp (from Halgren et al. 1986).

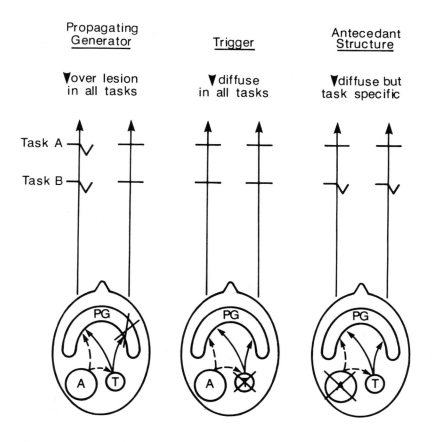

Fig. 5. Criteria for differentiating mechanisms of lesion effects. According to the terminology of Figure 4, an EP component may require antecedant (A) calculations that instruct a trigger (T) neuromodulatory structure to activate the actual generators that propagate (PG) to the scalp. A lesion in the trigger would be expected to produce a diffuse decrease in the EP component in all tasks *(center)*. A lesion in an antecedant structure would also produce a diffuse decrease in the EP component, but perhaps only in particular tasks *(right)*. Finally, a lesion that removes part of the propagating generator would change the topography of the EP component across all tasks *(left)*.

depth component may be evaluated to determine whether it volume conducts to produce all or part of the scalp component. A deeper level of analysis seeks to identify the precise origin, termination, and neurotransmitter and electrical properties of the generating synapses. It is possible to begin, but not to complete, this latter analysis in humans.

3. Sensory EPs

3.1. Auditory Evoked Potentials (AEP)

Auditory EPs are divided into Brainstem Auditory EPs (BAEPs: latency <10 ms), Middle Latency Auditory EPs (MLAEPs: latency 10–50 ms), and Long Latency Auditory EPs (LLAEP: latency 50–250 ms) (Fig. 6: Picton et al., 1974).

3.1.1. Brainstem Auditory EPs

First described by Jewett and Williston (1971) and Hecox and Galambos (1974), BAEPs have been found to have considerable clinical utility for noninvasively monitoring brainstem function and helping to localize brainstem lesions in humans (Picton, 1986; Spehlmann, 1985). BAEPs are decomposed into seven components (I–VII), each corresponding to a peak of relative positivity at the vertex (Cz). Negative peaks are indicated by an "N" after the preceding positive peak number (i.e., "IN", with "N" following "I"). Superimposed on these very brief peaks are slow potentials that may be relatively enhanced by appropriate filtering. Table 1 lists the putative generators of the BAEPs. The generators of these components are still controversial, and in many cases probably involve several regions. However, animal models (Legatt et al., 1986; Bullock, 1986; Velasco et al., 1984), direct brainstem recordings in humans (Velasco et al., 1982; Hashimoto et al., 1981), observations of patients with known lesions (Moller and Jannetta, 1986), and topographical studies (Hughes and Fino, 1985) have led to a convergence toward the putative generators listed in Table 1. Note that the highly synchronous activation of the auditory system permits the small fields generated by action-potential volleys and presynaptic depolarizations to be detected at the scalp.

Because of their low amplitude and high frequency, BAEPs require many trials (>1000) at a high frequency. They are very insensitive to behavioral state or anesthesia, and can thus be used

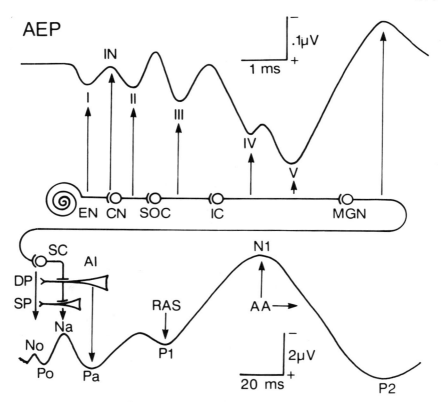

Fig. 6. Typical waveforms and putative generating structures for auditory EP components. Above: The nerve impulses beginning in the cochlea generate the brainstem AEPs (*see* Table 1 for abbreviations and additional putative generators). Below: Middle and long latency AEPs are thought to reflect sequential activation of the stellate cells (SC) in layer IV, then superficial (SP) and deep (DP) pyramidal cells of primary auditory cortex (AI), ascending reticular system (RS) influences, and spread to auditory association (AA) cortex (*see* Table 2 and text).

to distinguish toxic metabolic or drug-induced coma from that caused by brainstem lesions. Increased sound intensity does affect BAEP latency (40 μs/dB: Picton, 1986). Both contacts in standard vertex-to-ear or mastoid recording derivation are active, hence a noncephalic reference will yield waveforms with greater resemblance to those actually recorded in the brainstem (Moller and Jannetta, 1986).

Table 1
Putative Major Generators for Brainstem Auditory EP Components,
Adapted from Legatt et al., 1986*

Component	Latency, ms**	Putative Generators
?		Cochlear summating potential
I	1.5	Action potential in distal eighth nerve (EN)
IN		EN terminal depolarization
II	2.5	Ipsilateral cochlear nucleus (CN) outflow decussating in trapezoid body and ascending in the lateral lemniscus (LL)
IIN		EN terminal depolarization, ipsilateral superior olivary complex (SOC) outflow ascending in LL, activity in contralateral CN
III	3.5–5	Contralateral SOC outflow ascending in LL
IV	5	Ipsilateral SOC outflow ascending in LL, outflow of both inferior colliculi (IC) in the brachium of inferior colliculus (BIC)
V	5.5–8	Ipsilateral nucleus LL outflow ascending in LL, contralateral SOC outflow ascending in LL, activity of contralateral IC
VN		Outflow of both IC in BIC
VI		Outflow of both medial geniculate Nuclei (MGN) in radiations, activity of both IC
VII	8.5	Outflow of both MGN in radiations, activity of both IC
SN		Postsynaptic potentials in both CN and both IC

*For other, usually similar interpretations, see Buchwald, 1983; Boston and Moller, 1985; Moore, 1983; Starr, 1985.
**Latency depends on loudness.

3.1.2. Middle Latency Auditory EPs

MLAEPs (Fig. 6 and Table 2) are easily obscured by sonomotor responses of the scalp and neck musculature (Bickford et al., 1964; Harker et al., 1977; Ruhm et al., 1967; Streletz et al., 1977). However, their reality has been clearly demonstrated in curarized patients (Kileny et al., 1983) and animals (Kaga et al., 1980). Like BAEPs, MLAEPs change little with fast stimulation rates, changes in atten-

Table 2
Middle Latency Auditory EPs

Component	Latency, ms	Putative Generators
No	9–10	Presynaptic activity in thalamocortical afferents + postsynaptic potentials (PSPs) in lamina IV stellate cells
Po	14–15	Excitatory PSPs (EPSPs) in basal dendrites of layer III pyramidal cells
Na	19	Inhibitory PSPs (IPSPs) in layer III pyramids
Pa	30–35	EPSPs in layer V pyramids

tion, light sleep, or mild sedation. Apparently very similar neural generators are expressed as the in-phase EEG evoked by a tone that is amplitude modulated at 40 Hz (Galambos et al., 1981; Spydell et al., 1985).

Laminar and multiunit recordings have identified the primary auditory cortex in the monkey as containing the putative generators for various peaks in this latency range (Arezzo et al., 1975, 1986; *see* Table 2). This is supported by intracranial recordings from humans (Ruhm et al., 1967; Lee et al., 1984; Celesia, 1976), by the abolition of these components by bilateral primary auditory cortical lesions that cause cortical deafness (Graham et al., 1980; Özdamar and Kraus, 1983; Özdamar et al., 1982), and by the lack of effect of unilateral temporal lobe lesions (Kraus et al., 1982) or bilateral temporal association cortex lesions (Parving et al., 1980). The MLAEPs have a widespread frontocentral topography (Goff et al., 1977; Streletz et al., 1977; Picton et al., 1974), which may also be consistent with bilateral primary auditory cortex generators (Wood and Wolpaw, 1982). However, intracranial recordings indicate that the generators are complicated, with frontal contributions from 20 ms and lateral temporal from 25 ms in the monkey, suggesting multiple contributors to waves Pa *et seq.* in humans (Arezzo et al., 1975; Wolpaw and Penry, 1975; Wood and Wolpaw, 1982).

3.1.3. Long Latency AEPs

The LLAEPs are labelled P1–N1–P2, according to sequence and polarity at the vertex (site C_Z in Fig. 3, at the top of the head).

The first of the LLAEPs, the P1, straddles the division between middle and late auditory EPs, and is often considered as a MLAEP (under the label Pb: Kileny et al. 1983). It is classified here as a LLAEP because, unlike the MLAEP components Po, Na, and Pa (Picton et al., 1974; Mendel and Goldstein, 1971), the P1 is very sensitive to the level of consciousness of the subjects, being abolished by slow wave sleep and restored during REM sleep (Erwin and Buchwald, 1986). This property has facilitated the identification of an apparently homologous component in the cat "wave A" (Chen and Buchwald, 1986). This component is correlated in latency, recovery cycle, and sensitivity to barbiturates to a system suggested, on the basis of field potential and unit recording, to course through the midbrain and thalamic ascending reticular formation (Hinman and Buchwald, 1983). Wave A continues to be observed after hemispherectomy, suggesting that this is a subcortically generated wave in the cat (Buchwald et al., 1981). However, cortical generators activated by the ascending reticular system may contribute to the scalp P1 in humans. Furthermore, the MEG field topography suggests a tonotopic potential in this latency range generated in the primary auditory cortex (Arthur et al., 1987).

The remaining LAEPs (N1–P2) are also strongly modulated by sleep (Kevanishvili and Von Sprecht, 1979; Mendel et al., 1975; Ornitz et al., 1967; Osterhammel et al., 1973; Rapin et al., 1972). Superimposed on the N1–P2 is a negativity (Nd) strongly affected by attention (Picton and Hillyard, 1974; Goodin et al., 1983; Picton et al., 1976; Salamy and McKean, 1977; Schwent and Hillyard, 1975; Schwent et al., 1976; *see also* section 5). These components decline rapidly with increasing stimulus repetition rates (Davis et al., 1966; Nelson and Lassman, 1968; Schafer et al., 1981; Surwillo, 1977). The N1–P2 have a fairly widespread topography (Goff et al., 1977; Streletz et al., 1977) that is slightly larger over the contralateral scalp and may change with changes in interstimulus interval. The polarity inversion of the N1–P2 on the scalp over the region of the sylvian fissure suggested that its origin may lie in the inferior bank of that fissure. MEG recordings have suggested a similar localization (Arthur et al., 1987; Hari et al., 1982; Romani et al., 1982). However, further analysis found topographical evidence for additional generator(s) (Kooi et al., 1971; Scherg and Von Cramon, 1985); this has been supported by differences in the auditory N1–P2 when recorded from the scalp rather than directly from the region of the auditory cortex (Celesia, 1976). The effects of lesions suggest generators in the superior-posterior temporal lobe (Knight et al., 1980; 1988). Combined with the MEG, animal, and human intracranial data, these observations suggest multiple generators, including the primary auditory cortex as well as auditory and perhaps some multimodal association areas, possibly even including the frontal lobes (Peronnet et al., 1984; Hari et al., 1984b; Wood and Wolpaw, 1982). These multimodal generators apparently contribute also to the N1–P2s evoked by visual and somatosensory stimulation (Bancaud et al., 1953).

3.2. Somatosensory Evoked Potentials (SEP)

Like the AEPs, SEPs, include short-latency subcortical components (<20 ms), middle-latency components from the primary cortex supplemented by related areas (20–80 ms), and finally labile long-latency components overlapping with multimodal cognitive components (Fig. 7). The early components (<30 ms) are unaffected by repetition, attention, or sleep, whereas the later are affected to varying degrees (Allison, 1962; Goff et al., 1966; Velasco et al., 1980). In general, SEPs are produced by synaptic relays or tracts in the specific somatosensory pathway: dorsal column in the spinal cord, medial lemniscus in the brainstem, nucleus ventralis posterolateralis and postermedialis in the thalamus, and rolandic cortex (Spehlmann, 1985). Consequently, SEPs are generally abnormal after lesions that impair vibration and position sensation, but not after those that specifically impair pain and temperature sensation.

3.2.1. Methods

The standard stimuli for evoking SEP are .2-ms shocks to the median nerve at the wrist, 4–7 ×/s (American EEG Society, 1984). This stimulates a variety of sensory as well as motor axons, and produces a somewhat different SEP than do natural stimuli, which are much more difficult to administer and standardize (Pratt and Starr, 1981). The lower extremity is commonly stimulated at the knee (common perineal n.) or ankle (posterior tibial n.). Pudendal n. evoked SEP may be useful for investigating sexual disorders (Haldeman et al., 1982). SEPs to painful stimuli (mainly long-latency) have been evoked by radiant heat (Bromm et al., 1983; Carmon et al., 1976) or tooth-pulp stimulation (Chapman et al., 1979; Chudler, 1983; Cruccu et al., 1983). Long-latency EPs to rotational acceleration/deceleration have been reported, but their vestibular origin is in doubt (Durrant and Furman, 1988). The EPs evoked by odorous air introduced over the olfactory mucosa are apparently the results of a mixture of trigeminal nerve and olfactory bulb activations (Kobal and Hummel, 1988). Attention and stimulus rarity effects have been studied in the somatosensory modality (Desmedt, 1981), but with the exception of a study of active palpitation (Desmedt, 1977b), SEP to complex information have not been studied, for obvious reasons.

3.2.2. Components and Generators

The ascending action-potential volley following a median n. stimulus arrives at the brachial plexus with a peak latency of 9 ms and ascends in the dorsal columns, producing a peak at 11 ms (Desmedt, 1986, in humans; Emerson and Pedley, 1984; Arezzo et al., 1979 in monkeys; similar interpretations are found in Ertekin, 1978 and Maruyama et al., 1982). At 13 ms, a component can be recorded over the back that is generated by dorsal horn EPSPs to cutaneous group A afferents (Beall et al., 1977; Desmedt, 1986). At the same time, the first clearly identified scalp component, P13, occurs. This component is abolished by high cord hemisection (Mauguiere et al., 1983a), but survives thalamic lesions (Chiappa et al., 1980; Lueders et al., 1983; Nakanishi et al., 1978; Eisen, 1982; Mauguiere et al., 1983b; Yamada et al., 1983), suggesting a pre-thalamic origin. This is consistent with the P13's scalp (Desmedt and Cheron, 1980) and depth (Suzuki and Mayanagi, 1984; Tsuji et al., 1984) topography. Direct recordings in monkey and man indicate that this component is probably generated by the termination of dorsal column fibers in the cuneate nucleus (Moller et al., 1986). Depth recordings (Hashimoto, 1984) and lesions (Mauguiere et al., 1983c) indicate that the next scalp component, N18, is also generated subcortically. The broad topography of this component helps distinguish it from the subsequent cortical components.

The identity and precise generators of the earliest cortical SEP have been subjected to intense investigation. It is clear that the predominant potentials are a parietally negative–frontally positive potential peaking at about 20 ms, followed by a parietally positive–frontally negative potential peaking at about 30 ms (Fig. 7). It is also clear that in many patients the parietal and frontal peaks are not precisely synchronous, and that smaller peaks may be present between the parietal N20–P30 or frontal P20–N30. All peaks are

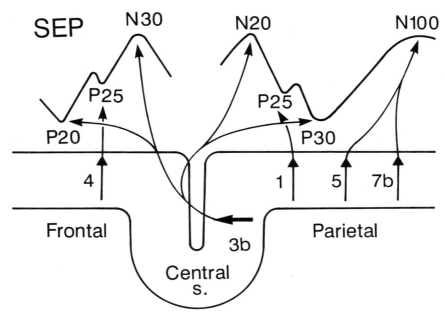

Fig. 7. Typical waveforms and putative generating structures for somatosensory EP components. At about 20 and 30 ms, the primary scalp components polarity-invert across the central sulcus and are thought to be mainly generated by a single dipole in the posterior bank of that sulcus.

predominately contralateral to the stimulated wrist at the scalp, and completely contralateral at the cortex (Wood et al., 1988). Two schools of thought have developed regarding these potentials. One school postulated a single generator for the parietal N20–P30 and frontal P20–N30 (Broughton, 1969; Broughton et al., 1981; Allison et al., 1980). The hypothesized generating dipole would be located in the posterior bank of the central sulcus, resulting in the opposite frontal vs parietal polarities. Other authors feel that the scalp (Deiber et al., 1986; Desmedt and Bourguet, 1985; Desmedt et al., 1987) and depth (Celesia, 1979; Papakostopoulos and Crow, 1980) topographies are inconsistent with a single generator. These authors tend to emphasize the latency differences, and therefore refer to the parietal N20–P27 and frontal P22–N30 (Desmedt, 1986; Desmedt and Bourguet, 1985). In its most extreme form, this point of view postulates one radial dipole in the crown of the postcentral gyrus, generating the parietal N20–P27, and another radial dipole in the crown of the precentral gyrus, generating the frontal P22–N30. The strongest evidence for separate generators is that some lesions have been reported to affect the parietal N20–P27, but not the frontal P22–N30, whereas other lesions affect the frontal, but not parietal, components (Mauguiere et al., 1983c; Slimp et al., 1986). Furthermore, the frontal P22, but not the parietal N20, is greatly decreased during active movement (Cheron and Borenstein, 1987).

Somatosensory stimuli also evoke clear magnetic field components in this latency range, localizable to the postcentral gyrus and somatopically organized (Huttunen et al., 1987; Hari and Kaukoranta, 1985). A combined study of the somatosensory magnetic field and electrical potential evoked 20–30 ms after median n. stimulation found that *most,* but not all, of both the magnetic and the electrical fields could be explained by a single tangential postcentral generator (Wood et al., 1985). Conversely, because the MEG and EEG are differentially sensitive to radially vs tangentially oriented dipole generators, these studies were able to demonstrate that the parietal negativity and frontal positivity at about 20 ms are highly unlikely to be generated by two coactive tangential generators of opposite polarity. Nonetheless, this study found evidence that a small part of the early cortical SEP could be a radially oriented dipole in the precentral and/or postcentral gyrus. Similar conclusions can be drawn from the lack of polarity inversions found in transcortical recordings from the perirolandic region (Allison et al., 1988). Furthermore, comparison of the linear separation of the frontal and parietal field maxima at about 20 ms, when recorded at the scalp, rather than directly from the cortical surface, are also consistent with a tangential principal generator in the somatosensory cortex adjacent to the rolandic fissure (area 3b: Wood, 1987). Finally, it has recently been reported that surgical excisions of the postcentral gyrus in both monkeys and humans abolish both the parietal N20–P30 and the frontal P20–N30, whereas neither are affected by precentral gyrus excisions (Wood, 1987). Since the lesions reported by Wood (1987) were focal excisions supported by pre- and postsurgical recordings, whereas those reported by Mauguiere et al. (1983c) were cerebrovascular and supported only by poststroke recordings, the balance of the evidence now indicates that the postcentral gyrus is necessary for both pairs of peaks. However, additional smaller peaks are probably caused by slightly later radial dipoles in the crowns of the postcentral and precentral gyri (areas 4 and 1). In fact, nearly all active investigators subscribe to this general view, with disagreements being concerned with the details of these smaller peaks and their nomenclature.

A preponderant generator in the posterior bank of the central sulcus (area 3b), with possible secondary contributions from other pre- and postcentral gyri sites, is also supported by laminar and unit recordings in monkeys (Gardner et al., 1984, 1986; Allison and Hume, 1981; Arezzo et al., 1981, 1986; Kulics and Cauller, 1986). These recordings also indicate that multiple cortical areas, including the premotor (area 6), precentral (4), postcentral (1, 2, and 3), medial postcentral (5), and lateral parietal (7b), are all activated with a latency of 24 ms or less and a duration of about 150 ms (Arezzo et al., 1986), suggesting that potentials after 30 ms have multiple generators in sensorimotor cortex. In particular, the human somatosensory N100 appears to be related to the late activity in medial postcentral (5) and lateral parietal (7b) areas. Overlapping primary and secondary somatosensory cortex generators are also suggested by the topography of somatosensory evoked magnetic fields in the 75–200 ms range (Hari et al., 1984a; Hari and Kaukoranta, 1985).

3.3. Visual EPs

3.3.1. Methods

VEPs are most effectively and consistently evoked by patterned stimuli. The background should remain dimly illuminated, in order to counteract the effects of stray light and promote more constant levels of dark adaptation. Stimuli are most commonly checkerboard patterns, with the white and black squares reversing every 500 ms. Reversal is generally used (rather than checkerboard onset from a diffusely illuminated field) because the lack of luminance changes is thought to evoke a more purely cortical response. The optimal spatial frequency for activation of the cortex receiving foveal projections (i.e., from the central 4–5° of the retina) is provided by checks that subtend about 12' of arc at the retina (Lesevre and Joseph, 1979; Spekreijse et al., 1973; Yiannikas and Walsh, 1983), whereas for more eccentric stimuli, 40' or larger checks are optimal (Harter and White, 1970; Regan and Richards, 1971). Usually, a compromise check-size is chosen.

Many other stimulus configurations are obviously possible, and this is a major advantage of the visual modality for cognitive EPs, particularly given the very powerful graphics capabilities of current inexpensive personal computers. The task presentation program causes a visual stimulus to be presented by writing that stimulus into a location in the part of memory corresponding to the desired location on the videoscreen. A circuit scans the block of memory devoted to the videoscreen, and writes it onto the screen, starting in the upper left-hand corner and proceeding line by line. Generally this process ("refreshing the screen") is repeated 60 × every second (in the US). Suppose that the stimulus (for example, a word) occupies only a small part of the videoscreen. Then the delay between the word being written into video memory and it being written onto the video screen will be between zero (if, when the word is written to memory, the scanner is positioned just before the position where the word is placed) and 16.7 ms (if the scanner has just passed the word's location). On some microcomputers, it is possible to time-lock stimulus presentation to the "videosynch pulse" at the onset of the sweep, resulting in a constant 8.3-ms delay for stimuli in the center of the monitor. This, however, will also time-lock the recordings to line current and thus cause the averages to reflect any 60-Hz noise present in the recordings. Randomizing stimulus presentation with respect to the videosynch will reduce line noise, but will smear the EPs by introducing a latency jitter of ± 8.3 ms (cf also van Lith et al., 1979; Sgro and Emerson, 1985). Whichever of these two evils the experimenter chooses, it should be noted, and the published latency of the peaks should be adjusted accordingly (cf van Lith et al., 1979).

A particularly elegant example of the power of visual stimuli to evoke high-order brain processes is seen in the VEPs recorded to random-dot stereograms (Lehmann and Julesz, 1978; Herpers et al., 1981; Julesz and Kropfl, 1982; Petrig et al., 1981). These stereograms are pairs of images of numerous small white dots arrayed like "snow" on a television screen. When viewed by each eye separately, the dots appear randomly arrayed. However, the dots in a certain area of the images are displaced by a constant amount between the images. Consequently, when the images are viewed convergently, this region appears to be at a different depth than the rest of the image. The onset of this displacement thus constitutes a "spatial" stimulus, where the binocular integration is known to occur cortically, unconfounded by any changes in simple visual parameters (luminance, contrast, contour, or spatial frequency).

Regan (1972, 1981) has reviewed the use of VEPs to help resolve current questions in visual psychophysics. The later (>200 ms) VEP components to complex stimuli (words, faces, drawings, and so forth) are very sensitive to the cognitive content and recent history of the evolving stimulus (*see* section 5). Rather than separately present individual words, some workers have recorded VEPs to the onset and offset of saccades during more natural reading tasks. The waveforms following the saccade are similar to those seen in response to individually presented words, suggesting that they are evoked by information delivery following fixation (Yagi, 1981; Marton et al., 1985a,b).

Flashes may also be used to evoke VEPs. However, the VEPs that they evoke are much smaller, given an equally intense stimulus, than are pattern VEPs. Furthermore, the flash VEPs are much more variable between subjects (Bodis-Wollner et al., 1979; Celesia, 1982). Part of this variability results from differences in age or pupillary diameter, but most is unexplained (Ciganek, 1975; Spehlmann, 1985). Like the pattern VEPs, the flash VEPs evoke a N75–P100–N135 complex. Flashes activate earlier stations of the visual pathway more effectively than do patterns, and several components preceding the N75–P100 complex have been reported (Cobb and Dawson, 1960; Cracco and Cracco, 1978; Pratt et al., 1982; Vaughan, 1966; Whittaker and Siegfried, 1983). However, these peaks are variable, and their generators have not yet been determined. Following about 250 ms, the flash VEP is often followed by synchronized α activity, especially if the subject's eyes are closed during stimulation, or he or she is drowsy (Barlow 1960). Reviews of the components of the flash EP may be found in Ciganek (1975), Kooi and Marshall (1979) and Vaughan (1966).

The "steady-state" VEP extracts EEG activity related to visual stimuli that are sinusoidally modulated in intensity or contrast (Picton et al., 1984; Regan 1972, 1982). The latency and amplitude of harmonies of the modulation frequency are extracted through a Fourier transform. This technique is often used in psychophysiological experiments, and in many cases can yield objectively quantified and reliable EEG or MEG measures in a shorter experimental session than can transient VEPs. However, these steady-state measures do not have as clearly defined a physiological generator as do the transient VEPs.

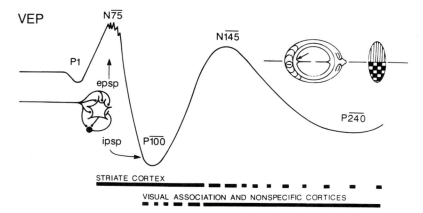

Fig. 8. Typical waveforms and putative generating structures for cortical visual EP components. Hemifield visual stimulation activates a dipole in the contralateral visual cortex that, because of its orientation, projects predominantly to the contralateral scalp (ipsilateral to the stimulus—*see* upper right corner of figure). As described in the text, the initial activation in layer IV of visual cortex is reflected by the N75, and the following inhibitory PSP by the P100. The P100, as well as later potentials, receives contributions from other cortical areas. A bar above the component designation is a commonly used convention for indicating that the latency is a modal value across subjects, rather than a reflection of the observation in an individual subject.

3.3.2. Components and Generators

In summary, the major components of both pattern-reversal and flash VEPs is a triphasic, occipitally dominant negative–positive–negative complex, peaking at 70–75, 90–110, and 130–145 ms, respectively (Fig. 8). The P100 can be quite large (100 μv), and when authors refer to an unidentified VEP, it is the P100, or the P100–N140 complex. Laminar EP and multiunit recordings in cats and monkeys (Kraut et al., 1985; Mitzdorf, 1986) suggest that the N70 represents synaptic depolarization of primary afferents and lamina IVC stellate cell EPSPs in striate cortex. Several authors have noted that superimposed on the human N70 are a series of high-frequency oscillations (Cracco and Cracco, 1978; Pratt et al., 1982; Whittaker and Siegfried, 1983; Vaughan and Hull, 1965). These are also seen in monkeys at the time of presynaptic depolarization of the primary afferents and lamina IV stellate cell EPSPs (Kraut et al., 1985). The following P100 appears to reflect inhibition in the thalamorecipient laminae, possibly mediated by GABA (Zemon et al., 1986). Earlier potentials (Allison et al., 1977) are thought by Kraut et al. (1985) to be subcortical, and later potentials from a combination of striate and extrastriate generators. In particular, a late, broad (200–310 ms) posterior temporal negativity evoked by complex visual stimuli (and associated with "template-matching") is decreased ipsilaterally by removal of the underlying inferotemporal cortex (Smith and Halgren, 1988b).

In general, these conclusions are supported by other studies. Direct recordings from the human occipital lobe suggest a calcarine cortex origin for the P100 and overlying fast wavelets (Darcey et al., 1980; Ducati et al., 1988). The N70–P100–N140 peaks are maximal occipitally (Vaughan, 1969). Furthermore, hemifield stimulation induces a P100 topography consistent with a calcarine generator (Darcey et al., 1980). This generator points toward the opposite cortex, resulting in the N70–P100–N140 to hemifield stimulation being maximal ipsilateral to the stimulated visual field, and thus contralateral to the activated cortex. The occipital scalp contralateral to the visual stimulus has peaks at the same latency, but of opposite polarity. The P100 is somewhat more symmetrical to foveal hemifield stimulation, presumably because the foveal projection includes the convexity of the occipital tip, which points toward the ipsilateral scalp (Blumhardt and Halliday, 1979; Blumhardt et al., 1978). The evoked magnetic field topography also is consistent with this interpretation (Brenner et al., 1981; Williamson and Kaufman, 1981) and even suggests retinotopic organization of the generators (Maclin et al., 1983). Finally, these VEP components are severely decreased by occipital lesions in humans (e.g., Chain et al., 1972; Streletz et al., 1981; reviewed by Harmony, 1984, pp. 60, 61), and in animals (Vaughan and Gross, 1969).

However, it is likely that at least the P100, and all subsequent peaks, receive contributions from multiple cortical regions. Thus, the monkey inferotemporal cortex responds to a meaningful visual stimulus with a 28-ms latency, following the striate cortex by only 8 ms (Ashford and Fuster, 1985). In the normal human, the occipital P100 is accompanied by a frontal negativity. The fact that this negativity does not have exactly the same latency as the occipital positivity, and is differently affected by brain lesions, suggests that multiple generators are active during this time period (Spitz et al.,

1986). These extrastriate generators may be related to the "vertex potentials" N1-P2 evoked by auditory and somaesthetic stimuli (Bancaud et al., 1953).

4. Movement Potentials

4.1. Methods

A series of EP components have been identified in the averaged EEG surrounding movements (Fig. 9: Kornhuber and Deecke, 1965; Gilden et al., 1966). Originally, "back-averaging" (or "opisthochronic" averaging) was accomplished by first tape-recording the EEG, with a trigger-pulse at the time of movement or electromyogram (EMG) onset, and then playing the recording backwards into a dedicated averager. General-purpose computers accomplish the same task by digitizing the signal into a buffer of the desired trace duration. When the signal reaches the end of the buffer, it is redirected to the beginning of the buffer until digitization is terminated by a trigger pulse. The sweep is then rotated so that the trigger is at its end. By delaying the trigger for a fixed period after the movement, postmovement EP components can also be resolved.

Most studies of movement potentials have required a simple keypress. Potentials preceding eye movements (Becker et al., 1973), simple phonation (Ertl and Schafer, 1967; Schafer, 1967), or speech (McAdam and Whitaker, 1971) have also been observed and may be strongly lateralized. However, extracerebral artifacts arising from respiration, perioral muscles, and especially the tongue, which has a large standing potential, are severe (Grozinger et al., 1977, 1980) and appear to account for most of the published prespeech potentials (Szirtes and Vaughan, 1977). Nonetheless, it is likely that speech-related potentials of cerebral origin do exist, inasmuch as they can be recorded from the pial surface (Fried et al., 1981). Potentials preceding and accompanying drawing and writing appear more promising *(see below)*.

4.2. Components

Components of movement EPs (Table 3) have been discussed by Deecke et al. (1976), Deecke and Kornhuber (1978), Vaughan

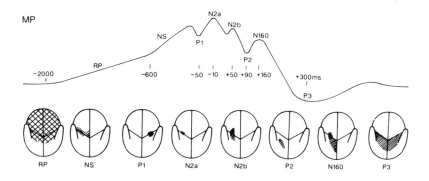

Fig. 9. Typical waveforms and putative generating structures for cortical movement potential components. The schematic topographical maps suggest that, as a movement approaches, is performed, and passes, the brain activation changes from diffuse, frontal, and bilateral; to focal, central, and contralateral; to diffuse, parietal and bilateral (*see* Table 3 and text for further discussion).

(1975), Vaughan et al. (1968), Gerbrandt (1977), and Shibasaki et al. (1980a). In general, Deecke and Kornhuber name their potentials according to their presumed function, Vaughan and Gerbrandt according to the polarity and numerical order of the peak, and Shibasaki according to the polarity and peak latency relative to the peak of the EMG (which occurs about 30 ms after EMG onset). The Readiness Potential (RP-Bereitschaftspotential=BP=Nl=NS'=N–90) is a widespread negativity beginning about 1 s before the movement (Kornhuber and Deecke, 1965). About 50–150 ms before the contraction, a small "Premotion Positivity" (=Pl=P–50) may be seen, followed by the "Motor Potential" (=MP=N2=N–10) close to EMG onset (Shibasaki and Kato, 1975), a slightly later positivity (=P2=P+90), and then a broader positivity (=P3=P+300), peaking about 300 ms after the movement. The N2 has been further subdivided into an N2a (probably corresponding to the Motor Potential) and a slightly later N2b (=Reafferente Potentiale=N+50). The smaller components occurring close to movement onset are quite variable across subjects, resulting in a confused and controversial nomenclature (Tamas and Shibasaki, 1985). Another negativity (N+160 of Shibasaki et al., 1980a) occurs riding on the downward slope of the P3.

Table 3

Component	Alternative Labels	Latency, ms	Topography
RP	Readiness potential Bereitschaft-spotential	–3000 or –1000–0*	Bilateral diffuse (central maximum)
NS'	N1	–700 or –300–0*	Contralateral central
P1	Premotor positivity P–50	–50	Ipsilateral central parietal
N2a	N–10	–10	Focal contralateral precentral
N2b	Reafferente poten-tiale N+50	+50	Slightly contralateral frontal
P2	P+90	+90	Contralateral parietal
N+160		+160	Contralateral parietal
P3	P+300	+300	Slightly contralateral diffuse (central maximum)

*These components do not have clear peaks, hence their onset and offset are indicated (the offset is uncertain because of overlapping potentials).

4.3. Topography

As might be expected, the movement potentials begin diffusely, related to psychological variables (i.e., cognitive), become progressively more focal and specific as the movement approaches, and then become more diffuse and possibly cognitive with increasing time after the movement (Figure 9). The RP, or at least the latter RP, is slightly larger over the hemisphere contralateral to the pressing hand, especially in right-handed subjects (Kutas and Donchin, 1980). This asymmetry is more prominent later in the epoch and in central recording sites. This has led to the subdivision of the RP into two components, an RP proper beginning 1–3 s prior to the movement, and an NS' (negative slope) superimposed on the RP and signaled by an inflection in the RP slope occurring about 500–700 ms prior to movement (Shibasaki et al., 1980a; Kutas and Donchin, 1977; Hillyard, 1973). The RP is maximal centrally (i.e., near Cz). It may appear positive at frontal sites if the ears or mastoids are used as a reference. However, recordings with noncephalic references indicate that both frontal and ear sites are actually negative (Deecke et al., 1973).

Unlike the other movement potentials, the P1 is larger ipsilateral to the moving hand and is maximal centroparietally (Shibasaki and Kato, 1975). The N2a is a small, sharp negativity, maximal over the precentral cortex contralateral to the movement and, indeed, may shift closer to the midline if the lower, rather than the upper, extremity is moved. The N2b is the most prominent and consistent component occurring in this latency range. Compared to the N2a, it is more frontal and frontopolar, and is only slightly larger contralateral to the moving hand (Shibasaki et al., 1980b). The next two components (P2 and N + 160) are maximal over the contralateral parietal lobe. The P3 is more diffuse, maximal centrally, and slightly larger contralateral to the movement (Shibasaki et al., 1980b).

Thus, contrasting topography and latency can be exploited to differentiate the MP components (*see* Table 3). The latencies given are for hand movements. Foot movements evoke potentials that are either earlier with respect to the movement (if they relate to pyramidal tract overflow) or later (if they reflect reafference). This property may be used to separate these components (Shibasaki et al., 1981). Similarly, differential recordings between ipsilateral and contralateral sites have been used by several authors to distinguish lateralized "motor" potentials from the preceding RP.

4.4. Generators—P1/N2/P2/P3

The topography of the P1 (ipsilateral and centroparietal), and the fact that it may be absent in bimanual movements, may suggest that it reflects inhibition in precentral neurons, functioning to suppress the movement that is a mirror image of that which is actually performed (Shibasaki and Kato, 1975). Moving more distant muscles increases the delay time from the P1–N2 until the movement (Gilden et al., 1966), suggesting a fairly direct link with the corticospinal discharge. Like the pyramidal tract discharge, the N2a is larger to extension that to flexion (Deecke et al., 1980). Kornhuber (1971) has suggested that the corticospinal discharge is reflected by the N2, with the P1 reflecting a preceding parietal discharge to the cerebellum, which in turn sets up the movements, in part by a projection back to the precentral cortex. This is supported by the finding that electrical stimulation of the deep cerebellar nuclei in primates produces a surface negativity in motor and premotor cortex (Sasaki, 1976–1977; Shibasaki et al., 1981). This effect is mediated via the thalamic nuclei VA and VL, where a premotion positivity has been reported in humans (Baba et al., 1976–1977; Straschill and Takahashi, 1980). A role of reafference is also suggested by the much *larger* and more complex potentials surrounding *passive* as opposed to *active* movements (Shibasaki et al., 1980b). Reafference from peripheral receptors (cf Papakostopoulos et al., 1975) has been considered unlikely, given the minimal effects of limb deafferentation on movement potentials in monkeys (Vaughan et al., 1970; Vaughan, 1975). However, Bioulac and Lamarre (1979) reported that the early (60 ms premovement) potentials in postcentral cortex (*see also* Soso and Fetz, 1980) were abolished by peripheral deafferentation.

Extensive studies of the origins of movement potentials have been conducted in the monkey, where a similar series of components is observed (Arezzo et al., 1977; Arezzo and Vaughan, 1975, 1980; Johnson, 1980). Laminar EP and multiunit recordings in these animal models, as well as occasional human recordings, tend to support the hypotheses outlined above. The part of the N2 that precedes EMG onset (termed N2a) appears to represent the discharge of deep pyramidal cells projecting into the corticospinal tract (Arezzo and Vaughan, 1980; Johnson, 1980). The precentral cortex is the apparent location of most of these cells. However, many monkey pyramidal cells lie in the postcentral gyrus (Fromm, 1983; Soso and Fetz, 1980), and epidural recordings in humans have recorded the N2 on both sides of the central fissure (Ganglberger et al., 1980; Lee et al., 1986). Transcortical recordings in both monkeys and humans have suggested that an additional area (in layer 6, adjacent to the supplementary motor cortex) also contributes.

Arezzo et al.'s (1977) data indicates that the monkey N2b, beginning just at movement onset, appears to be generated by PSPs evoked by afferents to either side of the central sulcus. The initial P2 (=P2a) is also caused by these afferents in areas 1, 2, and 5 (Arezzo and Vaughan, 1980). Later (90 ms after movement onset), the P2 (=P2b) is caused by PSPs in superficial sensorimotor cortex laminae, according to Arezzo and Vaughan (1980), or more broadly in contralateral parietal postcentral, precentral, and frontal cortex according to Johnson (1980). Direct cortical recordings in humans, although limited, tend also to suggest a broad contralateral generator (Pieper et al., 1980). Similarly, Johnson (1980) finds a diffuse contralateral generator for the N + 160 and a diffuse bilateral generator for the P3, whereas Arezzo and Vaughan (1980) find a focal generator in the depth of the central sulcus for the N + 160, and a bilateral postcentral and parietal (area 5) generator for the P3. Sakata et al. (1973) also found primate units in somatosensory cortex that fire at about 300 ms latency following movements. Finally, Pieper et al.'s (1980) recordings in the human suggest a bilateral area 5 generator for the P3 in parietal cortex.

The average magnetic fields accompanying simple keypresses also suggest a predominant generator in the contralateral precentral cortex (Deecke et al., 1982; Okada et al., 1982). Appropriate movements of the field along the precentral gyrus have been observed for foot/toe movements (Antervo et al., 1983; Deecke et al., 1983). Prespeech magnetic fields have been described (Hari et al., 1983; Weinberg and Brickett, 1983), but as with prespeech electrical fields, the appropriate controls to exclude extracerebral sources are unclear.

4.5. Generators—RP, NS[1]

In their studies, Arezzo and coworkers (1977) found that the major generator of the RP recorded at the scalp (as indicated by laminar EP and multiunit recordings) is activation of the deeper pyramids in the contralateral precentral cortex, rather than the subcortical structures (including thalamus, basal ganglia, and hippocampus) where potentials are also simultaneously recorded (Arezzo et al., 1987). Hashimoto et al. (1981) also find only contralateral field potentials during the RP. However, this activity extends beyond area 4 to area 6 (premotor cortex), often to areas 1 and 2 (postcentral), rarely to area 7 (parietral) and never to area 19 (prestriate). Johnson (1980) and Pieper et al. (1980) find even more extensive field potentials during the RP, including a small contribution of area 5 (parietal) ipsilateral to the movement. Unit recordings also support wide generation. Primate precentral neurons, including pyramidal tract cells, have long been known to fire up to 500 ms prior to EMG onset (Evarts and Tanji, 1976). Area 6 (premotor and supplementary motor cortex [SMC]) cells in primates (Pieper et al., 1980) and cats (Neafsey et al., 1978) fire at least as early, and probably earlier (Tanji and Kurata, 1982; Weinrich et al., 1984). The early SMC cell-firing differentiates among sensory stimuli that cue distinct movements (Tanji, 1984; Tanji et al., 1980). Similarly, cells in the dorsolateral frontal eye field (near the SMC) fire 500 ms prior to spontaneous saccades (Schlag and Schlag-Rey, 1987). The clear evidence for cell-firing in premotor and SMC during the RP suggests that the failure of some studies to find significant field potentials in these areas may be a consequence of task factors. Specifically, it seems possible that task performance might become so overlearned and automatized that premotor and SMC are no longer engaged.

Widespread neural activation has also been found in human intracranial recordings during the RP. Papakostopoulos et al. (1975) report a negativity on the surface of pre- and postcentral cortex during the RP. However, this is not apparent in their published waveforms. Groll-Knapp et al. (1980) report a slow premotor negativity and an early *positivity* on the surface of parietal and frontopolar cortex. However, their figure shows, instead, negative potentials in these areas. The subcortical recordings are more consistent. Many human hippocampal and parahippocampal gyrus neurons increase firing before movements. In well-controlled cognitive tasks, the firing may begin 200–300 ms prior to a key-press indicating the response to a word presented 600–800 ms previously (Halgren et al., 1978; Heit et al., in press). Hippocampal firing may increase up to 5 s prior to a spontaneous key-press (Halgren, in preparation). This is consistent with the strikingly increased firing of many rat hippocampal neurons, as well as large field potentials (θ rhythm, or rhythmic slow activity) immediately preceding and during a certain class of movements (O'Keefe and Nadel, 1978; Ranck, 1973; Vanderwolf et al., 1975; Buzsaki et al., 1983). These movements roughly correspond to what is termed "voluntary" in humans. Unit activity has also been found in the human n. reticularis thalami to precede the EMG by 100–700 ms in voluntary movements to verbal command (Raeva, 1986). Thalamic field potentials also occur during the RP. Groll-Knapp et al. (1980) reported these to be negative and to be especially large in the "nonspecific" nuclei (dorsalis medialis, center median). In sum, these human studies support the possibility of widespread RP generators, but systematic studies of cortical areas are lacking.

Indirect evidence in humans for RP generators outside the precentral cortex may be found in the effects of lesions on the RP.

First, lesions in humans often greatly reduce the RP without producing the pyramidal signs or clear weakness that would be expected were the precentral cortex involved (Shibasaki, 1975). Decreased RPs are common in many neurological diseases, especially Parkinson's (Deecke et al., 1977). Conversely, DOPA increases the early RP as well as its late peak (Dick et al., 1987). Small vascular or stereotaxic lesions of the motor thalamus may abolish the RP, sometimes temporarily, consistent with involvement of an ascending neuromodulatory system in triggering the RP. Deecke and Kornhuber (1978) pointed out that the striking decrease in the RP in Parkinson's patients is confined to the scalp overlying precentral cortex, with the vertex and anterior vertex RP nearly normal. Since these sites overlie the SMC, this finding suggests that the SMC also generates the RP. A role of the SMC in the preparation for and planning of voluntary movements (Wise, 1984) is supported by the akinetic mutism that may result from SMC lesions (Laplane et al. 1977) and by the increased SMC blood flow during the execution or even the planning of voluntary movements (Roland, 1985; Orgogozo and Larsen, 1979). The scalp topography of premovement potentials in humans (Goldberg et al., 1984) and primates (Hashimoto et al., 1981) also suggests that SMC activity precedes that in the precentral gyrus. Deecke et al. (1985) propose, on the basis of RP recordings in a wide variety of tasks, that the SMC is activated prior to voluntary movements of all kinds, regardless of whether they are executed by primary motor cortex or by other brain areas. The premotor cortex on the lateral surface of the frontal lobe (area 6) may also be activated during the preparation to move, when it plays a role that is unknown, but apparently distinct from that of the SMC (Goldberg, 1985; Wise, 1984).

4.6. Cognitive Correlates—RP

Even with simple movements, it has been found that the RP varies substantially with cognitive factors. For example, the amplitude of the NS (like subsequent components) increases with increased force of contractions (Wilke and Lansing, 1973; Kutas and Donchin, 1974), whereas a RP of maximum amplitude can be observed to the voluntary contraction of a single motor unit (Kato and Tanji, 1972). Similarly, the RP is much larger prior to movements that are self-initiated than prior to those that are triggered by a sensory stimulus (Kurtzberg and Vaughan, 1982; Kutas and

Donchin, 1980; Thickbroom et al., 1985b). RPs to self-initiated movements are larger if instructions emphasize spontaneity over planning (Libet et al., 1982). These data have led some authors to suggest that the RP may reflect brain processes underlying volition (Goldberg, 1985; Eccles, 1982). However, Libet et al.'s (1983a,b) data suggests that the RP begins long before the beginning of the subjective experience of wanting to move. In any case, it appears that when the patient expects the consequence of his movement to be more rewarding—or risky or interesting—a larger RP may be seen (Hink et al., 1982; McAdam and Seales, 1969; Becker et al., 1973). However, a recent abstract by Empson (1986) suggests that some of these effects might be related to response force, rather than to more "cognitive" variables. It should be remembered that pyramidal tract neurons begin firing about 500 ms before a movement *(see above)* and that diffuse motor modulation is known to occur prior to voluntary movements. The monosynaptic tendon reflex may be increased as much as 500 ms prior to movement onset (Bonnet 1981), and the EMG may decrease 90–150 ms prior to movement onset (Yabe et al., 1981).

The power of sensory-triggered EPs to reveal brain processes during cognition has been greatly enhanced as the inherent complexity of the sensory stimulus has been increased (e.g., *see* section 5.2 on N400). It seems likely that new premovement EP components related to cognition will also be revealed when the EPs preceding more complex movements can also be examined. The RP preceding a complex key-pressing sequence changes systematically during learning (Taylor, 1978). RPs preceding the most obvious movements with intrinsic meaning, speech, were noted above to be severely contaminated with extracerebral artifacts (Szirtes and Vaughan, 1977). However, Jung et al. (1982) found substantial RPs that preceded writing by 1–3 sec. In a recent study by Deecke et al. (1987), the subjects's pressing of a pen on a writing surface triggered a complex stimulus to be copied by the subject. On separate trials, the stimulus, in the left or right visual field, was a word or a drawing, and the pen was held in the left or right hand. Distinct scalp topographies related to all three task factors were observed.

In a previous study, Deecke et al. (1984) studied the RP preceding pen pressure that started a visual tracking task. The RP was largest over the right parietal lobe, suggesting that it might reflect a "directed attention potential" separable from the left frontocentral potential reflecting preparation to move. A correlation with attentive processes is also suggested by the observation that, when a stimulus evoked by a movement is clearly perceived, the RP preceding that movement tends to be larger (McAdam and Rubin, 1971).

During the actual tracking of movements, a sustained widespread negativity, punctuated by apparent P3s was observed (Deecke et al., 1984). Sustained negativities have also been found during sustained ramp movements (Grunewald-Zuberbier and Grunewald, 1978). This is similar to what is observed in most subjects while writing words to dictation, although in some subjects a sustained positivity is instead consistently observed (Jung et al., 1982). The negative potentials during mirror tracing were larger than those during direct tracing, and were larger to learned than unlearned movements, especially over the frontal lobes (Lang et al., 1984, 1987; Schreiber et al. 1983). In a variety of verbal writing tasks, regardless of the hand used, the left central area was more negative than the right in all of the right-handed subjects studied by Jung et al. (1984). Conversely, Desmedt (1977b) observed a right parietal negativity during tactile exploration of a (nonverbally) patterned surface. Although these studies are preliminary, they suggest that complex hand movements may elicit EPs related to cognition without unacceptable extracerebral artifacts.

Taken as a whole, these studies of potentials preceding complex movements suggest that the RP may actually represent the sum of various generators, whose location depends upon the type of processing leading to the movement (cf Rolls, 1983; Kornhuber, 1984). An intriguing possibility is that these components *preceding* complex movements are the same as the various processing negativities that *follow* complex stimuli (*see* section 5). However, the possibility that small systematic differences in extracerebral generators (tongue and retina) may contribute to these potentials, especially *during* the movement, has not been eliminated.

The RP is also evoked prior to a stimulus that releases a movement, when that stimulus has been cued 1–10s previously by a warning stimulus. In this situation, the RP is continuous with the other EP components constituting the contingent negative variation (or CNV). The generators and behavioral correlates of the CNV are discussed below (section 5.6.).

5. Cognitive EPs

5.1. Methods and Components

Since the mid-1960s, EPs have been recorded across a wide variety of time-locked cognitive tasks. Cognitive processing is synchronized across individual trials by initiating each trial with the brief exposure of a stimulus and requiring a rapid response according to instructions given to the subject prior to the task. Consequently, cognitive studies are most complete for stimuli that can be presented in a single brief exposure (e.g., words rather than stories), and for responses that are regular and rapid (e.g., recognition rather than recall). This limitation is not shared by probe-evoked potentials (reviewed by Papanicolaou and Johnstone, 1984, but not here). In this technique, EPs to irrelevant sensory stimuli are recorded during the performance of various cognitive tasks, under the assumption that the probe EPs will indirectly reflect the allocation of processing resources to the primary task.

Within the rather broad constraints of the stimulus–evaluation–response format, cognitive processing is accompanied by an initially modality-specific processing negativity that becomes widespread, followed by an equally diffuse closure positivity. Division of this sequence into components is difficult and controversial, because the components overlap each other very substantially in latency, topography, and response to task manipulations. The following division is broadly consistent with several recent reviews (Donchin et al., 1978; Ritter et al., 1983; Naatanen and Gaillard, 1983; Picton and Stuss, 1980; Renault, 1983), but nonetheless should not be considered as anything more than tentative.

In general, a task-relevant cognitive stimulus will first evoke a series of early peaks that are sensitive to sensory parameters and gross state of consciousness, but not to cognitive variables. Overlapping with and extending beyond the later sensory peaks are a series of "processing negativities" including the Nd, NA, N2, mismatch negativity, and N4 components (see Naatanen and Picton, 1986; Pritchard et al., in press; Ritter et al., 1984). Aspects of stimuli that can be rapidly detected (such as location in space) tend to be associated with the shorter-latency negativities. The NA is related to perceptual processing of a stimulus, regardless of its rarity (Ritter et al., 1982, 1983). The mismatch negativity is evoked by a stimulus that does not match preceding stimuli on simple sensory characteristics, regardless of whether that stimulus is attended or detected (Naatanen and Gaillard, 1983; Naatanen et al., 1982). The N2b is most easily evoked by attended events that are rare within the context of the task, including stimuli of any modality, stimulus omissions, and relevant semantic categories (e.g., names) (Naatanen and Gaillard, 1983; Picton and Stuss, 1980; Renault, 1983). The longest-latency processing negativity—the N4—is evoked by task-relevant words, faces, and meaningful line drawings (Kutas and Van Petten, 1987; Halgren and Smith, 1987; Bentin et al., 1985; Stuss et al., 1983; Smith and Halgren, 1987a,b).

These negativities are usually followed by a positivity associated with cognitive closure, and termed the P3, P300, or LPC ("late positive component") (Hillyard and Kutas, 1983; Hillyard and Picton, 1988; Picton and Stuss, 1980). Like the N2b described above, the P3 is associated with infrequent target stimuli in simple tasks. Indeed, the N2b–P3a usually occur together, perhaps with a preceding P165. The N2b–P3a is maximal at Cz or Fz. Overlapping with the P3a, but at somewhat longer latency, is the P3b component, maximal at Pz (Naatanen and Gaillard, 1983; Squires et al. 1975). In that the N2b–P3a and the P3b have very similar task correlates, they usually can be distinguished only by analyzing the scalp topography of EPs on single trials within a given subject (Renault, 1983) or across subjects on the same task (Naatanen et al., 1982; Squires et al., 1975: Courchesne et al., 1975). In these situations, the N2b–P3a complex appears to be substantially larger to nontarget stimuli that are, nonetheless, definitely distinct from the background, frequent stimuli. For example, when a subject is instructed to read a book and ignore a stream of tones, rare tones in the stream will still sometimes evoke an N2b–P3a (Squires et al., 1975). Similarly, in a visual oddball task, the stream of repeated rare (counted) and frequent slides were sometimes interrupted by a novel strange slide (Courchesne et al., 1975). Although the subject was instructed to ignore the novel slides, they still evoked a large, more frontal P3. Similar components are seen following saccades that terminate with word fixation (Marton et al., 1985 a,b). Like the processing negativity, the P3 latency varies across tasks, apparently because the duration of stimulus identification processes antecedent to cognitive closure varies with stimulus complexity (Kutas et al., 1977). Other cognitive components may be seen prior to an isolated voluntary movement (the readiness potential—section 4.6.), or between two stimuli when the response to the second is related to the content or timing of the first (CNV—section 5.6).

In summary, the exact number of distinct processing negativities or of closure positivities is unclear. The voltage distribution over the scalp ("topography") for some earlier processing negativities are clearly distinct, suggesting modality-specific generators (Ritter et al., 1984). Similarly, two P3 subcomponents have been found that are evoked together, but to different degrees, across tasks, trials, and subjects. An earlier, more fronto-midline component appears to be relatively more prominent to nontarget, unexpected stimuli in easy tasks, whereas a later, more posterior, and lateral component predominates when complex stimuli are definitively processed (Stapleton et al., 1987b).

However, subtle differences in scalp topography are limited in their ability to distinguish depth components (Fig. 2). On the one hand, identical scalp topographies may result from very different depth generators (Wood, 1982). Conversely, distinct topographies in two situations may result from differing relative activations of two coactive generators, rather than from two totally distinct generators (e.g., Stapleton and Halgren, 1987). Statistical attempts to factor out the effects of different components at each latency have been problematic (Wood and McCarthy, 1984). However, direct brain recordings and, sometimes, MEG can resolve these ambiguities.

5.2. Cognitive Correlates of the N4

Cognitive correlates of the N4 (or N400) have been reviewed recently by Halgren and Smith (1987), Kutas and Van Petten (1987), and Rugg et al. (1986). In the initial studies of Kutas and Hillyard (1980a), the N4 was observed to the terminal word of sentences when that word was not expected, given the preceding words in the sentence; however, the N4 was not evoked if the terminal word was syntactically or orthographically incongruent with those preceding it (Kutas and Hillyard, 1980c, 1983). Conversely, an N4 was evoked by words that formed a meaningful ending, as long as they were unusual (i.e., in Garden Path Sentences, Kutas and Hillyard, 1984b). This gave rise to the hypothesis that the N4 is actually evoked by "semantic incongruity," a special case of the hypothesized cognitive correlate of the N2–P3 with incongruity in general (e.g., Donchin, 1981). However, subsequent studies have found that the N4 is evoked in many situations that do not appear to involve incongruity with the established context. The evoking stimulus can be individually presented words, whether printed, spoken, or signed (McCallum et al., 1984; Kutas et al., 1987; Domalski et al., submitted). Effective tasks include reading, recognizing, naming, categorizing, and rhyming. A negativity with the same latency, similar topography, and (when possible to test) identical task-correlates is evoked by drawings of meaningful objects and by photographs of faces (Barrett et al., 1988; Smith et al., 1986; Smith and Halgren, 1987a; Stuss et al., 1983). It is apparently necessary that the stimulus be intrinsically meaningful within a complex associative cognitive system: complex abstract sounds and pictures have not been found to evoke an N4. In some cases, the N4 is not evoked by words if the discrimination required by the task depends solely upon the physical features of the stimulus (Rugg et al., 1988; Rugg and Nagy, 1987). Thus, it appears that the N4 is evoked by any stimulus capable of activating a widespread cerebral associative network, within any task that requires or permits such activation.

Some authors (e.g., Kutas and Van Petten, 1987) feel that the slight topographical differences observed between N4s are sufficient to assert that the N4 evoked by meaningful pictures is different than the N4 evoked by words, or that the N4 evoked by sentence terminal words is different from that evoked by isolated words in various semantic tasks. However, we have not observed differences in the intracranial voltage topography of the N4s evoked by various tasks (Smith et al., 1986). Furthermore, the scalp differences between these N4s are too small to constitute convincing evidence for substantially distinct generators, with one exception. This is between the N4s evoked by auditorily vs visually presented words within the same task (Domalski et al., submitted). Thus, it appears that there is a generic N4, with the precise neural substrate differing mainly in the modality of presentation.

The N4 and the P3 that follows it are exquisitely sensitive to the ease with which the stimulus is integrated into the current cognitive context. "Ease" in this case is operationally defined as being greater if a memory trace (remote, recent, or immediate) for that stimulus-contextual gestalt already exists. It appears that the N4 is emitted after an initial evaluation indicates that the stimulus belongs to a meaningful class (e.g. words, objects, or people), and that it terminates when that stimulus is integrated with the current context or when the attempt at integration fails. The existence of this pre-N4 screening for potential meaningfulness is suggested both by the N4's latency and by the special circumstances under which an N4 can be evoked by meaningless stimuli (Smith and Halgren, 1987b). The latency of the N4, about 250 ms, is about equal to the duration of saccadic eye fixations during reading. Although the postsaccade N4 has a shorter latency than the stimulus-evoked N4, and some preliminary processing of words occurs before they are fixated, this still suggests that perceptual identification of the stimulus precedes the N4 (Just and Carpenter, 1980; 1987). Letter-strings that cannot be pronounced evoke no N4. Thus, EPs evoked by nonpronounceable letter-strings diverge from EPs evoked by words at a latency of about 250 ms. This again suggests that some word-specific perceptual analysis has been completed by this time. However, *pronounceable* nonword letter-strings *do* evoke a large N4. Thus, this stage of perceptual identification preceding entry into the N4-type associative activation appears not to involve analysis for meaning, but only for the potential for meaning. In this sense, the face of an unknown person is similar to a word with an unknown referent. Electrophysiologically, it appears that the general meaning of a word is accessed at the same time that it is integrated with the current cognitive environment; that is, the effects of semantic and episodic context appear to operate on the same EP component—the N4.

In its purest form, the influence of remote lexical memory is apparent in the smaller N4 evoked by commonly used English words as compared to uncommon words (Smith and Halgren, 1987b). Remote semantic memory also influences the N4; if the terminal word in a sentence makes that sentence false, then a larger N4 will be evoked than if the sentence were true (Fischler et al., 1984). The N4 to semantically incongruous words at the ends of sentences is another example of this effect. The N4 to a target word is also decreased if it is preceded by words of the same category (Polich et al., 1983) or by a synonym (Bentin et al., 1985). These experiments illustrate the effects of the current context (Primary Memory). The strongest modulatory effects on the N4 are induced by contextual repetition in recent memory. Repetition of a word or face induces a large decrease of the N4, even if the repetition is not task-relevant (Halgren and Smith, 1987). The imposition of a delay of up to a minute or of distracting stimuli, between initial and subsequent presentation of the target word does not appreciably reduce the effect. The memory trace underlying this effect is not modality-specific: the repetition-induced N4 decrease persists when words are learned in one modality and tested in another (Domalski et al., submitted). However, the stimulus must be meaningful; delayed repetition of a pronounceable nonword has no effect on the size of the N4 it evokes (Smith and Halgren, 1987b).

5.3. Cognitive Correlates of the P3

Cognitive correlates of the P3 (or P300) have been reviewed many times (e.g., Donchin, 1981; Donchin et al., 1978; Pritchard, 1981; Rosler et al., 1986). The P3 is evoked by simple or complex attended stimuli in the auditory, visual, or somatosensory modalities. If the stimuli are simple and occurring at a rapid rate, then the P3 will occur at the time when a stimulus was expected, but did not occur. If the stimuli are complex and well-known, or if they are simple but occurring at slow rate (less than .3/s), then a P3 will occur to every stimulus. However, if the stimuli are simple, rapidly presented, and belong to two task-relevant categories, then stimuli belonging to the less frequently occurring category (termed "rare") will evoke a much bigger P3 than the stimuli belonging to the other category. Most of this effect results from sequence: to a first approximation, a rare tone will evoke a large P3 if and only if it is preceded by a series of frequency tones. Although the P3 is evoked in a large variety of tasks, the "auditory oddball" task has become a de facto standard, because its simplicity and reliability render it useful for clinical and developmental studies as well as for psychological analysis. The relation of the P3 to rarity within context, in the auditory oddball and related tasks, has led to hypothesized correlations of the P3 with "context updating" (Donchin and Coles, 1988) and "context closure" (Verleger, 1988).

An extension of the context-updating hypothesis posits that the P3 represents the updating of internal models of the external environment. The "memory-updating" hypothesis has been held to be generally consistent with the P3's variation across conditions in cognitive tasks that do not specifically probe memory (Donchin, 1981). That is, the P3 is generally larger in task situations that might be expected to be accompanied by memory updating, for instance, when a less-frequent stimulus follows a series of identical stimuli. However, as noted above, these studies have in most cases used very simple stimuli (e.g., tones) that are already well-learned and have little information content. Recently, several studies have used word-learning tasks to test specifically a related hypothesis. This "trace-formation hypothesis" posits that the amplitude of the P3 evoked by a stimulus reflects the strength of the memory trace formed at that time. These studies have compared the P3 evoked at initial exposure to words that either were, or were not, subsequently remembered. Indeed, they have found that under appropriate conditions words that are subsequently recalled (Karis et al., 1984; Paller et al., 1987) or recognized (Sanquist et al., 1980; Neville et al., 1986) evoke a larger-amplitude P3 on their initial input presentation than do words that are not subsequently remembered.

A stronger and more consistent effect on both the processing negativity N4 and the contextual closure P3 are their differences to repeated vs nonrepeated words in a recent memory recognition task. The N4 to a particular word is large when that word is first presented, and then declines when it is repeated. Conceivably, the decreased N4 could reflect either of two processes that have been hypothesized to underlie behavioral recognition performance: processing facilitation or retrieval of episodic context (Jacoby, 1983; Mandler, 1980). However, since this repetition-induced N4 decline is abolished by left anterior temporal lobe removal, and this removal impairs behavioral indices of contextual retrieval but not of processing facilitation, it follows that the N4 decline also probably represents contextual retrieval, rather than processing facilitation (Smith and Halgren, 1988a). Thus, the N4 appears to represent a modulation of medial temporal lobe (MTL) and probably associations cortex neurons that is large during trace formation and small during memory retrieval. Since the MTL N4 occurs in a structure that is necessary for cognitive memory, and at a time when that structure is making its contribution, it is likely that it represents an important process in this form of plasticity. That this potential is elicited in both semantic and episodic memory tasks indicates that some components of neural activity are common to these two types of tasks.

The P3 represents a later stage in cognitive processing with a less clear relation to memory formation and retrieval. Individuals can be found that in particular situations may exhibit larger P3s to words that are subsequently retrieved. However, this effect is not at all general—the size of the P3 at word input can be dissociated from its subsequent retrievability. A more robust finding is the larger P3 to recognized repeated words. This P3 is abolished by left anterior temporal lobe removal, suggesting that it reflects contextual retrieval (Halgren and Smith, 1987).

5.4. Generation of the P3

5.4.1. Component Identification

This subject has been reviewed previously (Wood et al., 1981; Halgren et al., 1982, 1983, 1986). Related reviews have discussed the generation of the P3 based on scalp evidence (Desmedt and Debecker, 1979; Desmedt, 1981; Simson et al., 1977a,b). Possible animal homologues of the P3 have been suggested (Arthur and Starr, 1984; Halgren et al., 1982; Buchwald and Squires, 1982; Buchwald, 1987; Wilder et al., 1981; Neville and Foote, 1984; Voorn et al., 1987) but will not be reviewed here. Generation of the P3 will be discussed in some detail, as an example of the issues and evidence that this analysis involves.

Before proceeding further, a note on terminology is important. We will use the term "scalp P3" to refer to the EP component that is positive over much of the scalp, but maximal in the midline at Cz or Pz (or occasionally Fz). The scalp P3 latency to peak is in the range of 240–700 ms, depending on the subject and task. EP components that occur in depth structures during the same behavioral situations and latency range as the scalp P3 will be referred to as the (structure) P3, even though their polarity may be negative. By this criterion, an MTL P3 occurs in many task situations in which the scalp P3 has been shown to occur (Stapleton and Halgren, 1987; McCarthy et al., 1989), including: (1) to a rare target tone in either the auditory, visual, or somaesthetic modality (Halgren et al., 1980; McCarthy and Wood, 1987; Squires et al., 1983); (2) to a rare nontarget if that tone belongs to a task-relevant category distinct from the preceding series of tones (Halgren et al., 1983); (3) to the omission of a tone from a series of tones presented at short, regular intervals; and (4) to visually presented male names when they were intermingled with more frequent female names (Wood et al., 1981; McCarthy and Wood, 1987).

The MTL EPs evoked by these tasks actually contain at least three components, distinguishable on the basis of their distinct (but overlapping) latency ranges, task correlates, and relative amplitudes across patients and sites (Stapleton and Halgren, 1987).

The earliest component is a fairly sharp negativity, peaking about 50 ms before the surface N2 recorded from the same patients and tasks. This MTL N2 is often most prominent in the amygdala, but negative potentials with very similar latencies and task correlates can be observed throughout the MTL. Positive MTL potentials with this latency are also observed, but only rarely. The next MTL component is also the largest. It follows the surface P3 by an average of 30 ms, and is termed the MTL P3. This component is usually largest in the anterior hippocampus and is negative there. In other MTL structures, at about the same latency, a positive potential with similar task correlates is recorded. A further component follows the MTL P3, but it has not yet been systematically studied. The MTL N2 is clearly smaller than the MTL P3 in the MTL and surrounding structures. However, as the surface is approached, the MTL P3 declines in amplitude more rapidly, often resulting in the MTL N2 being larger in amplitude than the MTL P3 at more superficial depth sites.

In their task correlates, both MTL N2 and MTL P3 bear a general resemblance to all the scalp components as defined above, but an exact correspondence to none. The strong enhancement of the MTL N2 to attended, as compared to ignored, rare tones distinguishes it from scalp N2 components. The MTL P3 is also much bigger to attended tones, suggesting that it corresponds to P3b. However, unlike P3b, the MTL P3 is about equal to rare target, as compared to rare distractor, tones. This lack of correspondence between the MTL P3 and subcomponents of the surface P3 might be partly owing to the MTL P3 being composed of subcomponents itself. In some but not all patients, two peaks are clearly apparent in the MTL P3, one preceding and one following the surface P3.

5.4.2. Local Generation

Conceivably, volume conduction from a distant generator could account for the MTL P3 (just as volume conduction accounts for the scalp P3). However, several sources of evidence strongly suggest that the MTL P3 is actually generated by activation of synapses lying within the MTL.

Many MTL neurons change their firing rate in the same task conditions and latency range as the MTL P3 (Halgren et al., 1983; Halgren et al., 1980). Clearly, synapses on MTL neurons must have been active to produce these firing-rate changes. The hippocampus is organized in such a manner that synaptic activation is likely to result in field potentials. Activation of an excitatory synapse on the distal part of the pyramidal cell's apical dendrite results in a net extracellular flow of positive ions from the soma toward the activated synapse (*see* Fig. 3B). Hippocampal (HC) pyramidal cell somata lie in a single layer and send their apical shafts in the same direction. Different synaptic pathways terminate onto these shafts in distinct layers (Lorente de No, 1934; Walaas, 1983). Consequently, the current-flows induced by activation of the individual synapses in a particular pathway will summate. The net current-flow results in a grossly recordable field potential, negative in the region of the active synapses and positive in the region of the pyramidal cell bodies. Activation of inhibitory synapses on the pyramidal somata may cause negative ions to flow from the apical dendrites, resulting ultimately in a similar extracellular field potential. Laminar analyses of HC field potentials evoked by the activation of known pathways in the animal HC have yielded voltage distributions consistent with these theoretical predictions (Leung, 1979; Andersen et al., 1971; Andersen et al., 1964; Spencer and Kandel, 1962).

In recordings from multiple contacts, the MTL P3 often is largest (approximately 200 μV) and negative medially in the HC, polarity-inverts at about the point where the lateral edge of the HC is estimated to lie, and declines in amplitude as the lateral temporal neocortex is approached (Stapleton and Halgren, 1987). In multiple-contact electrodes approaching the MTL from above (entering from the prefrontal neocortex) or from behind (entering from occipitoparietal neocortex), the depth P3 is sometimes observed to be first positive and then negative in the region of the MTL, and finally positive again as the probe passes beyond (Wood et al., 1981). MTL P3 topography and correlated unit activity thus appear consistent with local generation of the MTL P3, possibly by apical excitatory and/or somatic inhibitory synapses (cf, McCarthy et al., 1989). Those patients who receive MTL depth electrodes suffer from complex partial seizures, and consequently have extensive MTL scarring (Brown, 1973; Margerison and Corsellis, 1966). In our observations of 35 patients, 14 had no clear MTL P3 (Halgren et al., 1983; Squires et al., 1983). In a small number of patients, the MTL P3 is severely depressed on one side only (Squires et al., 1983). This is also consistent with local generation, inasmuch as unilateral MTL scarring is not uncommon in complex partial epilepsy (Margerison and Corsellis, 1966). Indeed, MTL P3 amplitude is correlated with the presence of an epileptic focus (Meador et al., 1989), and the histologically determined loss of hippocampal neurons (Wood et al., 1988). However, this observation clearly rules out a thalamic generator for the MTL P3, because a thalamic generator would conduct approximately equally to both MTLs.

Extracerebral mapping of evoked magnetic fields correlated with the scalp P3 have yielded mixed results. On the one hand, Okada and colleagues (Okada et al., 1983) found an apparent endogenous magnetic field generator in the MTL in a visual oddball task. In contrast, Richer and colleagues (Richer et al., 1983) found apparent endogenous magnetic field generators in the auditory association cortex during an auditory oddball task and in the visual association cortex in the visual oddball task.

5.4.3. Propagation to Surface

Taken as a whole, the evidence for local generation of the P3 recorded in the MTL is very strong. Whether or not this MTL P3 actually volume conducts to the surface to contribute substantially to the scalp P3 is, however, still unclear. That is, in the terminology of Fig. 3a, it is unclear whether the MTL P3 is an occult generator or a propagating generator.

If the scalp P3 is generated completely (or in part) by the MTL, then it should be eliminated (or reduced) by MTL lesions. Consistent with this possibility, the size of the P3 recorded at the surface (Fz/Cz) is, across patients, highly correlated with that recorded in the MTL (Halgren et al., 1986; Squires et al., 1983).

Most of one MTL is removed in anterior temporal lobectomy (ATL) for the treatment of epilepsy (Delgado-Escueta and Walsh, 1983). Neither left nor right ATL significantly affects the amplitude or scalp topography of the P3 evoked by rare, distractor, or omitted tones (Wood et al., 1982; Johnson and Fedio, 1986; Stapleton et al., 1987a). In contrast, left ATL (in right-handed subjects) *does* affect the P3 evoked by repeated words in a recent memory recognition task (Smith and Halgren, 1988a). Behavioral discrimination was also affected by left ATL, but only slightly, whereas the P3 in this task was completely abolished. Right ATL had no significant effect on the P3 or behavior.

These results would be expected if the same P3 generator were active in all tasks, with the left ATL being necessary to activate that generator in the recognition task. That is (in the terminology of Fig. 3A), it is possible that the antecedent structure varies among tasks, whereas the propagating structure is constant and lies outside the ATL (Fig. 4). This possibility is supported by the very similar MTL topographies of the P3s evoked to infrequent tones and to repeated words (Smith et al., 1986). Alternatively, P3 generators may differ across tasks, with the left ATL containing the P3 generator for repeated words, but not for infrequent tones.

Finally, it should be noted that the lack of significant changes in scalp topography or amplitude of the infrequent-tone P3 after ATL removal does not prove that the MTL makes *no* contribution to this potential. The MTL lies only about 25 mm from the midline (total head diameter, about 170 mm [Talairach et al., 1967]), and the orientation of the MTL generator is unknown. Therefore, it is unclear how much scalp P3 asymmetry would have been expected from MTL removal, even if the scalp P3 were generated in the MTL. If the equivalent MTL dipole pointed toward the opposite scalp, then unilateral removal of an MTL generator could conceivably produce a larger scalp P3 on the side of removal. It is also difficult to estimate the effects of the skull defect produced by the neurosurgeon in order to gain access to the temporal lobe. The skull has much lower conductance than the brain and scalp, and thus provides a barrier to the flow of current from an intracerebral generator to the scalp (Wood, 1982). By providing a preferential path for current flow, a skull defect can affect potentials over the entire scalp (Nunez, 1981). For example, suppose that one MTL is removed, leaving a vertically oriented dipole in the contralateral MTL. Then current from the remaining dipole might shunt through the contralateral skull defect, drawing current away from the ipsilateral scalp.

Most of the patients in a recent study by Syndulko and coworkers (Syndulko et al., 1984) had bilateral brain damage and no skull defect. However, because these patients were selected on the basis of clinically severe global amnesia, not all of them could be expected to have damaged MTL (Squire, 1982). Nonetheless, it is of interest that all the patients in this study showed a P3 potential in the auditory oddball task, albeit often of decreased amplitude and increased latency. Furthermore, confirmed bilateral MTL removal in monkeys does not markedly influence the late surface positivity evoked by rare stimuli in an oddball task (Paller et al., 1984).

Thus, studies have consistently found that unilateral MTL damage does not markedly alter the infrequent-tone P3 topography in humans and that bilateral MTL damage does not eliminate this scalp P3 in humans or the apparently homologous potential in monkeys. Possible confounding influences, especially of skull defects, prevent us from concluding that the MTL makes no contribution to this scalp P3. However, these studies clearly imply that at least part of the surface P3 must be generated outside the MTL.

Limited depth recording studies have begun to localize these additional P3 generators. The depth P3 in the middle temporal gyrus (Stapleton and Halgren, 1987) or inferior parietal/superior occipital cortex (Wood et al., 1981; Smith et al., 1988) appears to be positive and smaller than that in the MTL. Instances of negative P3 have been recorded in the thalamus (Goff et al., 1980; Groll-Knapp et al., 1980; Velasco, personal communication; Yingling and Hosobuchi, 1984), supplementary motor and orbitofrontal cortices (Smith et al., 1988; submitted), and possibly on the medial surface of the parietal lobe (Prim et al., 1983). However, large amplitude and steep voltage gradients in these structures have not been reported. In general, further confirmation that these potentials correspond to the scalp P3 across tasks is required.

Recently, Wood and McCarthy (Wood and McCarthy, 1985; McCarthy and Wood, 1987) have reported evidence of locally generated potentials in the P3 range for infrequent tones at many, but not all, frontal cortex recording sites. Although smaller than the MTL P3, this frontal P3 is probably more widely distributed and is certainly closer to the scalp, and thus may make a substantial contribution to the scalp P3 (cf Klee and Rall, 1977). However, the P3 has been found to be fairly normal in patients with frontal lobe lesions (Knight, 1984). These lesions did affect the change of the P3 in response to novel stimuli. Because the P3 was affected bilaterally by unilateral lesions, Knight (Knight, 1984) concluded that the frontal lobe functioned in the detection of and response to novelty, rather than as a generator of P3 itself (i.e., as an "antecedent structure" in the terminology of Figs. 3A and 4). Similarly, Knight (in press) found that lesions in the temporoparietal junction decreased the P3 to infrequent tones. Again, unilateral lesions produced a bilaterally symmetrical decrease, suggesting that the temporoparietal cortex functions as an antecedent structure to the P3 generator in this task.

The most straightforward method for evaluating whether or not the MTL P3 propagates to the scalp is to recreate within the MTL the same voltage distribution as is observed during the MTL

P3 and to determine whether or not potentials can then be recorded from the scalp. To reproduce the MTL voltage distribution exactly using implanted electrodes would require thousands of stimulation sites in as yet unknown locations. Smith and coworkers (Smith et al., 1983), using only two MTL electrodes found that interelectrode currents resulted in a potential that attenuated by a factor of about 10 or 11 to 1 when recorded from the scalp over the temporal lobe, rather than from the amygdala. Inasmuch as this is actually less attenuation than is often seen between the P3s recorded at these sites, this study indicates that the MTL P3 is the right order of magnitude to propagate to the scalp.

Another approach is to look for physiological situations that reproduce the MTL voltage distribution found in the MTL during the P3, but that are unlikely to involve structures outside the MTL. Focal epileptiform MTL spikes in humans are usually followed by a stereotyped slow wave lasting 300–600 ms, also localized to the MTL (Altafullah et al., 1986). The MTL voltage topography of this typical slow wave (TSW) was essentially identical in polarity and relative amplitude to that of the MTL P3, suggesting that the two are generated by synaptic activation of the same MTL neurons. Simultaneous unit recording indicated that, like the slow waves following interictal hippocampal EEG spikes in animal models of epilepsy (Spencer and Kandel, 1969), the TSW probably represents a prolonged IPSP. Thus, these results are consistent with the P3 representing inhibitory synapses on hippocampal pyramidal cell somata (but *see* Fig. 3B). If we assume that the TSW has essentially the same MTL voltage distribution as the MTL P3, then the TSW should volume conduct to the scalp with the same surface topography, and with the same amount of attenuation, as the MTL P3. In fact, a positive potential was reliably recorded at the vertex during the TSW, presumably representing passive volume conduction of the TSW to the scalp. However, the P3 attenuated about one-half as much from MTL to vertex as the TSW attenuates between identical sites, implying that the scalp P3 receives substantial contributions from both MTL and extra-MTL generators. Extra-MTL generators are also suggested by recordings from multicontact electrodes passing from the lateral temporal neocortex to the hippocampus. In these recordings, the positivity during the MTL P3 does not drop off as rapidly at the lateral cortical contacts as it does for the TSW.

5.5. Generation of the N4

In addition to the endogenous components associated with the P3 (N2b–P3a–P3b–SW), recent evidence suggests that a potential corresponding to the scalp N4 is also generated in the human MTL (Smith et al., 1986). The scalp N4 is evoked at a latency-to-peak of about 400 ms by tasks requiring associative activation related to semantic meaning, such as deciding whether or not a string of letters is a word or finding the word portrayed by a line drawing *(see above)*. In these tasks, a (usually negative) potential component is also evoked in the MTL, with latency, morphology, and task correlates similar to those of the scalp N4. This same component was also reliably elicited during verbal tasks requiring secondary memory for their performance, when it decreased in amplitude to repeated items during memory testing. In some recordings, the MTL N4 was very large (up to 300 µV), reversed polarity over short distances in the hippocampus and parahippo-campal gyrus, and attenuated in amplitude at more lateral recording sites. The memory task also evoked an MTL P3 following the N4 and increasing in amplitude to repeated words. The MTL N4 and P3 had clearly distinct depth distributions. Thus, the MTL N4 component observed in these tasks is probably of local origin, but generated by different synapses from those involved with the MTL P3.

Like the P3, the amplitude of the scalp N4 is not significantly decreased by unilateral ATL that removes the MTL (Smith and Halgren, 1989). Thus, the N4 must have other generators in addition to the MTL. The N4 has a widespread scalp topography, suggesting generation in multiple lobes in both hemispheres (Kutas et al., 1988b).

However, recent studies have suggested that essential antecedent processing leading to the N4 to visually presented words is localized to the posterior left hemisphere (Halgren 1989). Lesions in this region to the angular gyrus have long been known to impair reading, with relatively preserved nonlinguistic visual processing and understanding of spoken language (Hecaen and Albert, 1978). Positron emission tomography (PET) demonstrates increased glucose metabolism in the left angular gyrus during visual word/nonword discrimination if the stimuli are only presented once, but not if they are repeated many times (Nenov et al., submitted). The nonrepeated stimuli also evoked a large N4, but the repeated did not. Furthermore, across subjects, the size of the N4 evoked by nonrepeated stimuli was significantly correlated with the metabolic activation of the left angular gyrus. Kutas et al. (1988a) studied the N4 evoked by visually presented sentence-terminal words in patients who had received a total section of the corpus collosum and anterior commissure. In patients with left-hemisphere language, an N4 was recorded over both hemispheres to words presented to the left hemisphere; words presented to the right hemisphere did not evoke an N4. These data suggest that when an area near the left angular gyrus recognizes a stimulus as a possible word, it activates a brainstem trigger that, in turn, leads to the generation of the N4 in multiple regions of both hemispheres.

5.6. Contingent Negative Variation

5.6.1. Methods and Components

A large negativity occurs over the scalp during the interval between two stimuli, when the first stimulus (S1) conditions the reaction to the second (S2) (Walter et al., 1964). It is now appreciated that the CNV is somewhat of a misnomer: the early CNV resembles the slow wave (SW) that can also be observed following isolated significant stimuli, and the late CNV resembles the RP seen before isolated movements—thus, the CNV is largely non-contingent (Rohrbaugh et al., 1976, 1978, 1980; Donchin et al., 1972; Sanquist et al., 1981; Loveless and Sanford, 1973; McCallum and Curry, 1981; Kutas and Donchin, 1977). It remains possible that a sustained negativity exists between S1 and S2, and the following discussion will attempt to focus on possible task correlates and generators of this sustained negativity. However, it must be borne in mind that in many experiments described below, the experimental design and/or the measurement techniques did not allow the various components to be definitely distinguished. *Components* of the CNV are best resolved when the S1–S2 interval is greater than 4 s. The early CNV is then seen to have a modality-specific distribution, being maximal frontocentrally to auditory stimuli and centro-parieto-occipitally to visual stimuli (Gaillard and Naatanen, 1976; Simson et al., 1977b). This early negativity probably corresponds to what is termed "SW," "SNWl," or "O wave" in other contexts, and peaks about 400–800 ms after S1 (Squires et al., 1975: Loveless, 1979; Ritter et al., 1984). The late CNV, occurring in the 1–3 s prior to S2, resembles the RP in topography, being maximal centrally, present frontally, and minimal parieto-occipitally (Cohen, 1969; Gaillard, 1980). Like the RPs that occur without a preceding stimulus, the late CNV has a topography that may vary with the task requirements (Kutas and Donchin, 1980). Specifically, a more focally central late CNV has been reported in tasks in which S1 induces a motor set released by S2 (Otto and Leifer, 1973; Syndulko and Lindsley, 1977; Vaughan, 1969, 1975). One study found a left frontal CNV when S2 provoked a verbal response (Zimmermann and Knott, 1974). However, no CNV assymmetry was observed in a study comparing the CNVs evoked during anticipation of words (requiring a verbal judgement) vs lines (requiring a spatial judgement) (Marsh and Thompson, 1973).

CNVs can also be observed in the S1–S2 interval when no overt motor response follows S2, for example, when S2 is a cue to think of a word related to S1 (Walter et al., 1964; Cohen and Walter, 1966) or when S2 provides feedback (Weinberg, 1973). In fact, CNVs are evoked in paradigms that require quite varied behavioral activity during the S1–S2 interval, including (1) holding a motor response in readiness, (2) preparing for a perceptual judgement, (3) anticipation of a positive or negative reinforcer, and (4) preparation to make a cognitive decision regarding S2, taking into account S1 (Hillyard, 1973). Across these tasks, it appears that the late CNV can be separated into a largely motor central component (comparable to the NS': *see* Table 3) and a largely cognitive frontal component (Jarvilehto and Fruhstorfer, 1970). Brunia and Damen (1988) have used task contingencies to separate the late CNV into a movement-preparation component (maximal contralateral to the moving hand), stimulus-anticipation component (maximal over the right hemisphere).

CNV amplitude is quite consistent for a given subject, task, and conditions, but is highly variable across many task and individual factors (Cohen, 1969; Harmony, 1984; Low et al., 1967; Naitoh et al., 1971; Walter, 1965, 1975). For example, the CNV has been reported to be larger when S2 is noxious, near threshold, or requires a relatively large muscular response (Irwin et al., 1966). The CNV is larger if S2 usually, but not always, follows S1 (>85% of the trials) (McCallum, 1979). It appears that the CNV is maximal at moderate levels of arousal (Low and Swift, 1971; Hamilton et al., 1973; Timsit-Berthier et al., 1977).

The elusive sustained potential in the S1–S2 interval, above and beyond the SW RP, may have some relationship to the "infra-slow potentials" or "sustained slow potentials" (Davis, 1965; McCallum, 1979). These may be slow oscillations (.1–.01 Hz: Alad-jalova, 1964; Gombi et al., 1973;), or they may be potential shifts, especially at the transition from sleep or drowsiness to alert waking (Caspers, 1974; Karrer et al., 1973; Rowland, 1968; Sano et al., 1967). These slow potentials are sometimes difficult to differentiate from electrodermal changes or sustained eye movements (Don-chin, 1973; Hillyard and Galambos, 1970; Picton and Hillyard, 1972). Indeed, skin potentials are a possible problem whenever the post-S1 recording epoch exceeds 2 s, and evoked eye movements may occur with a latency of about 250 ms. Intracranial recordings in rats establish that very large sustained potentials (100s of μV) are generated by the brain (Gerbrandt and Fowler, 1980). In humans, controls for electrodermal responses include abrading the skin until the electrode impedance is low (certainly less than 3 Kohm), using needle electrodes, or applying atropine topically (thus block-ing the innervation of the sweat glands).

The timing, task and individual correlates, and apparent fron-tal location of the CNV has led to it being assigned various hypothesized psychological roles, including: expectancy (Walter, 1964; Weinberg et al., 1976), motivation (Irwin et al., 1966; McA-dam and Seales, 1969), volition (McAdam et al., 1966), conation (Low et al., 1966), and arousal (McAdam, 1969). Such hypotheses are of limited utility until the neural process that the CNV represents is defined and the role of that process in the neural interactions leading to these psychological phenomena is ex-plicated.

5.6.2. Generators

(*See also* McSherry, 1973; Rebert, 1973b; Rockstroh et al., 1982).

Widespread field potentials are observed inside the human brain, simultaneous with the scalp CNV. Cortical surface record-ings are negative parietally, centrally, and frontally (Papakosto-poulos and Crow, 1976; Groll-Knapp et al., 1980). These cortical CNVs are similar in distribution to the P3 and RP, but they are not identical. In particular, the CNV is relatively more anterior than the P3 in most tasks. Subcortically, the CNV is positive in grey matter anterior to the thalamus, negative posterior to the thalamus, and small in the white matter (McCallum et al., 1973; McCallum and Papakostopoulos, 1976; Tsubokawa et al., 1976/1977; Tsubokawa and Moriyasu, 1978). Within the thalamus itself, negative CNVs are recorded in the midline nuclei (center median, dorsomedial, and medial subthalamic), whereas only transient potentials are present in motor nuclei (VA, VOP).

Widespread CNVs are also recorded in lower mammals, even rats (Pirch, 1980). In monkeys, cortical CNVs are found frontally, occipitally, and centrally (Donchin et al., 1971; Rebert, 1972; Stamm and Rosen, 1972; McSherry and Borda, 1973). This CNV is maximal in frontal cortex, *not* precentral. Subcortically, many structures anterior to the thalamus (e.g., caudate, preoptic, amygdala) are positive, whereas many posterior (e.g., posterior hypothalamus, mesencephalic reticular formation) are negative (Rebert, 1972, 1977, 1980). Within the monkey thalamus, midline nuclei are negative, whereas other nuclei (e.g., the pulvinar) show little.

In general, negative slow potentials are accompanied by increases in local unit firing rates (Caspers et al., 1979, 1980; Rebert, 1973a; Boyd et al., 1982; Skinner and Yingling, 1977). The behavioral correlates of prefrontal unit firing have been studied during the CNV in S1–S2–R paradigms, when the task is to compare S1 and S2 (delayed match to sample) or to delay the response to S1 until S2 appears (delayed response) (Boyd et al., 1982; Fuster, 1980; Fuster, 1973; Fuster and Alexander, 1973; Rosenkilde et al., 1981; Niki, 1974; Niki et al., 1972; Suzuki and Azuma, 1977). In a given area, different cells will fire during the original (cue) stimulus, the delay, the second (imperative) stimulus, and the postresponse reinforcement. During the delay, some cells will fire differentially according to different aspects of the cue, and others according to different aspects of the intended response (Fuster et al., 1982; Niki and Watanabe, 1976). The analogy between the dorsolateral frontal firing pattern and that seen in dorsomedial thalamus (Fuster and Alexander, 1973), inferotemporal cortex (Fuster and Jervey, 1981), hippocampal formation (Halgren, in preparation), supplementary motor cortex (Tanji et al., 1980), and the frontal eye fields (Bruce and Goldberg, 1985) is striking and suggests that similar mechanisms and functions are involved (cf Rockstroh et al., 1982)

Widespread neural generation of the CNV is further supported by the effects of lesions. Localized or even widespread cortical lesions in humans usually decrease the CNV recorded at the overlying scalp, but not grossly over normal cortex (McCallum and Cummins, 1973; Cohen, 1975; Zappoli et al., 1975, 1976), although widespread effects on the early CNV (possibly equivalent to the slow wave) have been reported after frontal lesions (Lutzenberger et al., 1980). In contrast, widespread effects on the CNV may occur after small diencephalic lesions (Low and Purves, 1975; Low 1979). Within the human thalamus itself, moderate decreases in CNV amplitude are seen after lesions of the centermedian, but not the ventralis lateralis nucleus (Tsubokawa et al., 1976/1977; Tsubokawa and Moriyasu, 1978). Conversely, the CNV is affected by stimulation of midline, but not motor, thalamic nuclei. Further evidence for a widespread generator activated by a diffuse system originating in the brainstem is the observation of bilateral CNVs after a unilateral warning cue in split-brain patients (Gazzaniga and Hillyard, 1973).

The system involved has been studied in lower mammals. It has long been known that direct electrical stimulation of the mesencephalic reticular formation evokes a diffuse negative cortical slow potential (Arduini et al., 1957; Arduini, 1958; Moruzzi, 1972; Skinner and Yingling, 1977). This system also appears to be necessary for the cortical negative slow potential evoked by novel or painful sensory stimuli. In contrast, inferior thalamic lesions in cats block the slow negativities evoked to conditioned S1s, but not those evoked by novel and/or painful stimuli (Skinner, 1971). This, and other evidence, led Skinner and Yingling (1976, 1977) to propose that the CNV is generated in each cortical region because of sustained excitatory influences from its associated thalamic nucleus (for example, from Medialis Dorsalis to the prefrontal cortex). These specific thalamic nuclei are inhibited by n. Reticularis thalami, which in turn is inhibited (they propose) by the mesencephalic reticular formation (MRF). MRF activation thus leads to cortical CNV by releasing afferent thalamic nuclei from inhibition by n. Reticularis thalami. Prefrontal control over the n. Reticularis is thus hypothesized to direct attention by activating the relevant thalamocortical circuits (as reflected in the CNV and sustained cellular firing) (Skinner and Yingling, 1977). Desmedt and Debecker (1979) also suggested that the CNV results from MRF activation under prefrontal control and reflects directed attention. They further suggest that the P3 results when this MRF drive is released at the time of cognitive closure, that is, when cognitive processing on a given topic is completed and the focus of attention is shifted. However, situations in which P3 occurs without a preceding CNV, and in which CNVs occur without a subsequent P3, have been described (Ruchkin and Sutton, 1979). Recent observations in rats suggest that inferior thalamic lesions may have abolished the CNV by injuring the cholinergic neurons in the nucleus basalis (Pirch et al., 1983, 1986; Rigdon and Pirch, 1986). Unilateral lesions of these cells produce a large decrease in the ipsilateral CNV, these cells respond differentially during the CNV, and blocking their effects at the cortex (with subdural atropine) decreases the ipsilateral CNV. It appears most likely that the CNV reflects a gross summation of neural activation within the neocortex. Various forms of neural activation result in increased extracellular potassium concentration. This concentration parallels slow-potential amplitude in several situations (Caspers et al., 1979, 1980). Glial cells are thought to help remove excess extracellular potassium from the vicinity of the active neurons. The extracellular potassium is passively and actively absorbed into the glia, where it diffuses internally. Through their gap junctions, glial cells are thought to form a synctium that has a major orientation perpendicular to the cortical surface and that extends into the white matter; this may result in an effective dipole current, with the negative pole in the grey matter and the positive pole in the white. Consistent with this view, the glial membrane potential has been found to closely reflect extracellular potassium concentration (Somjen, 1973, 1979), as well as local slow-potential magnitude (Karahashi and Goldring, 1966; Speckmann et al., 1978). As would be expected from its mainly passive role following neural activation, the glial depolarization may lag slightly after the slow-potential onset (Grossman et al., 1969, Grossman and Hampton, 1968, 1970). Further evidence for a glial role is the observation that slow potentials sometimes do not invert in polarity within the grey matter (e.g., Castellucci and Goldring, 1970). It must be emphasized that many processes at the synaptic and metabolic levels accompany the CNV (e.g., Bessom et al., 1970; Skinner and King, 1980; Skinner et al., 1978), and their role in CNV generation remains to be determined. However, the conclusion that the CNV probably reflects general neural activation suggests that it has been underutilized as a monitor of patterns of cortical activation in the S1–S2 interval.

5.7. Interpretation of Cognitive EPs

Much of the evidence regarding the intracerebral generation of the human scalp P3 is, as yet, preliminary. This question is further complicated by the evidence reviewed above for multiple endogenous components both at the scalp and in the MTL. Some or all of these MTL endogenous components are actually generated in the MTL. It is possible that inhibitory synapses on hippocampal pyramidal somata help generate the MTL P3. The MTL P3 probably volume conducts to the scalp, producing part, but not all, of the scalp P3. Thus far, the most likely candidate for an extra-MTL generator is the frontal lobe. The frontal P3 has somewhat shorter latency than the MTL P3, implying that its contribution to the scalp may be partly separated on the basis of latency. The possibility that the frontal and MTL P3s may also be differentiated across tasks is suggested by scalp topography, but lacks confirmation from direct depth recordings. Possible additional P3 generators could either be weak and widely distributed, or strong but in a structure as yet inadequately sampled by depth electrodes. Current evidence regarding the generation of the N4 is far less complete than for the P3. Again, however, the evidence is most consistent with generation partly within and partly outside the MTL. The CNV also appears to be diffusely generated.

We are thus presented with the notion that multiple cognitive EP components are generated within the MTL and, conversely, that multiple cerebral structures contribute to the generation of individual cognitive EP components. That is, it appears that, rather than representing activation of different structures, multiple cognitive EP components represent multiple sequential and overlapping modes of activation extending across structures (Fig. 10). What might appear to be a simple sequence from sensory to cognitive potentials, is sequential at most in indicating the onset of activation of specific, then secondary sensory, associational, and limbic structures, and only at the shortest latencies. By 100 ms after stimulus onset, all of these areas are involved, and remain involved for an extended period. This view is consistent with the diffuse and overlapping projections of several synaptic systems thought to influence large masses of forebrain neurons synchronously. For example, the basal forebrain (substantia innominata/septal) cholinergic neurons, the locus coerulus noradrenergic neurons, and the midbrain raphe serotonergic neurons all project to both the hippocampus and neocortex in lower mammals (Walaas, 1983; Jones and Moore, 1977; Fuxe and Jonsson, 1974). These quantitatively small projections from brainstem nuclei have a powerful influence on the EEG (Vanderwolf, 1975; Vanderwolf and Baker,

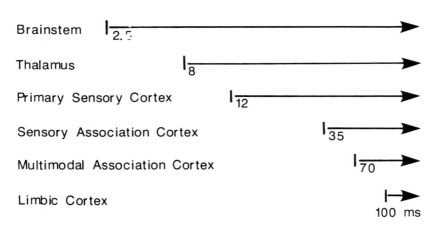

Fig. 10. The *Sequential Model* holds that each EP component reflects activation in a different structure and that the sequence of components in a given EP represents sequential activation of structures from brainstem to thalamus, primary, association, and limbic cortices. Although this is true for the actual onset of EP components, in that activity is conducted from periphery to center, each structure does not turn off when the subsequent structure is turned on. Thus, by 100 ms after stimulus onset, very large parts of the brain at all levels of the neuraxis are active and contributing to the observed scalp potentials.

1986; Vanderwolf et al., 1985), as do the midline thalamic nuclei (Buser, 1987; Steriade and Deschenes, 1984). Inhibiting circuits intrinsic to cortical regions may also be sources of modulation and ERP generation (cf Altafullah et al., 1986). The inhibitory modulation may be activated either by local activity or by diffuse external modulatory inputs (e.g., Buzsaki, 1984).

Overall, the hippocampal formation might receive a higher density of these diffuse modulatory systems than the neocortex. Even given an equal density of synaptic input to hippocampus and neocortex, the ideal geometric arrangement of hippocampal synaptic and dendritic elements for field-potential generation could account for its relatively large role in producing scalp-recorded potentials. In addition, the hippocampal formation, by virtue of its widespread reciprocal connections with the highest levels of association neocortex (Van Hoesen, 1982), is ideally suited to modulate the sequential modes of information processing engaged in by neocortical neurons.

Alternatively, it is possible that cognitive EPs, and especially processing negativities, are generated in a manner analogous to sensory EPs, i.e., directly by millions of specific interactions of cerebral neurons as they form associations to a complex stimulus within a particular context. The particular set of synapses generating the negativities to different stimuli would in some cases be unresolvable at the scalp, because the active synapses to each stimulus are intermingled in the brain, and thus have overlapping projections at the scalp. In this view, processing negativities would be considered as constituting the overall envelope of focal transactions during associative activation. This situation is known to occur, for example, in the visual cortical response to reversal of a checkerboard. Whereas distinct groups of synapses are activated at the two reversals (positive-to-negative image, or negative-to-positive), the groups are intermingled; hence at a distance (i.e., the scalp), the evoked potentials appear identical.

Thus, the N4–P3 may be directly generated by: (1) synapses carrying specific information; (2) diffuse modulatory synaptic systems from the brainstem (cholinergic, noradrenergic, serotonergic, and the like); and/or (3) intrinsic inhibitory modulatory systems. Current evidence does not permit choosing among these three possibilities for the generator of either the processing negativity or the closure positivity. In any case, the apparent generality across tasks and structures of these potentials is consistent with their reflecting the neural activity modulating the construction and dissolution of mental gestalts. The small number of EP components observed across tasks may be an important empirical demonstration that only three or four modes of cortical processing are used to accomplish the whole variety of gestalt-cognitive (i.e., whole-brain) operations. Alternatively, the small number of ERP components might represent the limited power of scalp recordings for separating intracerebral events.

6. Uses of EPs

Compared to long-latency EPs, short-latency EPs have generally clearer neural generators and lower normal variability, and can be more easily evoked in uncooperative, or even asleep or comatose, subjects. Consequently, they have more highly developed clinical utility for the measurement of sensory capacities in infants, for detecting lesions along sensory paths, and for monitoring the integrity of these paths during surgery (please *see* the reviews in Chiappa, 1983). Except for the possible use of the P3 in differentiating depression from dementia (Goodin et al., 1978; Syndulko et al., 1982), the late EP components (N2, N4, P3, SW) have been little used for diagnosis (however, *see* Curry et al., 1986). The "vertex potentials" (N1–P2) between the early sensory and late cognitive EP components are robust and fairly easy to record in neurologic or psychiatric patients, but also have widespread generators sensitive to cognitive variables or general brain dysfunction. A very large normative database has allowed N1–P2 amplitude and topography to be used as part of an EEG/EP battery to detect such conditions as minimal brain dysfunction in children (Harmony, 1984; John et al., 1977).

Assuming that cognitive EPs each have multiple generators, it is not likely that cognitive potentials will be useful for localizing pathology, except in the special case of small modulatory "triggers" or specialized antecedent structures (Figs. 4,11). For most structures, pathology is already being localized with remarkable and increasing precision using CT, PET, and MRI. Rather than competing with these imaging technologies, it seems likely that cognitive EPs will be used as a complementary, noninvasive probe for biochemical pathology by testing the integrity of synaptic systems that extend across many structures. The P3 increases in latency and decreases in amplitude during normal aging (Ford and Pfefferbaum, 1980). About 80% of patients with dementia from various causes display a P3 latency more than two standard deviations longer than their age-matched controls. P3 amplitude is also smaller in those with dementia (Syndulko et al., 1982; Squires et al., 1980). Epileptics with complex partial seizures, but normal mental abilities, may also have severely abnormal P3 amplitude (Squires et al., 1983). Among the other clinical populations that have been reported to have decreased scalp endogenous potential amplitude are hyperactive children (Prichep et al., 1976; Loiselle et al., 1980), chronic alcoholics (Begleiter et al., 1980; Porjesz et al., 1980; Pfefferbaum et al., 1979), and schizophrenics (Verleger and Cohen, 1978; Roth et al., 1980).

Identification of the P3s generating a synaptic pathway will allow the conclusion that this pathway is activated in an abnormally weak or late manner in the above diseases. This, in turn, suggests possible therapeutic drugs as well as a diagnostic technique

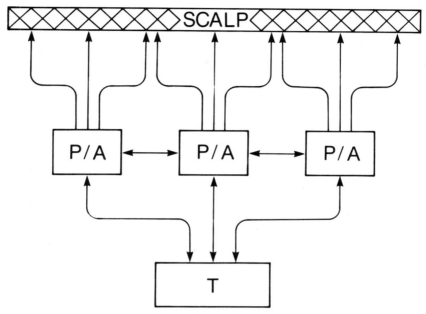

Fig. 11. Cognitive EP components recorded at the scalp seem to be generated in multiple brain structures. These structures are thus propagating generators (P) in the terminology of Fig. 4. Each of these same structures may, in particular tasks, perform some computation that is necessary for the EP component to appear anywhere. In these tasks, that structure would thus be antecedant (A) to the other generators. It is likely that many cognitive EP components result from the activation of a diffusely projecting neuromodulatory trigger (T) structure. Apparently, T is under the control of different P/A structures in different tasks. Thus, cognitive EPs may represent a mechanism whereby an individual structure can, if it is particularly competent in a given task, pace and synchronize the mode of information-processing in other structures.

for titrating their effectiveness in restoring normal function. In addition, the ability of cognitive EPs to reveal different component processes in the stimulus-to-response path of difficult cognitive tasks may lead to their use in differentiating modes of breakdown, such as that of reading in dyslexics.

In contrast to their clinical role, smaller than that of the early EPs, the late EPs have been used more extensively for scientific studies. This is presumably because the sensory pathways observed by early EPs can better be studied in animal models. In contrast, the late potentials are influenced by cognitive variables, and thus offer phenomena with both neural and cognitive aspects, which may be used to link these realms. The use of late EPs is the only method available for linking membrane/receptor events through electrophysiology to cognition, *as it occurs*. EP recordings are furthermore noninvasive, have practically no risks, and require relatively inexpensive equipment (as such things go). On the other hand, it is important to emphasize their intrinsic limitations. EPs do not permit one to observe the actual neural transactions that process information, only the envelope of millions or billions of such transactions. This envelope may reflect an active modulation of the neurons active in a task, imposed by a strategic center controlling the sequence and location of brain structures contributing to a task. Presumably, this would be the result of thalamocortical synchronizing mechanisms under frontal control (e.g., Skinner and Yingling, 1977), or to monoaminergic or cholinergic cortical projections, mainly under the control of limbic cortex. Alternatively, this envelope may be a passive emergent consequence of many neural transactions under no general synchronizing or active modulating influence. This is unknown.

In any case, EPs appear to observe the active and/or emergent modulation of components of neuronal information processing, and their consequences on the onset, duration, size, and type of subsequent modulation. Many neural processes, even those reflecting widespread modulation, will not be reflected in scalp potentials because of inappropriate generator geometries or inadequate synchronization (Wood, 1982, 1987; Halgren et al., 1986). Only future studies will reveal if Nature was kind enough to allow an important process (as opposed to a frivolous epiphenomenon) to be recorded at the scalp. Even an epiphenomenon would be useful to the degree to which it is correlated with an important process. The timing and cognitive task correlates of the late EP components are consistent with their reflection of important modulatory processes.

Furthermore, active modulation appears to be very important for neural function. Field potentials are not only very widespread and large in the mammalian brain, but also, they often have a very strong correlation with the firing of neurons in "association" areas (e.g. Creutzfeldt et al., 1966; Fox and Ranck, 1981, 1986; Buzsaki et al., 1983). Finally, the human nervous system is characterized by the vast numbers of influences (current sensation and past experience) that interact in forming a percept or choosing a "voluntary" behavior. Formal systems of elements interacting in this manner have been found to achieve better solutions when their interactions are modulated (Gardner-Medwin, 1976; Ackley et al., 1985; Halgren and Smith, 1987; Nenov et al., 1990).

Acknowledgments

Research from my laboratory reported in this review was conducted in collaboration with June Stapleton, Michael Smith, Gary Heit, and Irfan Altafullah, and was supported by the US National Institutes of Health and the Veterans Administration. Special thanks to Susan Leon Pietsch for manuscript preparation and to Jean-Michel Badier for discussions on MEG, dipole localization, and SEP generation.

Abbreviations

ADC	Analog-to-Digital Converter
AEP	Auditory Evoked Potential
ANOVA	Analysis of Variance
ATL	Anterior Temporal Lobectomy
BAEP	Brainstem Auditory EP
CNV	Contingent Negative Variation EP component
CT	Computed Tomography
dB	Decibel
EEG	Electroencephalogram
EMG	Electromyogram
EOG	Electro-oculogram
EP	Evoked Potential
EPSP	Excitatory Postsynaptic Potential
ERG	Electroretinogram
FFT	Fast Fourier Transform
LLAEP	Long Latency Auditory EP
MEG	Magnetoencephalogram
MLAEP	Middle Latency Auditory EP
MRF	Mesencephalic Reticular Formation
MRI	Magnetic Resonance Imaging

MTL	Medial Temporal Lobe
N4	N400 EP component
NS	Negative Slope EP component
P3	P300 EP component
PCA	Principal Components Analysis
PET	Positron Emission Tomography
PSP	Postsynaptic Potential
RP	Readiness Potential
SEP	Somatosensory Evoked Potential
SMC	Supplementary Motor Cortex
S:N	Signal-to-Noise Ratio
SW	Slow Wave EP component
TSW	Typical Slow Wave
VEP	Visual Evoked Potential

References

Ackley D. H., Hinton G. E., and Sejnowski T. J. (1985) A learning algorithm for Boltzmann Machines. *Cognit. Science* **9**, 147–169.

Aladjalova N. A. (1964) Slow electrical processes in the brain, *Prog. Brain Res.*, vol. 7 Elsevier, Amsterdam,

Allison R. and Hume A. L. (1981) A comparative analysis of short-latency somatosensory evoked potentials in man, monkey, cat and rat. *Exp. Neurol.* **72**, 592–611.

Allison T. (1962) Recovery functions of somatosensory evoked responses in man. *Electroencephalogr. Clin. Neurophysiol.* **14**, 331–343.

Allison T., Goff W. R., Williamson P. D., and Van Gilder J. C., (1980) On the neural origin of early components of the somatosensory evoked potential, in *Clinical Uses of Cerebral, Brainstem and Spinal Somatosensory Evoked Potentials* (Desmedt J. E., ed.) (*Prog. Clin. Neurophysiol.*, vol. 7), Karger, Basel, pp. 51–68.

Allison T., Matsumiya Y., Goff G. D., and Goff, W. R. (1977) The scalp topography of human visual evoked potentials. *Electroencephalogr. Clin. Neurophysiol.* **43**, 185–197.

Allison T., McCarthy G., Wood C. C., Darcey T. M., Spencer D. D., and Williamson P. D. (1988) Human sensorimotor cortex potentials evoked by stimulation of the median nerve. I. Cytoarchitectonic areas generating short-latency potentials. *J. Neurosurg.* (in press).

Altafullah I., Halgren E., Stapleton J., and Crandall P. H. (1986) Interictal spike–wave complexes in the human medial temporal potentials. *Electroencephalogr. Clin. Neurophysiol.* **63**, 503–516.

American EEG Society (1984) Guidelines for clinical evolved potential studies. *J. Clin. Neurophysiol.* **1**, 3–53.

Andersen P., Bliss T. V. P., and Skrede K. K. (1971) Lamellar organization of hippocampal excitatory pathways. *Exp. Brain Res.* **13**, 208–221.

Andersen P., Eccles J. C., and Loyning Y. (1964) Location of post-synaptic inhibitory synapses on hippocampal pyramids. *J. Neurophysiol.* **27**, 592–607.

Antervo A., Hari R., Katila T., Pautenaen T., Seppanen M., and Tuomisto T. (1983) Cerebral magnetic fields preceding self-paced plantar flexions of the foot. *Acta Neurol. Scand.* **68**, 213–217.

Arduini A. (1958) Enduring potential changes evoked in the cerebral cortex by stimulation of brainstem reticular formation and thalamus, in *Reticular Formation of the Brain* (Jasper, H. H., Proctor, L. D., Knighton, R. S., Noshay, W. C., and Costello, R. T., eds.), pp. 333–354.

Arduini A., Mancia M., and Mechelse K. (1957) Slow potential changes in the cerebral cortex by sensory and reticular stimulation. *Arch. Ital. Biol.* **95**, 127–138.

Arezzo J. L. and Vaughan H. G., Jr. (1975) Cortical potentials associated with voluntary movements in the monkey. *Brain Res.* **88**, 99–104.

Arezzo J. C. and Vaughan H. G., Jr. (1980) Intracortical sources and surface topography of the motor potential and somatosensory evoked potential in the monkey, in *Motivation, Motor and Sensory Process of the Brain: Electrical Potentials, Behaviour and Clinical Use* (Kornhuber H. H. and Deecke L., eds.) (*Prog. Brain Res.*, vol. 54), Elsevier, Amsterdam, pp. 77–83.

Arezzo J. C., Vaughan H. G., Jr., and Legatt A. D. (1981) Topography and intracranial sources of somatosensory evoked potentials in the monkey II. Cortical components. *Electroencephalogr. Clin. Neurophysiol.* **51**, 1–18.

Arezzo J. C., Legatt A. D., and Vaughan H. G., Jr. (1979) Topography and intracranial sources of somatosensory evoked potentials in the monkey I. Early components. *Electroencephalogr. Clin. Neurophysiol.* **46**, 155–172.

Arezzo J. C., Pickoff A., and Vaughan H. G., Jr. (1975) The sources and intracerebral distribution of auditory evoked potentials in the alert rhesus monkey. *Brain Res.* **90**, 57–73.

Arezzo J. C., Tenke C. E., and Vaughan H. G., Jr. (1987) Movement-related potentials within the hippocampal formation of the monkey. *Brain Res.* **401**, 79–86.

Arezzo J. C., Vaughan H. G., Jr., and Koss B. (1977) Relationship of neuronal activity to gross movement-related potentials in monkey pre- and postcentral cortex. *Brain Res.* **132**, 362–369.

Arezzo J. C., Vaughan H. G., Jr., Kraut M. A., Steinshneider M., and Legatt A. D. (1986) Intracranial generators of event-related potentials in the monkey, in *Evoked Potentials* (Cracco R. and Bodis-Wollner I., eds), Alan R. Liss, New York, pp. 141–154.

Arthur D. L. and Starr A. (1984) Task-relevent late positive component of the auditory event-related potentials in monkeys resembles P300 in humans. *Science* **223**, 186–188.

Arthur D. L., Flynn E. R., and Williamson S. J. (1987) Source localization of long-latency auditory evoked magnetic fields in human temporal cortex. *Current Trends in Event-Related Potential Research* (Johnson, R., Jr., Rohrbaugh J. W., and Parasuraman, R., eds.) *(EEG Suppl. 40)*, Elsevier, Amsterdam, 429–439.

Ary J. P., Klein S. A., and Fender D. H. (1981b) Location of source of evoked scalp potentials: Corrections for skull and scalp thickness. *IEEE Trans. Biomed. Eng.* **28(6)**, 447–452.

Ary J. P., Darcey T. M., and Fender D. H. (1981) Locating electrical sources in the human brain. *IEEE Trans. Biomed. Eng.* **28**, 1–5.

Ashford J. W. and Fuster J. M. (1985) Occipital and inferotemporal responses to visual signals in the monkey. *Exp. Neurol.* **90**, 444–466.

Aunon J. I., McGillem C. D., and Childers D. G. (1981) Signal processing in evoked potential research: Averaging and modeling. *CRC Crit. Rev. Biol.* **5**, 323–367.

Baba G., Asano T., Nakamura S., and Orimoto T. (1976–77) Readiness potential recorded from the scalp and depth leads. *Appl. Neurophysiol.* 39, 268–271.

Bancaud J. (ed.) (1975) *Stereoencephalography* (Remond A. ed.) (*Handbook of Electroencephalography and Clinical Neurophsiology,* vol. 10B), Elsevier, Amsterdam.

Bancaud J., Bloch V., and Paillard J. (1953) Contributions EEG a l'etude des potentiels evoques chez l'homme au niveau du vertex. *Rev. Neurol. (Paris)* **89**, 399–418.

Barlow J. S. (1960) Rhythmic activity induced by photic stimulation in relation to intrinsic alpha activity of the brain in man. *Electroencephalogr. Clin. Neurophysiol.* **12**, 317–326.

Barlow J. S. and Remond A. (1981) Eye movement artifact nulling in EEGs by multichannel on-line EOG subtraction. *Electroencephalogr. Clin. Neurophysiol.,* **52**, 418–423.

Barrett S. E., Rugg M. D., and Perrett D. I. (1988) Event-related potentials and the matching of familiar and unfamiliar faces. *Neuropsychologia* **26**, 105–117.

Barth D. S., Sutherling W., Broffman J., and Beatty J. (1986) Magnetic localization of a dipolar current source implanted in a sphere and human cranium. *Electroencephalogr. Clin. Neurophysiol.*, **63**, 260–273.

Beall J. E., Applebaum A. E., Foreman R. D., and Willis W. D. (1977) Spinal cord potentials evoked by cutaneous afferents in the monkey. *J. Neurophysiol.* **40**, 199–211.

Becker W., Hoehne O., Iwase K., and Kornhuber H. H. (1973) Cerebral and ocular muscle potentials preceding voluntary eye movements in man, in Event-Related Potentials of the Brain: Their Relations to Behavior (McCallum W. C. and Knott J. R., eds) (*Electroencephalogr. Clin. Neurophysiol.*, Suppl. 33) Elsevier, Amsterdam, pp. 99–104.

Begleiter H., Porjesz B., and Tenner M. (1980) Neuroradiological neurophysiological evidence of brain deficits in chronic alcoholics. *Acta. Psychiatr. Scand. Suppl. 286*, **62**, 3–14.

Bentin S., McCarthy, G., and Wood C. C. (1985) Event-related potentials, lexical decision and semantic priming. *Electroencephalogr. Clin. Neurophysiol.* **60**, 343–355.

Bertrand O., Perrin F., and Pernier J. (1985) A theoretical justification of the average reference in topographic evoked potential studies. *Electroencephalogr. Clin. Neurophysiol.*, **62**, 462–464.

Bessom J. M., Woody C. D., Aleonard P., Thompson H. K., Albe-Fessard D., and Marshall W. H. (1970) Correlations of brain d-c shifts with changes in cerebral blood flow. *Am. J. Physiol.* **218**, 284–291.

Bickford R. G. (1972) Physiological and clinical studies of micro-reflexes. *Electroencephalogr. Clin. Neurophysiol.* **31**, 93–108.

Bickford R. G., Jacobson J. L., and Cody D. T. R. (1964) Nature of average evoked potentials to sound and other stimuli in man. *Ann. NY Acad. Sci.* **112**, 204–223.

Bioulac B. and Lamarre Y. (1979) Activity of post-central cortical neurons of the monkey during conditioned movements of the deafferented limb. *Brain Res.* **172**, 427–438.

Blom J. L. and Anneveldt J. (1982) An electrocap tested. *Electroencephalogr. Clin. Neurophysiol.* **54**, 591–594.

Blumhardt L. D. and Halliday A. M. (1979) Hemisphere contributions to the composition of the pattern-evoked potential waveform. *Exp. Brain Res.* **36**, 53–69.

Blumhardt L. D., Barrett G., Halliday A. M., and Kriss A. (1978) The effect of experimental "scotomata" on the ipsilateral and contralateral responses to pattern-reversal in one half-field. *Electroencephalogr. Clin. Neurophysiol.* **15**, 376–392.

Bodis-Wollner I., Hendley C. D., Mylin L. H., and Thornton J. (1979) Visual evoked potentials and the visuogram in multiple sclerosis. *Ann. Neurol.* **5,** 40–47.

Bonnet M. (1981) Comparison of monosynaptic tendon reflexes during preparation for ballistic or ramp movement. *Electroencephalogr. Clin. Neurophysiol.* **51,** 353–362.

Boston J. R. and Moller A. R. (1985) Brainstem auditory-evoked potentials. *Crit. Rev. Biomed. Eng.* **13,** 97–123.

Boyd E. H., Boyd E. S., and Brown L. E. (1982) Precentral cortex unit activity during the M-wave and contingent negative variation in behaving squirrel monkeys. *Exp. Neurol.* **75,** 535–554.

Brazier M. A. (1984) Pioneers in the discovery of evoked potentials. *Electroencephalogr. Clin. Neurophysiol.* **59,** 2–8.

Brenner D., Williamson S. J., and Kaufman L. (1975) Visually evoked magnetic fields of the human brain. *Science* **190,** 480–482.

Brenner D., Okada Y., Maclin E., Williamson S. J., and Kaufman L. (1981) Evoked magnetic fields reveal different visual areas in human cortex, in *Biomagnetism* (Erne S. N., Hahlbohm H. -D., and Lubbig H., eds.), Walter de Gruyter, New York, pp. 431–444.

Bromm B., Neitzel H., Tecklenburg A., and Treede R. D. (1983) Evoked cerebral potential correlates of C-fibre activity in man. *Neurosci. Lett.* **43,** 109–114.

Broughton R. J. (1969) Discussion, in *Average Evoked Potentials* (NASA SP-19) (Lindsley B. and Donchin E., eds.), US Government Printing Office Washington, DC, pp. 79–84.

Broughton R., Rasmussen T., and Branch C. (1981) Scalp and direct cortical recordings of somatosensory evoked potentials in man (Circa 1967). *Can. J. Psychol.* **35,** 136–158.

Brown W. J. (1973) Structural substrates of seizure foci in the human temporal lobe, in *Epilepsy: Its Phenomena in Man* (Brazier M. A. B., ed.), Academic, New York, pp. 339–374.

Bruce C. J. and Goldberg M. E. (1985) Primate frontal eye fields. I. Single neurons discharging before saccades. *J. Neurophysiol.* **53,** 603–635.

Brunia C. H. M. and Damen E. J. P. (1988) Distribution of slow brain potentials related to motor preparation and stimulus anticipation in a time estimation task. *Electroencephalogr. Clin. Neurophysiol.* **69,** 234–243.

Buchwald J. (1983) Generators, in *Bases of Auditory Brain-stem Evoked Responses* (Moore E. J. ed.), Grune & Stratton, New York, pp. 157–195.

Buchwald J. S. (1987) Animal models of event-related potentials. In: *Event-Related Potentials of the Brain*, (Rohrbaugh J., Parasuraman R., and Johnson R., eds.) New York, (in press).

Buchwald J. S. and Squires N. S. (1982) Endogenous potentials in the cat, in *Conditioning Representation of Involved Neural Function* (Woody C., ed.), Plenum, New York, pp. 503.

Buchwald J. S., Hinman C., Norman R. J., Huang C. M. and Brown K., A. (1981) Middle- and long-latency auditory evoked responses recorded from the vertex of normal and chronically lesioned cats. *Brain Res.* **205**, 91–109.

Bullock T. H. (1986) Interspecific comparison of brainstem auditory evoked potentials and frequency following responses among vertebrate classes, in *Evoked Potentials* (Cracco R., and Bodis-Wollner I., eds.), Alan R. Liss, New York, pp. 141–154.

Buser P. (1987) Thalamocortical mechanisms underlying synchronized EEG activity, in *A. Textbook of Clinical Neurophysiology* (Halliday A. M., Butler S. R., Paul R., eds.) Wiley, New York, pp. 595–622.

Buzsaki G. (1984) Feed-forward inhibition in the hippocampal formation. *Prog. Neurobiol.* **22**, 131–153.

Buzsaki G., Leung L. S., and Vanderwolf C. H. (1983) Cellular bases of hippocampal EEG in the behaving rat. *Brain Res. Rev.* **6**, 139–171.

Carmon A., Mor J., and Goldberg, J. (1976) Evoked cerebral response to noxious thermal stimuli in humans. *Exp. Brain Res.* **25**, 103–107.

Caspers H. (1974) DC potentials recorded directly from the cortex, in *Handbook of Electroencephalography and Clinical Neurophysiology*, vol. 10 (A. Remond, ed.), Elsevier, Amsterdam. pp. 5–80.

Caspers H., Speckmann E.-J., and Lehmenkuhler A. (1979) Effects of CO_2 in cortical field potentials in relation to neuronal activity, in *Origin of Cerebral Field Potentials* (Speckmann E. -J. and Caspers H. eds.), G. Thieme, Stuttgart, pp. 151–163.

Caspers H., Speckmann E. -J., and Lehmenkuhler A. (1980) Electrogenesis of cortical DC potentials. *Prog. Brain Res.* **54**, 3–15.

Castellucci V. F. and Goldring S. (1970) Contribution to steady potential shifts of slow depolarization in cells presumed to be glia. *Electroencephalogr. Clin. Neurophysiol.* **28**, 109–118.

Caton R. (1875) The electric currents of the brain. *Brit. Med. J.* **2**, 278–278.

Celesia G. G. (1976) Organization of auditory cortical areas in man. *Brain* **99**, 403–414.

Celesia G. G. (1979) Somatosensory evoked potentials recorded directly from human thalamus and Sm I cortical area. *Arch. Neurol.* **36**, 399–405.

Celesia G. G. (1982) Clinical applications of evoked potentials. In: *Electroncephalography: Basic Principles, Clinical Applications and Related Fields,* (Niedermeyer E. and Lopes da Silva F., eds.), Urban and Schwarzenberg, Baltimore, pp. 665–684.

Chain F., Lesevre N., Leblanc M., Remond A., and Lhermitte F. (1972) Etude topographique des responses evoquées visuelles dans un cas de lobectomie occipitale. *Rev. Neurol. (Paris)* **126,** 372–378.

Chapman C. R., Chen A. C. N., and Harkins S. W. (1979) Brain evoked potentials as correlates of laboratory pain: A review and perspective, *Adv. Pain Res. Ther.* **3,** 791–803.

Chen B. M. and Buchwald J. S. (1986) Midlatency auditory evoked responses: Differential effects of sleep in the cat. *Electroencephalogr. Clin. Neurophysiol.* **65,** 373–382.

Cheron G. and Borenstein S. (1987) Specific gating of the early somatosensory evoked potentials during active movement. *Electroencephalogr. Clin. Neurophysiol.* **67,** 537–548.

Chiappa K. H. (ed.) (1983) *Evoked Potentials in Clinical Medicine.* (Raven, New York).

Chiappa K. H., Choi S. K., and Young R. R. (1980) Short-latency somatosensory evoked potentials following median nerve stimulation in patients with neurological lesions, in *Clinical Uses of Cerebral, Brainstem and Spinal Somatosensory Evoked Potentials* (Desmedt J. E., ed.) (*Prog. Clin. Neurophysiol.,* vol. 7), Karger, Basel, pp. 264–281.

Childers D. and Durling A. (1975) *Digital Filtering and Signal Processing* (West Publishing, St. Paul, New York).

Chudler E. H. (1983) The assessment of pain by cerebral evoked potentials, *Pain* **16,** 221–244.

Ciganek L. (1975) Visual evoked responses, in *Handbook of Electroencephalography and Clinical Neurophysiology,* vol. 8A (Remond A., ed.), Elsevier, Amsterdam, pp. 33–59.

Clark W. A. (1958) Average response computer (ARC-1). *Quart. Progr. Rep.,* Research Laboratory of Electronics, M.I.T., Cambridge, MA, 114–117.

Cobb W. A. and Dawson G. D. (1960) The latency and form in man of the occipital potential evoked by bright flashes. *J. Physiol. (Lond.)* **152,** 108–121.

Cohen D. and Cuffin B. N. (1983) Demonstration of useful differences between magnetoencephalogram and electroencephalogram. *Electroencephalogr. Clin. Neurophysiol.* **56,** 38–51.

Cohen J. (1969) Very slow brain potentials relating to expectancy: The CNV, in *Averaged Evoked Responses* (Donchin E. and Lindsley D. B., eds.), NASA, Washington DC, pp. 143–163.

Cohen J. (1975) The CNV in cases of hemispheric vascular lesions. *Electroencephalogr. Clin. Neurophysiol.* **38,** 542.

Cohen J. and Walter W. G. (1966) The interactin of responses in the brain to semantic stimuli. *Psychophysiology* **2,** 187–196.

Courchesne E., Hillyard S. A. and Galambos R. (1975) Stimulus novelty, task relevance and the visual evoked potential in man. *Electroencephalogr. Clin. Neurophysiol.* **39,** 131–143.

Cracco R. Q. and Bodis-Wollner I. (eds.) (1986) *Evoked potentials.* (Liss, New York).

Cracco R. Q., and Cracco J. B. (1978) Visual evoked potential in man: Early oscillatory potentials. *Electroencephalogr. Clin. Neurophysiol.* **45,** 731–739.

Creutzfeldt O. D., Watanabe S., and Lux H. D. (1966) Relations between EEG phenomena and potentials of single cortical cells. I. Evoked responses after thalamic and epicortical stimulation. *Electroencephalogr. Clin. Neurophysiol.* **20,** 1–18.

Cruccu G., Fornarelli M., Inghilleri M., and Manfredi M. (1983) The limits of tooth pulp evoked potentials for pain quanitation. *Physiol. Behav.* **31,** 339–342.

Cuffin B. N. (1986) Effects of measurement errors and noise on MEG moving dipole solutions *IEEE Trans. Biomed. Eng.* **BME-33,** 854–861.

Curry S. H., Woods D. L., Low M. D. (1986) Applications of cognitive ERPs in neurosurgical and neurological patients. In: *Cerebral Psychophysiology: Studies in Event-Related Potentials (EEG Suppl. 38),* McCallum W. C., Zappoli R., and Denoth F., eds.) Elsevier, Amsterdam, pp. 469–484.

Darcey T. M. (1979) Methods for localization of electrical sources in the human brain and applications to the visual system. Ph.D. thesis, California Institute of Technology, Pasadena.

Darcey T. M., Ary J. P. and Fender D. H. (1980) Spatiotemporal visually evoked scalp potentials in response to partial-field patterned stimulation. *Electroencephalogr. Clin. Neurophysiol.* **50,** 348–355.

Darcey T. M., Wieser H. G., Meles H. P., Skrandies W. and Lehmann D. (1980) Intracerebral and scalp fields evoked by visual stimulation. *Electroencephalogr. Clin. Neurophysiol.* **49,** 111P.

Davis P. A. (1939) Effects of acoustic stimuli on the waking human brain. *J. Neurophysiol.* **2,** 494–499.

Davis H. (1965) Slow cortical responses evoked by acoustic stimuli. *Acta Otolaryngol.* **59,** 179–185.

Davis H. and Hirsh S. K. (1977) Brain stem electric response audiometry (BSERA). *Acta Otolaryngol.* **83,** 136–139.

Davis H., Mast T., Yoshie N., and Zerlin S. (1966) The slow response of the human cortex to auditory stimuli: Recovery process. *Electroencephalogr. Clin. Neurophysiol.* **21,** 105–113.

Dawson G. D. (1950) Cerebral responses to nerve stimulation in man. *Brit. Med. Bull.* **6,** 326–329.

Deecke L. and Kornhuber H. H. (1978) An electrical sign of participation of the mesial supplementary motor cortex in human voluntary finger movement. *Brain Res.* **159,** 473–376.

Deecke L., Eisinger H. and Kornhuber H. H. (1980) Comparison of Bereitschaftspotential, pre-motor positivity, and motor potential preceding voluntary flexion and extension movements in man, in *Motivation, Motor and Sensory Processes of the Brain: Electrical Potentials, Behavior and Clinical Use* (Kornhuber H. H. and Deecke L., eds.) *(Prog. Brain Res.* vol. 54) Elsevier/North Holland, Amsterdam, pp. 171–176.

Deecke L., Grozinger G., and Kornhuber H. H. (1976) Voluntary finger movements in man: Cerebral potentials and theory. *Biol. Cybern.* **23,** 99–119.

Deecke L., Weinberg H., and Brickett P. (1982) Magnetic fields of the human brain accompanying voluntary movement. Bereitschaftsmagnetfeld. *Exp. Brain Res.* **48,** 144–148.

Deecke L., Boschert J., Weinberg H. and Brickett P. (1983) Magnetic fields of the human brain (Bereitschaftsmagnetfeld) preceding voluntary foot and toe movements. *Exp. Brain Res.* **52,** 81–86.

Deecke L., Englitz H. G., Kornhuber H. H., and Schmitt G. (1977) Cerebral potentials preceding voluntary movement in patients with bilateral or unilateral Parkinson akinesia, in Attention, Voluntary Contraction and Event-related Cerebral Potentials (Desmedt, J. E. ed), *(Prog. Clin. Neurophysiol.,* Vol. 1) Karger, Basel, pp. 151–163.

Deecke L., Becker W., Grozinger B., Scheid P., and Kornhuber H. (1973) Human brain potentials preceding voluntary limb movements, in Event-Related Slow Potentials of the Brain: Their Relations to Behavior (McCallum W. C. and Knott J. R., eds.) *(Electroencephalogr. Clin. Neurophysiol. Suppl. 33),* Elsevier, Amsterdam, pp. 87–94.

Deecke L., Heise B., Kornhuber H. H., Lang M., and Lang W. (1984) Brain potentials associated with voluntary manual tracking. *Ann. NY Acad. Sci.* **374,** 361–372.

Deecke L., Kornhuber H. H., Lang W., Lang M., and Schreiber H. (1985) Timing function of the frontal cortex in sequential motor and learning tasks. *Hum. Neurobiol.* **4,** 143–154.

Deecke L., Uhl F., Spieth F., Lang W., and Lang M. (1987) Cerebral potentials preceding and accompanying verbal and spatial tasks, in *Current Trends in Event-Related Potential Research (EEG Suppl. 40)*

(Johnson R., Jr., Rohrbaugh J. W., and Parasuraman R., eds.) Elsevier, Amsterdam, pp. 17–23.

Deiber M. P., Giard M. H., and Mauguiere F. (1986) Separate generators with distinct orientations for N20 and P22 somatosensory evoked potentials to finger stimulation? *Electroencephalogr. Clin. Neurophysiol.* **65**, 321–334.

Delgado-Escueta A. V., and Walsh G. O. (1983) The selection process for surgery of complex partial seizures: Surface EEG and depth electrography. *Res. Publ. Assoc. Res. Nerv. Ment. Dis.* **61**, 295–326.

Desmedt J. E. (ed.) (1977a) *Attention, Voluntary Contraction, and Event-Related Cerebral Potentials* Karger, Basel.

Desmedt J. E. (1977b) Active touch exploration of extrapersonal space elicits specific electrogenesis in the right cerebral hemisphere of intact right-handed man. *Proc. Natl. Acad. Sci. USA* **74**, 4037–4040.

Desmedt J. E. (ed.) (1979) *Cognitive Components in Cerebral Event-Related Potentials and Selective Attention* Karger, Basel.

Desmedt J. E. (1981) Scalp-recorded cerebral event-related potentials in man as point of entry into the analysis of cognitive processing, in *The Organization of the Cerebral Cortex* (Schmitt F. O., Worden F. G., Edelman G., and Dennis S. D., eds.), MIT, Cambridge, Massachusetts pp. 441–473.

Desmedt J. E. (1986) Generator sources of SEP in man, in *Evoked Potentials* (Cracco R. and Bodis-Wollner I., eds.), pp. 235–245.

Desmedt J. E. and Bourguet M. (1985) Color imaging of parietal and frontal somatosensory potential fields evoked by stimulation of median or posterior tibial nerve in man. *Electroencephalogr. Clin. Neurophysiol.* **62**, 1–19.

Desmedt J. E. and Cheron G. (1980). Somatosensory evoked potentials to finger stimulation in healthy octogenarians and in young adults: Wave forms, scalp topography and transit times of parietal and frontal components. *Electroencephalogr. Clin. Neurophysiol.* **50**, 404–425.

Desmedt J. E. and Debecker J. (1979) Wave form and neural mechanisms of the decision P350 elicited without pre-stimulus CNV or readiness potential in random sequences of near-threshold auditory clicks and finger stimuli. *Electroencephalogr. Clin. Neurophysiol.* **47**, 648–670.

Desmedt J. E., Nguyen T. H., and Bourguet M. (1987) Bit-mapped color imaging of human evoked potentials with reference to the N20, P22, P27 and N30 somatosensory responses. *Electroencephalogr. Clin. Neurophysiol.* **68**, 1–19.

Dick J. P. R., Cantello R., Buruma O., Gioux M., Benecke R., Day B. L., Rothwell J. C., Thompson P. D., and Marsden C. D. (1987) The bereitschaftspotential, L-DOPA and Parkinson's disease. *Electroencephalogr. Clin. Neurophysiol.* **66,** 263–274.

Domalski P., Smith M. E., and Halgren E. Cross-modal repetition effects on the N4 (submitted).

Donchin E. (1973) Methodological issues in CNV research. A review, in *Event-Related Slow Potentials of the Brain: their Relations to Behavior* (McCallum W. C. and Knott J. R., eds.) *(Electroencephalogr. Clin. Neurophysiol. Suppl. 33),* Elsevier, Amsterdam, pp. 3–17.

Donchin E. (1981) Surprise! . . . Surprise? *Psychophysiologr.* **18,** 493–513.

Donchin E. and Coles G. H. (1988) Precommentary on Verlager's critique of the context updating model. *Behav. Brain Sci.,* 11, 357–375

Donchin E. and Heffley E. F., III (1978) Multivariate analysis of event-released potential data: A tutorial review, in *Multidisciplinary perspectives in event-related brain potential research* (EPA-600/9-77-043) (Otto D. A., ed.), US Government Printing Office, Washington DC pp. 555–572.

Donchin E., Ritter W. and McCallum W. C. (1978) Cognitive psychophysiology: The endogenous components of the ERP, in *Brain and Information: Event-Related Potentials, Annals of the New York Academy of Sciences* (Callaway E., Tueting, P., and Koslow S., eds.), New York Academy of Sciences, New York, pp. 349–411.

Donchin E., Gerbrandt L. K., Leifer L., and Tucker L. (1972) Is the contingent negative variation contingent on a motor response? *Psychophysiology* **9,** 178–188.

Donchin E., Otto D., Gerbrandt L. K., and Pribram K. H. (1971) While a monkey waits: Electrical events recorded during the foreperiod of a reaction time study. *Electroencephalogr. Clin. Neurophysiol.* **31,** 115–127.

Donchin E., Callaway R., Cooper R., Desmedt J. E., Goff W. R., Hillyard S. A., and Sutton S. (1977) Publication criteria for studies of evoked potentials (EP) in man. (J. E. Desmedt, ed.) *(Prog. Clin. Neurophysiol.* vol. 1), 1–11.

Doyle D. J. and Hyle M. L. (1981) Bessel filtering of brain stem auditory evoked potentials. *Electroencephalogr. Clin. Neurophysiol.* **51,** 446–448.

Ducati A., Fava E., and Motti E. D. F. (1988) Neuronal generators of the visual evoked potentials: intracerebral recording in awake humans. *Electroencephalogr. Clin. Neurophysiol.* **71,** 89–99.

Duffy F. H. (ed.) (1986) *Topographic Mapping of Brain Electrical Activity.* (Butterworths, Boston).

Durrant J. D. and Furman J. M. R. (1988) Long-latency rotational evoked potentials in subjects with and without bilateral vestibular loss. *Electroencephalogr. Clin. Neurophysiol.* **71,** 251–256.

Eccles J. C. (1982) The initiation of voluntary movements by supplementary motor area. *Arch. Psychiatr. Nervenkr.* **231,** 423–441.

Eisen A. (1982) The somatosensory evoked potential. *Can. J. Neurol. Sci.* **9,** 65–77.

Elbert T., Lutzenberger W., Rockstroh B., and Birbaumer N. (1985) Removal of ocular artifacts from the EEG—a biophysical approach to the EOG. *Electroencephalogr. Clin. Neurophysiol.,* **60,** 455–463.

Elul R. (1972) The genesis of the EEG. *Int. Rev. Neurobiol.* **15,** 227–272.

Emerson R. G. and Pedley T. A. (1984) Generator sources of median somatosensory evoked potentials. *J. Clin. Neurophysiol.* **1,** 203–218.

Empson J. A. C. (1986) Response force, motivation, and the EEG readiness potential. *Psychophysiol. 1986.* **23,** 433–434.

Ertekin C. (1978) Comparison of the human evoked electrospinogram recorded from the intrathecal, epidural and cutaneous levels. *Electroencephalogr. Clin. Neurophysiol.* **44,** 683–690.

Ertl J. and Schafer E. W. (1967) Cortical activity preceding speech. *Life Sci.* **6,** 473–479.

Erwin R. and Buchwald J. S. (1986) Midlatency auditory evoked responses: differential effects of sleep in the human. *Electroencephalogr. Clin. Neurophysiol.* **65,** 383–392.

Evarts E. V. and Tanji J. (1976) Reflex and intended responses in motor cortex pyramidal tract neurons of monkey. *J. Neurophysiol.* **39,** 1069–1080.

Fischler I., Bloom P. A., Childers D. G., Arroyo A. A., and Perry N. W. (1984) Brain potentials during sentence verification: late negativity and long-term memory strength. *Neuropsychologia.* **22,** 559–568.

Ford J. M. and Pfefferbaum A. (1980) The utility of brain potentials in determining age-related changes in central nervous system and cognitive functioning, in *Aging in the 1980's: Psychological Issues,* (Poon L. W., ed.), American Psychological Association, Washington DC, pp. 115–124.

Fox S. E. and Ranck J. B., Jr. (1981) Electrophysiological characteristics of hippocampal complex-spike cells and theta cells. *Exp. Brain Res.* **41,** 399–410.

Fox S. E., Wolfson S., and Ranck J. B., Jr. (1986) Hippocampal theta rhythm and the firing of neurons in walking and urethane anesthetized rats. *Exp. Brain Res.* **62,** 495–508.

Freeman W. J. (1975) *Mass Action of the Nervous System* (Academic, New York).

Freeman W. J. (1978) Models of the dynamics of neural populations, in *Contemporary Clinical Neurophysiology* (Cobb W. A. and Van Duijn H., eds.) *(EEG Suppl. No. 34),* Elsevier, Amsterdam.

Fromm C. (1983) Contrasting properties of pyramidal tract neurons located in precentral or postcentral areas and of corticorubral neurons in the behaving monkey. *Adv. Neurol.* **39,** 329–345.

Fuster J. M. (1973) Unit activity in prefrontal cortex during delayed-response performance: Neuronal correlates of transient memory. *J. Neurophysiol.* **36,** 61–78.

Fuster J. M. (1980) *The Prefrontal Cortex* (Raven, New York).

Fuster J. M. and Alexander G. E. (1973) Firing changes in cells of the nucleus medialis dorsalis associated with delayed response behavior. *Brain Res.* **61,** 79–91.

Fuster J. M. and Jarvey J. P. (1981) Inferotemporal neurons distinguish and retain behaviorally relevant features of visual stimuli. *Science* **212,** 952–955.

Fuster J. M., Bauer R. H., and Jervey J. P. (1982) Cellular discharge in the dorsolateral prefrontal cortex of the monkey in cognitive tasks. *Exp. Neurol.* **77,** 679–694.

Fuxe K. and Jonsson G. (1974) Further mapping at central 5-hydroxytryptamine neurons: Studies with the neurotoxic dihydroxytryptamines. *Adv. Biochem. Psychopharmacol.* **10,** 1–12.

Gaillard A. W. K. (1980) Cortical correlates of motor preparation, in *Attention and Performance VIII* (Nickerson, R. S., ed.), Erlbaum, Hillsdale, New Jersey.

Gaillard A. W. and Naatanen R. (1976) Modality effects on the contingent negative variation in a simple reaction-time task, in *The Responsive Brain* (McCallum, W. C. and Knott, J. R. ed.), Wright, Bristol, pp. 40–45.

Galambos R., Makeig S., and Tamachoff P. J. (1981) A 40-Hz auditory potential recorded from the human scalp. *Proc. Natl. Acad. Sci. USA* **78,** 2643–2647.

Ganglberger J. A., Haider M., Knapp E., and Schmid H. (1980) Subdural recordings of the cortex motor potentials. In: *Motivation, Motor and Sensory Processes of the Brain: Electrical Potentials, Behavior and Clinial Use* (Kornhuber, H. H., Deecke, L., eds.) (*Prog. Brain Res.* vol. 54) Elsevier/North Holland, Amsterdam. pp. 57–61.

Gardner E. P., Costanzo R. M., Hamalainen H. A., Warren S., and Young W. (1986) Facilitation and inhibition in somatosensory cortex: Comparison of the single unit responses and somatosensory evoked potentials (SEP), in *Evoked Potentials* (Cracco R. and Bodis-Wollner I., eds.), Alan R. Liss, New York, pp. 141–154.

Gardner E. P., Hamalaihen H. A., Warren S., Davis J., and Young W. (1984) Somatosensory evoked potentials (SEPs) and cortical single unit responses elicited by mechanical tactile stimuli in awake monkeys. *Electroencephalogr. Clin. Neurophysiol.* **58,** 537–52.

Gardner-Medwin A. R. (1976) The recall of events through the learning of associations between their parts. *Proc. R. Soc. London Biol.* **194,** 375–402.

Gasser T., Sroka L., Mocks J. (1986) The correction of EOG artifacts by frequency dependent and frequency independent methods. *Psychophysiology* 23, 704–712.

Gazzaniga M. S. and Hillyard S. A. (1973) Attention mechanisms following brain bisection, in *Attention and Performance,* vol. 4 (Kornblum, S., ed.), Academic, New York, pp. 221–238.

Gerbrandt L. K. (1977) Analysis of movement potential components, in *Attention, Voluntary Contraction and Event-Related Cerebral Potentials.* (Desmedt J. E., ed.) (*Progress in Clinical Neurophysiol,* vol 1), Karger, Basel, pp. 174–188.

Gerbrandt L. K. and Fowler J. R. (1980) Arousal-related sustained potentials in neocortex and hippocampus of rats. *Prog. Brain Res.* **54,** 109–116.

Gevins A. S. (1984) Analysis of the electromagnetic signals of the human brain: Milestones, obstacles, and goals. *IEEE Trans. Biomed. Engin.* **BME-31,** 833–850.

Gevins A. S. and Aminoff M. J. (1987) Brain electrical activity: Clinical applications and methods of computer analysis. *Encyclopedia of Medical Devices and Instrumentation,* (Webster, J. G. ed.), Wiley, New York, pp. 1084–1107.

Gevins A. S., and Cutillo B. A. (1987) Signals of cognition, in Application of Computational Analysis to Electroencephalography *Handbook of Electroencephalography and Clinical Neurophysiology* vol. 2, (Lopes da Silva F., Van Leeuwen W. S., and Remond A., eds.), Elsevier, Amsterdam, pp. 335–381.

Gevins A. S. and Remond A. (eds.) (1987) Methods of analysis of brain electrical and magnetic signals, in *Handbook of Electroencephalography and Clinical Neurophysiology,* Revised Series, vol. 1, (Elsevier, Amsterdam).

Gevins A. S., Morgan N. H., Bressler S. L., Doyle J. C., and Cutillo B. A. (1986) Improved event-related potential estimation using statistical pattern classification. *Electroencephalogr. Clin. Neurophysiol.* **64,** 177–186.

Gevins A. S., Bressler S. L., Cutillo B. A., Doyle J. C., Morgan N. H., and Zeitlin G. M. (1984) Neurocognitive pattern analysis of an auditory and visual numeric motor control task, Part 1: Development of methods. A.F.O.S.R. Final Report, Contract No. F49620-82-K-0008.

Gevins A. S., Doyle J. C., Cutillo B. A., Schaffer R. E., Tannehill R. S. and Bressler S. L. (1985) Neurocognitive pattern analysis of a visuospatial task: low-frequency evoked correlations. *Psychophysiology,* **22,** 32–43.

Gevins A. S., Schaffer R. E., Doyle J. C., Cutillo B. A., Tannehill R. L., and Bressler S. L. (1983) Shadows of thoughts: Rapidly changing, asymmetric brain-potential patterns of a brief visuomotor task. *Science*, **220**, 97–99.

Gevins A. S., Cutillo B. A., Bressler, S. L., Morgan N. H., White R. M., Illes, J., and Greer D. S. (1989) Event-related covariances during a bimanual visuomotor task: II. Preparation and feedback *Electroencephalogr. Clin. Neurophysiol.* **74**, 147–160.

Gilden L., Vaughan H. H., Jr., and Costa L. D. (1966) Summated human EEG potentials associated with voluntary movements. *Electroencephalogr. Clin. Neurophysiol.* **20**, 433–438.

Glaser E. M. and Ruchkin D. S. (1979) *Principles of neurobiological signal analysis.* (Academic, New York).

Gloor P. (1985) Neuronal generators and the problem of localization in electroencephalography: Application of volume conductor theory to electroencephalography. *J. Clin. Neurophysiol.* **2**, 327–354.

Goff G. D., Matsumiya T., Allison T., and Goff W. R. (1977) The scalp topography of human somatosensory and auditory evoked potentials. *Electroencephalogr. Clin. Neurophysiol.* **42**, 57–76.

Goff W. R. (1974) Human average evoked potentials: Procedures for stimulating and recording, in *Bioelectric Recording Techniques Part B, EEG and Human Brain Potentials* (Thompson R. F. and Patterson M. M. eds.), Academic, New York, pp. 101–156.

Goff W. R., Allison T., and Vaughan H. G., Jr. (1978) The functional neuroanatomy of event-related potentials, in *Event-Related Brain Potentials in Man.* (Callaway E., Tueting P., and Koslow S. H., eds.), Academic, New York, pp. 1–79.

Goff W. R., Allison T., Shapiro A., and Rosner B. S. (1966) Cerebral somatosensory responses evoked during sleep in man. *Electroencephalogr. Clin. Neurophysiol.* **21**, 1–9.

Goff W. R., Williamson P. D., Van Gilder J. C., Allison T., and Fisher T. C. (1980) Neural origins of long-latency evoked potentials recorded from the depth and cortical surface of the brain in man, in *Clinical Uses of Cerebral, Brainstem, and Spinal Somatosensory Evoked Potentials* (Desmedt J. E., ed), *(Prog. Clin. Neurophysiol.,* vol. 7) Krager, Basel, pp. 126–145.

Goldberg G. (1985) Supplementary motor artea structure and function: Review and hypotheses. *Behav. Brain Sci.* **8**, 567–616.

Goldberg G., Kwan H. C., Borrett D., and Murphy J. T. (1984) Topography of the movement-associated scalp potential suggests initiation of spontaneous movement by the supplementary motor area. *Arch. Phys. Med. Rehabil.* **65**, 662.

Gombi R., Cooper R., Papakostopoulos D., and Crow H. J. (1973) Measurement of slowly changing potentials in the human brain. *Electroencephalogr. Clin. Neurophysiol.* **34**, 109.

Goodin D. S., Squires K. C., and Starr A. (1978) Long latency event-related components of the auditory evoked potential in dementia. *Brain* **101**, 635–648.

Goodin D. S., Squires K. C., and Starr A. (1983) Variations in early and late event-related components of the auditory evoked potential with task difficulty. *Electroencephalogr. Clin. Neurophysiol.* **55**, 680–686.

Graham J., Greenwood R., and Lecky B. (1980). Cortical deafness. A case report and review of the literature. *J. Neurol. Sci.* **48**, 35–49.

Groll-Knapp E., Ganglberger J., Haider M., and Schmid H. (1980) Stereoelectroencephalographic studies on event-related slow potentials in the human brain, in *Electroencephalography and Clinical Neurophysiology* (Lechner H. and Aranibar A., eds), Execpta Medica, Amsterdam, pp. 746–760.

Grossman R. G. and Hampton T. (1968) Depolarization of cortical glial cells during electrocortical activity. *Brain Res.* **11**, 316–324.

Grossman R. G. and Hampton T. (1970) Relationship of cortical glial cell depolarization to electrocortical surface wave activity. *Electroencephalogr. Clin. Neurophysiol.* **28**, 95–96.

Grossman R. G., Whiterids L., and Hampton T. L. (1969) The time course of evoked depolarization of cortical glial cells. *Brain Res.* **14**, 401–415.

Grozinger B., Kornhuber H. H., and Kriebel J. (1977) Human cerebral potentials preceding speech production, phonation, and movements of the mouth and tongue, with reference to respiratory and extracerebral potentials, in *Language and Cerebral Specialization in Man: Cerebral ERPs* (Desmedt J. E., ed.), Karger, Basel, pp. 87–103.

Grozinger B., Kornhuber H. H., Kriebel J., Szirtes J., and Westphal K. T. P. (1980) The Bereitschaftspotential preceding the act of speaking. Also an analysis of artifacts, in *Motivation, Motor and Sensory Processes of the Brain: Electrical Potentials, Behaviour and Clinical Use.* (H. H. Kornhuber and L. Deecke, eds.) (*Progress in Brain Research* vol. 54), Elsevier, Amsterdam, pp. 798–804.

Grunewald-Zuberbier E. and Grunewald G. (1978) Goal-directed movement potentials of human cerebral cortex. *Exp. Brain Res.* **33**, 135–138.

Grynszpan F. and Geselowitz D. B. (1973) Model studies of the magnetocardiogram. *Biophys. J.* **13**, 911–926.

Haldeman S., Bradley W. E., Bhatia N. N., and Johnson B. K. (1982) Pudendal evoked responses. *Arch. Neurol.* **39**, 280–283.

Halgren E. Firing of human hippocampal units in relation to voluntary movements (in preparation).

Halgren E. (1989) Insights from evoked potentials into the neuropsychological mechanisms of reading. In *Neurobiology of Cognition* (Scheibel A. and Weschsler A., eds.), Guilford, New York, in press.

Halgren E. and Smith M. E. (1987) Cognitive evoked potentials as modulatory processes in human memory formation and retrieval. *Hum. Neurobiol.* **6,** 129–140.

Halgren E., Babb T. L., and Crandall P. H. (1978) Activity of human hippocampal formation and amygdala neurons during memory testing. *Electroencephalogr. Clin. Neurophysiol.* **45,** 585–601.

Halgren E., Squires N. K., Wilson C. L., and Crandall P. H. (1982) Brain generators of evoked potentials: the late (endogenous) components. *Bull. Los Angeles Neurol. Soc.* **47,** 108–123.

Halgren E., Stapleton J. M., Smith M., and Altafullah I. (1986) Generators of the human scalp P3(s), in *Evoked Potentials* (Cracco R. and Bodis-Wollner I., eds.), pp. 269–286. Alan R. Liss New York

Halgren E., Squires N. K., Wilson C. L., Rohrbaugh J. W., Babb T. L., and Crandall P. H. (1980) Endogenous potentials generated in the human hippocampal formation and amygdala by infrequent events. *Science* **210,** 803–805.

Halgren E., Wilson C. L., Squires N. K., Engel J., Jr., Walter R. D., and Crandall P. H. (1983) Dynamics of the human hippocampal contribution to memory, in *Neurobiology of the Hippocampus,* (Seifert W., ed.) Academic, London, pp. 529–572.

Hamilton C. E., Peters J. F., and Knott J. R. (1973) Task initiation and amplitude of the CNV. *Electroencephalogr. Clin. Neurophysiol.* **34,** 587–592.

Hari R. and Ilmoniemi R. J. (1986) Cerebral magnetic fields. *CRC Crit. Rev. Biomed. Eng.* **14,** 93–126.

Hari R. and Kaukoranta E. (1985) Neuromagnetic studies of somatosensory system: Principles and examples. *Prog. Neurobiol.* **24,** 233–256.

Hari R. and Lounasmaa O. V. (1989) Recording and interpretation of cerebral magnetic fields. *Science* **244,** 432–436.

Hari R., Kaila K., Katila T., Tuomisto T., and Varpula T. (1982) Interstimulus interval dependence of the auditory vertex response and its magnetic counterpart: Implications for their neural generation. *Electroencephalogr. Clin. Neurophysiol.* **54,** 561–569.

Hari R., Reinikainen K., Kaukoianta E., Hamalaninen M., Slmonemi R., and Peuttlinen A. (1984a) Somatosensory evoked cerebral magnetic fields from SI and SII in man. *Electroencephalogr. Clin. Neurophysiol.* 57, 254–263.

Hari R., Hamalalainen M., Ilmoniemi R., Kaukoranta E., Reinikainen K., Salminen J., Alho K., Naatanen R., and Sams M. (1984b) Responses of the primary auditory cortex to pitch changes in a sequence of tone pips: neuromagnetic recordings in man. *Neurosci. Lett.* **50**, 127–132.

Hari R., Antervo A., Katila T., Poutanen T., Seppanen M., Tuomisto T., and Varpula T. (1983) Cerebral magnetic fields associated with voluntary limb movements in man. *Il Nuovo Cimento* **2**, 484–494.

Harker L. A., Hosick E., Voots R. J., and Mendel M. I. (1977) Influence of succinylcholine on middle component auditory evoked potentials. *Arch. Otolaryngol.* **103**, 133–137.

Harmony T. (1984) *Neurometric Assessment of Brain Dysfunction in Neurological Patients* (Erlbaum, Hillsdale, New Jersey).

Harner P. F. and Sannit T. (1974) *A Review of the International Ten-Twenty System of Electrode Placement* (Grass Instrument Company, Quincy, Massachusetts).

Harter M. R. and White C. T. (1970) Evoked cortical responses to checkerboard patterns: Effect of check-size as a function of visual acuity. *Electroencephalogr. Clin. Neurophysiol.* **28**, 48–54.

Hashimoto I., Ishiyama Y., Yoshimoto T., and Nemoto S. (1981) Brainstem auditory-evoked potentials recorded directly from human brain-stem and thalamus. *Brain* **104**, 841–859.

Hashimoto I. (1984) Somatosensory evoked potentials from the human brainstem: Origins of short-latency potentials. *Electroencephalogr. Clin. Neurophysiol.* **57**, 221–227.

Hashimoto S., Gemba H., and Sasaki K. (1981) Distribution of slow cortical potentials preceding self-paced hand and hindlimb movements in the premotor and motor areas of monkeys. *Brain Res.* **224**, 247–259.

He B., Musha T., Okamoto Y., Homma S., Nakajima Y., and Sato T. (1987) Electric dipole tracing in the brain by means of the boundary element method and its accuracy. *IEEE Trans. Biomed. Eng.* **BME-34**, 406–414.

Hecaen H. and Albert M. L. (1978) *Human Neuropsychology*, Wiley, New York.

Hecox K. and Galambos R. (1974) Brain stem auditory evoked response in human infants and adults. *Arch. Otolaryngol.* **99**, 30–33.

Heit G., Smith M. E., and Halgren E. Human medial temporal-lobe neuronal firing during memory tasks. *Brain*, in press.

Heringa A., Stegeman D. F., Uijen G. J. H., and de Weerd J. P. C. (1982) Solution methods of electrical field problems in physiology. *IEEE Trans. Biomed. Eng.* **BME-29**, 34–42.

Herpers M. J., Caberg H. B., and Mol J. M. F. (1981) Human cerebral potentials evoked by moving dynamic random dot stereograms. *Electroencephalogr. Clin. Neurophysiol.* **52**, 50–56.

Hillyard S. A. (1973) The CNV and human behavior. A review, in *Event-Related Slow Potentials of the Brain: Their Relations to Behavior* (McCallum W. C., and Knott J. R., eds.) *(Electroencephalogr. Clin. Neurophysiol. Suppl. 33)*, Elsevier: Amsterdam. pp. 161–171.

Hillyard S. A. and Galambos R. (1970) Eye movement artifact in the CNV. *Electroencephalogr. Clin. Neurophysiol.* **28**, 173–182.

Hillyard S. A. and Kutas M. (1983) Electrophysiology of cognitive processing. *Annu. Rev. Psychol.* **34**, 33–61.

Hillyard S. A. and Picton T. W. (1988) Electrophysiology of congnition, in: *Handbook of Physiology: The Nervous System V*, American Physiological Society: Bethesda, Maryland, pp. 519–584.

Hink R. F., Kohler H., Deecke L., and Kornhuber H. H. (1982) Risk-taking and the human Bereitschaftspotential. *Electroencephalogr. Clin. Neurophysiol.* **53**, 361–373.

Hinman C. L. and Buchwald J. S. (1983) Depth evoked potential and single unit correlates of vertex midlatency auditory evoked responses. *Brain Res.* **264**, 57–67.

Hjorth B. (1976) Localization of foci in the scalp field, in *Quantitative Analytic Studies in Epilepsy*, (Kellaway O. and Peterson I., eds.) Raven, New York, pp. 483–492.

Hosek R. S., Sances A., Jodat R., and Larson S. (1978) The contribution of intracerebral currents to the EEG and evoked potentials. *IEEE Trans. Biomed. Eng.* **5**, 405–413.

Hughes J. R. and Fino J. J. (1985) A review of generators of the brainstem auditory evoked potential: Contribution of an experimental study. *J. Clin. Neurophysiol.* **2**, 355–381.

Huttunen J., Hari R., and Leinonen L. (1987) Cerebral magnetic responses to stimulation of ulnar and median nerves. *Electroencephalogr. Clin. Neurophysiol.* **66**, 391–400.

Irwin D. A., Knott J. R., McAdam D. W., and Rebert C. S. (1966) Motivational determinants of the contingent negative variation. *Electroencephalogr. Clin. Neurophysiol.* **21**, 538–543.

Jacoby L. L. (1983) Perceptual enhancement: persistent effects of an experience. *J. Exp. Psychol. (Learn. Mem. Cogn.)* **9**, 21–38.

Jarvilehto T. and Fruhstorfer H. (1970) Differentiation between slow cortical potentials associated with motor and mental acts in man. *Exp. Brain Res.* **11**, 309–317.

Jasper H. H. (1958) The ten-twenty electrode system of the International Federation. *Electroencephalogr. Clin. Neurophysiol.* **10**, 371–375.

Jewett D. L. and Wiliston J. S. (1971) Auditory-evoked far fields averaged from the scalp of humans. *Brain* **94**, 681–696.

John E. R., Ruchkin, D. S., and Vidal, J. J. (1978) Measurement of event-related potentials, in *Event-Related Brain Potentials in Man*, (Callaway E., Tueting P., Koslow S. H., eds.), Academic, New York, pp. 93–138.

John E. R., Karmel B. Z., Corning W. C., Easton, P., Brown, D., Ahn, H., John, M., Harmony, T., Prichep, L., Toro, A., Gerson, I., Bartlett, F., Thatcher, R., Kaye, H., Valdes, H., and Schwartz, E. (1977) Neurometrics. Numerical taxonomy identifies different profiles of brain. *Science* **196**, 1393–1410.

Johnson R. (1980) Event-related potentials accompanying voluntary movement in Rhesus monkeys, in *Motivation, Motor and Sensory Processes of the Brain: Electrical Potentials, Behavior and Clinical Use.* (Kornhuber, H. H., and Deecke, L., eds.) (*Prog. Brain Res.*, vol. 54) Elsevier/North Holland, Amsterdam, pp. 70–73.

Johnson R., Jr. and Fedio, P. (1986) P300 activity in patients following unilateral temporal lobectomy: A preliminary report, in *Cerebral Psychophysiology: Studies in Event-Related Potentials (EEG Suppl. 38)*, McCallum W. C., Zappoli R., and Denoth F. eds.) Elsevier, Amsterdam. pp. 552–554.

Johnson R. Jr., Rohrbaugh J. W., and Parasuraman R. (eds.) (1987) Current trends in event-related potential research, in *Electroencephalogr. Clin. Neurophysiol. Suppl. 40*, Elsevier, Amsterdam.

Jones B. E. and Moore R. Y. (1977) Ascending projections of the locus coeruleus in the rat. II. Autoradiographic study. *Brain Res.* **127**, 23–53.

Julesz B. and Kropfl W. (1982) Binocular neurons and cyclopean visually evoked potentials in monkey and man. *Ann. NY Acad. Sci.* **388**, 37–44.

Jung R., Altenmuller E., and Natsch B. (1984) Zur Hemispharendominanz fur Sprache and Rechnen: Elektrophysiologische Korrelate einer Linksdominanz bei Linkshandern. *Neuropsychologia.* **22**, 755–775.

Jung R., Hufschmidt A., and Moschallski W. (1982) Langsame hirnpotentiale beim schreiben: Die wechselwirkung von schreibhand und sprachdominanz bie rechtshandern. *Arch. Psychiatr. Nervenkr.* **232**, 305–324.

Just M. A. and Carpenter P. A. (1980) A theory of reading: From eye fixations to comprehension. *Psychol. Rev.* **87(4)**, 329–354.

Just M. A. and Carpenter P. A. (1987) *The Psychology of Reading and Language Comprehension*, Allyn and Bacon, Newton, MA.

Kaga K., Hink R. F., Shinoda Y., and Suzuki J. (1980) Evidence for a primary cortical origin of middle latency auditory evoked potentials in cats. *Electroencephalogr. Clin. Neurophysiol.* **50**, 254–266.

Karahashi Y. and Goldring S. (1966) Intracellular potentials from "idle" cells in cerebral cortex of cat. *Electroencephalogr. Clin. Neurophysiol.* **20,** 600–607.

Karis D., Fabiani M., and Donchin D. (1984) "P300" and memory: Individual differences in the von Restorff effect. *Cogn. Psychol.* **16,** 177–216.

Karrer R., Cohen J., and Tueting P. (eds.) (1984) Brain and information: Event-related potentials. *Ann. NY Acad. Sci.,* **425,**

Karrer R., Kohn H., and Ivins J. (1973) Large steady potential shifts accompanying phasic arousal during CNV recording in man, in *Event-Related Slow Potentials of the Brain: Their Relations to Behavior* (McCallum W. C. and Knott J. R., eds.) *(Electroenceph. Clin. Neurophysiol. Suppl. 33),* Elsevier, Amsterdam, pp. 119–124.

Kato M. and Tanji J. (1972) Cortical motor potentials accompanying voluntary controlled single motor unit discharge in human finger muscle. *Brain Res.* **47,** 103–110.

Kaufman L. and Williamson S. J. (1986) The neuromagnetic field, in *Evoked Potentials,* (Cracco R. C., and Bodis-Wollner B., eds.), Alan R. Liss, New York, pp. 85–98.

Kavanagh R. N., Darcey T. M., Lehmann D., and Fender D. H. (1978) Evaluation of methods for three-dimensional localization of electrical sources in the human brain. *IEEE Trans. Biomed. Eng.,* **25,** 421–429.

Kenvanishvili Z. S. and Von Sprecht H. (1979) Human slow auditory evoked potentials during natural and drug-induced sleep. *Electroencephalogr. Clin. Neurophysiol.* **47,** 280–288.

Kileny K., Dobson D., and Gelfand E. E. (1983) Middle-latency auditory evoked responses during open-heart surgery with hypothermia. *Electroencephalogr. Clin. Neurophysiol.* **55,** 268–276.

King D. W., So E. L., Marcus R., and Gallagher B. B. (1986) Techniques and applications of sphenoidal recording. *J. Clin. Neurophysiol.* **3,** 51–65.

Klass D. W. and Bickford R. G. (1960) Glossokinetic potentials appearing in the electroencephalogram. *Electroencephalogr. Clin. Neurophysiol.* **12,** 188.

Klee J. and Rall W. (1977) Computed potentials of cortically arranged populations of neurons. *J. Neurophysiol.* **40,** 644–666.

Knight R. T. (1984) Decreased response to novel stimuli after prefrontal lesions in man. *Electroencephalogr. Clin. Neurophysiol.* **59,** 9–20.

Knight R. T. Neural mechanisms of event related potentials evidence from lesion studies, in *Eighth International Conference of Event Related Potentials of the Brain,* (Rohrbaugh J., Johnson R., Jr., and Parasuranam R., eds.) Oxford Univ. Press, Oxford. (in press)

Knight R. T., Hillyard S. A., Woods D. L., and Neville H. J. (1980) The effects of frontal and temporal-parietal lesions on the auditory evoked potential in man. *Electroencephalogr. Clin. Neurophysiol.* **50,** 112–124.

Knight R. T., Scabini D., Woods D. L., and Clayworth C. (1988) The effects of lesions of superior temporal gyrus and inferior parietal lobe on temporal and vertex components of the human AEP. *Electroencephalogr. Clin. Neurophysiol.* **70,** 499–509.

Kobal G. and Hummel C. (1988) Cerebral chemosensory evoked potentials elicited by chemical stimulation of the human olfactory and respiratory nasal mucosa. *Electroencephalogr. Clin. Neurophysiol.* **71,** 241–250.

Koles Z. J., Kasmia A., Paranjape R. B., and McLean D. R. (1989) Computed radial-current topography of the brain: patterns associated with the normal and abnormal EEG. *Electroencephalogr. Clin. Neurophysiol.* **72,** 41–47.

Kooi K. A. and Marshall R. E. (1979) *Visual Evoked Potentials in the Central Disorders of the Visual System* (Harper and Row, Philadelphia).

Kooi K. A., Tipton A. C., and Marshall R. E. (1971) Polarities and field configurations of the vertex components of the human auditory evoked response: A reinterpretation. *Electroencephalogr. Clin. Neurophysiol.* **31,** 166–169.

Kornhuber H. H. (1971) Motor functions of cerebellum and basal ganglia: the cerebellocortical saccadic (ballistic) clock, the cerebellonuclear hold regulator, and the basal ganglia ramp (voluntary speed smooth movement) generator. *Kybernetik* **8,** 157–162.

Kornhuber H. H. (1984) Attention, readiness for action and the stages of voluntary decision—Some electrophysiological correlates in man. *Exp. Brain Res.* **Suppl. 9,** 420–429.

Kornhuber H. H. and Deecke L. (1965) Hirnpotentialanderungen bei Wilkurbewegungen und passiven Bewegungen des Menschen: Bereitschaftspotential und reafferente Potentiale. *Pflugers Arch.* **284,** 1–17.

Kramer A. F. (1985) The interpretation of the component structure of event-related brain potentials: An analysis of expert judgements. *Psychophysiology* **3,** 334–344.

Kraus N., Ozdamar O., Hier D., and Stein L. (1982) Auditory middle latency responses (MLRs) in patients with cortical lesions. *Electroencephalogr. Clin. Neurophysiol.* **54,** 275–287.

Kraut M. A., Arezzo J. C., and Vaughan H. G., Jr. (1985) Intracortical generators of the flash VEP in monkeys. *Electroencephalogr. Clin. Neurophysiol.* **62,** 300–312.

Kulics A. T. and Cauller L. J. (1986) Cerebral cortical somatosensory evoked responses, multiple unit activity and current source-densities: Their interrelationships and significance to somatic sensation as revealed by stimulation of the awake monkey's hand. *Exp. Brain Res.* **62,** 46–60.

Kurtzberg D. and Vaughan H. G. (1982) Topographic analysis of human cortical potentials preceding self-initiated and visually triggered saccades. *Brain Res.* **243,** 1–9.

Kutas M. and Donchin E. (1974) Studies of squeezing: Handedness, responding hand, response force and asymmetry of the readiness potential, *Science* **186,** 545–548.

Kutas M. and Donchin E. (1977) The effect of handedness, of responding hand and of response force on the contralateral dominance of the readiness potential, in *Attention, Voluntary Contraction and Event-Related Cerebral Potentials* (Desmedt, J. E. ed.) *(Prog. Clin. Neurophysiol., Vol. 1),* Karger, Basel, pp. 189–210.

Kutas M. and Donchin E. (1980) Preparation to respond as manifested by movement-related brain potentials. *Brain Res.* **202,** 95–115.

Kutas M. and Hillyard S. A. (1980a) Reading senseless sentences: Brain potentials reflect semantic incongruity. *Science* **207,** 203–205.

Kutas M. and Hillyard S. A. (1980c) Event-related brain potentials to semantically inappropriate and surprisingly large words. *Biol. Psychol.* **11,** 99–116.

Kutas M. and Hillyard S. A. (1983) Event-related brain potentials to grammatical errors and semantic anomalies. *Mem. Cogn.* **11,** 539–550.

Kutas M. and Hillyard S. A. (1984b) Brain potentials during reading reflect word expectancy and semantic association. *Nature* **307,** 161–163.

Kutas M., Hillyard S. A., and Gazzaniga M. S. (1988) Processing of semantic anomaly by right and left hemispheres of commissurotomy patients. Evidence from event-related brain potentials. *Brain* **111,** 553–576.

Kutas M., McCarthy G., and Donchin E. (1977) Augmenting mental chronometry: The P300 as a measure of stimulus evaluation time. *Science* **197,** 792–795.

Kutas M., Neville H. J., and Holcomb P. J. (1987) A preliminary comparison of the N400 response to semantic anomalies during reading, listening, and signing, in: *The London Symposia (EEG Suppl. 39),* (Ellingson R. J., Murray N. M. F., Halliday A. M. eds.) Elseiver, Amsterdam, pp. 325–330.

Kutas M., Van Petten C., and Besson M. (1988) Event-related potential asymmetries during the reading of sentences. *Electroencephalogr. Clin. Neurophysiol.* **69**, 218–233.

Kutas M. and Van Petten C. (1987) Event-related brain potential studies of language, in *Advances in Psychophysiology* (Ackles P. K., Jennings J. R. and Coles M. G. H., eds.), JAI Press, Greenwich, Connecticut.

Lagerlund T. D. and Sharbough F. W. (1989) Computer simulation of the generation of the electroencephalogram. *Electroencephalogr. Clin. Neurophysiol.* **72**, 31–40.

Lang W., Lang M., Uhl F., Kornhuber A. (1987) Slow negative potential shifts in a verbal concept formation task, in: (Johnson R., Jr., Rohrbaugh J. W., and Parasuraman R., eds), *Current Trends in Event-Related Brain Potential Research (Electroencephalogr. Clin. Neurophysiol., Suppl. 40)* Elsevier, Amsterdam, pp. 335–340.

Lang W., Lang M., Heise B., Deecke L., and Kornhuber H. H. (1984) Brain potentials related to voluntary hand tracking, motivation, and attention. *Hum. Neurobiol.* **3**, 235–240.

Laplane D., Talairach J., Meininger V., Bancaud J., and Orgogozo J. M. (1977) Clinical consequences of corticectomies involving the supplementary motor area in man. *J. Neurol. Sci.* **34**, 310–314.

Lee B. L., Luders H., Lesser R. P., Dinner D. S., and Morris H. H. (1986) Cortical potentials related to voluntary and passive finger movements recorded from subdural electrodes in humans. *Ann. Neurol.* **20**, 32–37.

Lee Y. S., Lueders H., Dinner D. S., Lesser R. P., Hahn J., and Klemm G. (1984) Recording of auditory evoked potentials in man using chronic subdural electrodes. *Brain* **107**, 115–131.

Legatt A. D., Arezzo J. C., and Vaughan H. G., Jr. (1986) Short-latency auditory evoked potentials in the monkey. II. Intracranial generators. *Electroencephalogr. Clin. Neurophysiol.* **64**, 53–73.

Lehmann D. and Julesz B. (1978) Lateralized cortical potentials evoked in humans by dynamic random-dot stereograms. *Vision Res.* **18**, 1265–1271.

Lehmann D. and Skrandies W. (1984) Spatial analysis of evoked potentials in man—A review. *Prog. Neurobiol.* **23**, 227–250.

Lehtonen J. B. and Koivikko M. J. (1971) The use of non-cephalic reference electrode in recording cerebral evoked potentials in man. *Electroencephalogr. Clin. Neurophysiol.* **31**, 154–156.

Lesevre N. and Joseph J. P. (1979) Modifications of the pattern-evoked potential (PEP) in relation to the stimulated part of the visual field (clues for the most probable origin of each component). *Electroencephalogr. Clin. Neurophysiol.* **47**, 183–203.

Leung L. S. (1979) Potentials evoked by alvear tract in hippocampal CA1 region of rats. II. Spatial field analysis. *J. Neurophysiol.* **42**, 1571–1589.

Libet B., Wright E. W., Jr., and Gleason C. A. (1982) Readiness-potentials preceding unrestricted "spontaneous" vs. preplanned voluntary acts. *Electroencephalogr. Clin. Neurophysiol.* **54**, 322–335.

Libet B., Gleason C. A., Wright E. W., Jr., and Pearl D. K. (1983a) Time conscious intention to act in relation to onset of cerebral activities (readiness-potential): The unconscious initiation of a freely voluntary act. *Brain* **106**, 623–642.

Libet B., Wright E. W., Jr. and Gleason C. A. (1983b) Preparation-or intention-to-act in relation to pre-event potentials recorded at the vertex. *Electroencephalogr. Clin. Neurophysiol.* **56**, 367–372.

Loiselle L., Stamm J. S., Marinsky S., and Whipple S. C. (1980) Evoked potential and behavioral signs of attentive dysfunction in hyperactive boys. *Psychophysiology* **17**, 193–201.

Lopes da Silva F. and van Rotterdam A. (1982) Biophysical aspects of EEG and MEG generation, in: *Electroencephalography: Basic Principles, Clinical Application and Related Fields* (Niedermeyer E., Lopes da Silva F., eds), Urban & Schwarzenberg, Baltimore, 15–26.

Lopes da Silva F. H., Storm van Leeuwen W., and Remond A. (1986) Clinical applications of computer analysis of EEG and other neurophysiological signals, in *Handbook of Electroencephalography and Clinical Neurophysiology, Revised Series,* vol. 2 (Elsevier, Amsterdam).

Lorente de No R. (1934) Studies on the structure of the cerebral cortex. II. Continuation of the study of the ammonic system. *J. Psychol. Neurol.* **45**, 113–177.

Lorente de No. R. (1947) A study of nerve physiology, in *Studies from Rockefeller Inst. Med. Res.,* vol. 132, pt. II, New York, Rockefeller Institute of Medical Research.

Loveless N. (1979) Event-related slow potentials of the brain as expressions of orienting function, in *The Orienting Reflex in Humans* (Kimmel H. D., van Olst E. H., Orlebeke J. F., eds.), Erlbaum, Hillsdale, New Jersey, pp. 77–100.

Loveless N. E. and Sanford A. J. (1973) The CNV baseline: Considerations of internal consistency of data. *Electroencephalogr. Clin. Neurophysiol. Suppl.* **33**, 19–23.

Low M. D. (1979) Event-related potentials and the electroencephalogram in patients with proven brain lesions, in *Cognitive Components in*

Cerebral Event-Related-Potentials and Selective Attention (Desmedt J. E., ed.), Karger, Basel, pp. 258–264.

Low M. D. and Purves S. J. (1975) Sensory evoked potentials, CNV and the EEG in patients with proven brain lesion. *Electroencephalogr. Clin. Neurophysiol.* **39**, 208.

Low M. D. and Swift S. J. (1971) The contingent negative variation and the resting DC potential of the human brain: effects of situational anxiety. *Neuropsychol.* **9**, 203–208.

Low M. D., Borda R. P., Frost J. D., and Kelleway P. (1966) Surface negative slow potential shift associated with conditioning in man. *Neurology (NY)* **16**, 771–782.

Low M. D., Coats A. C., Rettig G. M., and McSherry J. W. (1967) Anxiety, attentiveness-alertness: A phenomenological study of the CNV. *Neuropsychol.* **5**, 379–384.

Lueders, H., Lesser R., Hahn J., Little J., and Klem G. (1983) Subcortical somatosensory evoked potentials to median nerve stimulation. *Brain* **106**, 341–372.

Lutzenberger W., Birbaumer N., Elbert T., and Rockstroh B. (1980) Self-regulation of slow cortical potentials in normal subjects and patients with frontal lobe sessions. *Prog. Brain Res.* **54**, 427–430.

Lux R. L., Smith C. R., Wyatt R. F., and Abildskov J. A. (1978) Limited lead selection for estimation of body surface potential maps in electrocardiography. *IEEE Trans. Biomed. Eng.* **25**, 270–276.

McAdam D. W. (1969) Increases in CNS excitability during negative cortical slow potentials in man. *Electroencephalogr. Clin. Neurophysiol.* **26**, 216–219.

McAdam D. W. and Rubin E. H. (1971) Readiness potential, vertex positive wave, contingent negative variation, and accuracy of perception. *Electroencephalogr. Clin. Neurophysiol.* **30**, 511–517.

McAdam D. W. and Seales D. M. (1969) Bereitschaftspotential enhancement with increased level of motivation. *Electroencephalogr. Clin. Neurophsyiol.* **27**, 73–75.

McAdam D. W. and Whitaker H. A. (1971) Language production: Electroencephalographic localization in the normal human brain. *Science* **172**, 499–502.

McAdam D. W., Irwin D. A., Robert C. S., and Knott J. R. (1966) Conative control of the contingent negative variation. *Electroencephalogr. Clin. Neurophysiol.* **21**, 194–195.

McCallum W. C. (1979) Cognitive aspects of slow potential changes, in *Prog. Clin. Neurophysiol.*, vol. 6 (Desmedt J. E., ed.), Karger, Basel, pp. 151–171.

McCallum W. C. and Cummins B. (1973) The effects of brain lesions on the contingent negative variation in neurosurgical patients. *Electroencephalogr. Clin. Neurophysiol.* **35,** 449–456.

McCallum W. C. and Curry S. H. (1981) Late slow wave components of auditory evoked potentials: Their cognitive significance and interaction. *Electroencephalogr. Clin. Neurophysiol.* **51,** 123–137.

McCallum W. C. and Papakostopoulos D. (1976) Distribution of CNV and other slow potential changes in human brainstem structures, in *The Responsive Brain* (McCallum W. C. and Knott J. R., eds.), Wright, Bristol, pp. 205–210.

McCallum W. C., Farmer S. F., and Pocock P. K. (1984) The effects of physical and semantic incongruities on auditory event-related potentials. *Electroencephalogr. Clin. Neurophysiol.* **59,** 477–488.

McCallum W. C., Papakostopoulos D., Gombi R., Winter A. L., Copper R., and Griffith H. B. (1973) Event related slow potential changes in human brain stem. *Nature* **252,** 465–467.

McCarthy G. and Wood C. C. (1985) Scalp distributions of event-related potentials: An ambiguity associated with analysis of variance models. *Electroencephalogr. Clin. Neurophysiol.,* **62,** 203–208.

McCarthy G. and Wood C. C. (1987) Intracranial recordings of endogenous ERPs in humans, in *The London Symposia* (Ellingson R. J., Murray N. M. F., Halliday, A. M., eds.) *(EEG Suppl. 39),* Elsevier, Amsterdam, pp. 331–337.

McCarthy G., Wood C. C., Williamson P. D., and Spencer D. D. (1989) Task-dependent field potentials in human hippocampal formation. *J. Neuroscience,* in press.

McGillem C. D., Aunon J. I., and Pomalaza C. A. (1985) Improved waveform estimation procedures for event-related potentials. *IEEE Trans. Biomed. Eng.* **BME-32,** 371–379.

MacKay D. M. (1983) On-line source-density computation with a minimum of electrodes. *Electroencephalogr. Clin. Neurophysiol.,* **56,** 696–698.

MacKay D. M. (1984) Source density analysis of scalp potentials during evaluated action. *Exp. Brain Res.* **54,** 73–94.

Maclin E., Okada Y. C., Kaufman L., and Williamson S. J. (1983) Retinotopic map on the visual cortex for eccentrically placed patterns: first noninvasive measurement. *Il Nuovo Cimento* **2,** 410–419.

McSherry J. W. (1973) Physiological Origins. A review, in *Event-Related Slow Potentials of the Brain: Their relations to Behavior* (McCallum W. C. and Knott J. R., eds.), *(Electroencephalogr. Clin. Neurophysiol., Suppl. 33)* pp. 53–61.

McSherry J. W., and Borda R. P. (1973) The intracortical distribution of the CNV in rhesus monkey, in Event-related slow potentials of the brain: their relations to behavior (McCallum W. C. and Knott J. R., eds.) *(Electroencephalogr. Clin. Neurophysiol., Suppl. 33)*, pp. 69–74.

Mandler G. (1980) Recognizing: the judgement of previous occurrence. *Psychol. Rev.* **87**, 23–81.

Margerison J. H. and Corsellis J. A. N. (1966) Epilepsy and the temporal lobes. *Brain* **89**, 499–530.

Marquardt D. W. (1964) Confidence region calculations. *IBM Share Program Catalog No. 3094*, Appendix Exhibit B.

Marsh G. R. and Thompson L. W. (1973) Effect of verbal and non-verbal psychological set on hemispheric asymmetries in the CNV, in *Event-Related Slow Potentials of the Brain: Their Relations to Behavior* (McCallum W. D., and Knott J. R., eds.) *(Electroenceph. Clin. Neurophysiol. Suppl. 33)*, Elsevier, Amsterdam, pp. 195–200.

Marton M., Szirtes J., and Breuer P. (1985a) Electrocortical signs of word categorization in saccade-related brain potentials and visual evoked potentials. *Int. J. Psychophysiol.* **3**, 131–144.

Marton M., Szirtes J., Donauer N., and Breuer P. (1985b) Saccade-related brain potentials in semantic categorization tasks. *Biol. Psychol.* **20**, 163–184.

Maruyama Y., Shimoji K., Shimizu H., Kuribayashi H., and Fujioka H. (1982) Human spinal cord potentials evoked by different sources of stimulation and conduction velocities along the cord. *J. Neurophysiol.* **48**, 1098–1107.

Matsuo F., Peters J. F., and Reilly E. L. (1975) Electrical phenomena associated with movements of the eyelid. *Electroencephalogr. Clin. Neurophysiol.* **38**, 507–511.

Mauguiere F., Courjon J., and Schott B. (1983a) Dissociation of early SEP components in unilateral traumatic section of the lower medulla. *Ann. Neurol.* **13**, 309–313.

Mauguiere F., Desmedt J. E., and Courjon J. (1983b) Neural generators of N18 and P14 far field somatosensory evoked potentials: Patients with lesion of thalamus or of thalamo-cortical radiations. *Electroencephalogr. Clin. Neurophysiol.* **56**, 283–292.

Mauguiere F., Desmedt J. E., and Courjon J. (1983c) Astereognosis and dissociated loss of frontal or parietal components of somatosensory evoked potentials in hemispheric lesions: Detailed correlations with clinical signs and computerized tomography scanning. *Brain* **106**, 271–311.

Meador K. J., Loring D. W., King D. W., Gallagher B. B., Gould M. J., Flanigan H. F., and Smith J. R. (1989) Limbic evoked potentials predict site of epileptic focus. *Neurol.* **37,** 494–497.

Meifs J. W. H., Bosch F. G. C., Peters M. J., and Lopes da Silva F. H. (1987) On the magnetic field distribution generated by a dipolar current source situated in a realistically shaped compartmental model of the head. *Electroencephalogr. Clin. Neurophysiol.* **66,** 286–298.

Mendel M. I. and Goldstein R. (1971) Early components of the averaged electroencephalic response to constant level clicks during all-night sleep. *J. Speech Hear. Res.* **14,** 829–840.

Mendel M. I., Hosick E. C., Windman T., Davis H., Hirsh S. K., and Dinges D. F. (1975) Audiometric comparison of the middle and late components of the audit auditory evoked potentials awake and asleep. *Electroencephalogr. Clin. Neurophysiol.* **38,** 27–33.

Mitzdorf U. (1985) Current source-density method and application in cat cerebral cortex: Investigation of evoked potentials and EEG-phenomena. *Physiol. Rev.* **65,** 37–100.

Mitzdorf U. (1986) The physiological causes of VEP: Current source density analysis of electrically and visually evoked potentials, in *Evoked Potentials* (Cracco R. and Bodis-Wollner I., eds.), Alan R. Liss, New York, pp. 141–154.

Moller A. R. and Jannetta P. J. (1986) Simultaneous surface and direct brainstem recordings of brainstem auditory evoked potentials (BAEP) in man, in *Evoked Potentials* (Cracco R. and Bodis-Wollner I., eds.), Alan R. Liss, New York, pp. 227–234.

Moller A. R., Jannetta P. J., and Burgess J. E. (1986) Neural generators of the somatosensory evoked potential. Recording from the cuneate nucleus in man and monkeys. *Electroencephalogr. Clin Neurophysiol.* **65,** 241–248.

Moore E. J. (ed.) (1983) *Brain-stem Evoked Response* (Grune and Stratton, New York).

Morgan N. H. and Gevins A. S. (1986) Wigner distributions of human event-related brain potentials. *IEEE Trans. Biomed. Eng.* **BME-33,** 854–861.

Moruzzi G. (1972) The sleep waking cycle. *Ergebn. Physiol.* **64,** 1–165.

Naatanen R. and Gaillard A. W. K. (1983) The orienting reflex and the N2 deflection of the event-related potential (ERP), in *Tutorials in ERP Research: Endogenous Components* (Gaillard A. W. K. and Ritter W., eds.), Elsevier/North-Holland, Amsterdam, p. 119.

Naatanen R. and Picton T. W. (1986) N2 and automatic versus controlled processes, in *Cerebral Psychophysiology: Studies in Event-Related Poten-*

tials *(EEG Suppl. 38)* (McCallum W. C., Zappoli, R., Denoth F., eds.), Elsevier, Amsterdam, pp. 169–186.

Naatanen R., Simpson M., and Loveless N. E. (1982) Stimulus deviance and evoked potentials. *Biol. Psychol.* **14,** 53–98.

Naitoh P., Johnson C. L., and Lubin A. (1971) Modification of surface negative slow potential (CNV) in the human brain after total sleep loss. *Electroencephalogr. Clin. Neurophysiol.* **30,** 17–22.

Nakanishi T., Shimada Y., Sakuta M., and Toyokura Y. (1978) The initial positive component of scalp-recorded somatosensory evoked potentials in normal subjects and in patients with neurological disorders. *Electroencephalogr. Clin. Neurophysiol.* **45,** 26–34.

Neafsey E. J., Hull C. D., and Buchwald N. A. (1978) Preparation for movement in the cat. I. Unit activity in the cerebral cortex. *Electroencephalogr. Clin. Neurophysiol.* **44,** 706–713.

Nelson D. A. and Lassman F. M. (1968) Effects of intersignal interval on the human auditory evoked response. *J. Acoust. Soc. Am.* **44,** 1529–1532.

Nenov V. I., Read W., Halgren E., and Dyer M. G. (1990) The effects of threshold modulation on recall and recognition in a sparse auto-associative memory: Implications for hippocampal physiology (submitted).

Nenov V. I., Halgren E., Smith M. E., Badier J. M., Ropchan J. R., Blahd W. H., and Mandelkern M. (1989) Metabolic localization of brain potentials to words (submitted).

Neville N. J. and Foote S. L. (1984) Auditory event-related potentials in the squirrel monkeys: parallels to human late wave responses. *Brain Res.* **289,** 107–116.

Neville H. J., Kutas M., Chesney G., and Schimdt A. C. (1986) Event-related brain potentials during initial encoding and recognition memory of congruous and incongruous words. *J. Mem. Lang.* **25,** 75–92.

Niki H. (1974) Prefrontal unit activity during delayed alternation in the monkey. II. Relation to absolute versus relative direction of response. *Brain Res.* **68,** 197–204.

Niki H. and Watanabe M. (1976) Prefrontal unit activity and delayed response: Relation to cue localization versus direction of response. *Brain Res.* **105,** 79–88.

Niki H., Sakai M., and Kubota K. (1972) Delayed alternation performance and unit activity of the caudate head and medial orbitofrontal gyrus in the monkey. *Brain Res.* **38,** 343–353.

Nunez P. L. (1981) *Electric Fields of the Brain* Oxford Univ. Press, New York.

Nunez P. L. (1986) The brain's magnetic field: Some effects of multiple sources on localization methods. *Electroencephalogr. Clin. Neurophysiol.* **63**, 75–82.

Nunez P. L. (1987) Removal of reference electrode and volume conduction effects by spatial deconvolution of evoked potentials using a three-concentric sphere model of the head, in *The London Symposia* (R. J. Ellingson, N. M. F. Murray, A. M. Halliday, eds.) *(EEG Suppl. 39)*, Elsevier, Amsterdam, pp. 143–147.

Okada Y. (1982) Discrimination of localized and distributed current dipole sources and localized single and multipole sources, in *Biomagnetism: Applications and Theory.* (Weinberg H., Stroink G., Katila T., eds.), Pergamon, New York, pp. 266–272.

Okada Y. C., Kaufman L., and Williamson S. J. (1983) The hippocampal formation as a source of the slow endogenous potentials. *Electroencephalogr. Clin. Neurophysiol.* **55**, 417–426.

Okada Y. C., Williamson S. J., and Kaufman L. (1982) Magnetic field of the human sensorimotor cortex. *Int. J. Neurosci.* **17**, 33–38.

O'Keefe J. and Nadel L. (1978) *The Hippocampus as a Cognitive Map* (Clarendon, Oxford).

Orgogozo J. M. and Larsen B. (1979) Activation of the supplementary motor area during voluntary movement suggests it works as supramotor area. *Science* **206**, 847–850.

Ornitz E. M., Ritvo E. R., Carr E. M., Panman L. M., and Walter R. D. (1967) The variability of the auditory averaged evoked response during sleep and dreaming in children and adults. *Electroencephalogr. Clin. Neurophysiol.* **22**, 514–524.

Osselton J. W. (1965) Acquisition of EEG data by bipolar, unipolar and average reference methods: A theoretical comparison. *Electroencephalogr. Clin. Neurophysiol.*, **19**, 527–528.

Osterhammel P. H., Davis H., Wier C. C., and Hirsh S. K. (1973) Adult auditory evoked vertex potentials in sleep. *Audiology* **12**, 116–128.

Otto D. A. and Leifer L. J. (1973) The effects of modifying response and performance feedback parameters on the CNV in humans. *Electroencephalogr. Clin. Neurophysiol. Suppl.* **33**, 29–37.

Owens J. H. and Davis H. (eds.) (1985) *Evoked Potential Testing: Clinical Applications.* Grune and Stratton, Orlando

Ozdamar O. and Kraus N. (1983) Auditory middle-latency responses in humans. *Audiology* **22**, 34–49.

Ozdamar O., Kraus N., and Curry F. (1982) Auditory brain stem and middle latency responses in a patient with cortical deafness. *Electroencephalogr. Clin. Neurophysiol.* **53**, 224–230.

Paller K. A., Kutas M., Shimamura A. P., and Squire L. R. (1987) Brain responses to concrete and abstract words reflect processes that correlate with later performance on a test of stem-completion priming. *Current Trends in Event-Related Potential Research (EEG Suppl., 40)* (Johnson R., Jr., Rohrbaugh J. W. and R. Parasuraman, eds.), Elsevier, Amsterdam, pp. 360–365.

Paller K. A., Zola-Morgan S., Squire L. R., and Hillyard S. A. (1984) Monkeys with lesions of hippocampus and amygdala exhibit event-related brain potentials that resemble the human P300 wave. *Soc. Neurosci. Abstr.* **10,** 849

Panter C., Hoke M., Lehnertz K., Lutkenhoner B., Anogianakis G., and Wittkowski W. (1988) Tonotopic organization of the human auditory cortex revealed by transient auditory evoked magnetic fields. *Electroencephalogr. Clin. Neurophysiol.* **69**, 160–170.

Papakostopoulos D. and Crow H. J. (1976) Electrocorticographic studies of the contingent negative variation and "P300" in man, in *The Responsive Brain* (McCallum W. C. and Knot J. R., eds.), Wright, Bristol, pp. 205–210.

Papakostopoulos D. and Crow H. J. (1980) Direct recording of the somatosensory evoked potentials from the cerebral cortex of man and the difference between precentral and postcentral potentials. *Prog. Clin. Neurophysiol.* **7**, 15–26.

Papakostopoulos D., Cooper R., and Crow H. J. (1975) Inhibition of cortical evoked potentials and sensation by self-initiated movement in man. *Nature* **258**, 321–324.

Papanicolaou A. C. and Johnstone J. (1984) Probe evoked potentials: Theory, method and applications. *Int. J. Neurosci.* **24**, 107–131.

Parving A., Salomon G., Elberling C., Larsen B., and Lassen N. A. (1980) Middle components of the auditory evoked response in bilateral temporal lobe lesions. *Scand. Audiol.* **9**, 161–167.

Peronnet F., Giard M. H., Bertrand O., and Pernier J. (1984) The temporal component of the auditory evoked potential: A reinterpretation. *Electroencephalogr. Clin. Neurophysiol.* **59**, 67–71.

Perrault N. and Picton T. W. (1984a) Event-related potentials recorded from the scalp and nasopharynx. I. N1 and P2. *Electroencephalogr. Clin. Neurophysiol.* **59**, 177–194.

Perrault N. and Picton T. W. (1984b) Event-related potentials recorded from the scalp and nasopharynx. II. N2, P3 and slow wave. *Electroencephalogr. Clin. Neurophysiol.* **59**, 261–278.

Petrig B., Julesz B., Kropfl W., Baumgartner G., and Anliker M. (1981) Development of stereopsis and cortical binocularity in human infants: Electrophysiological evidence. *Science* **213**, 1402–1405.

Pfefferbaum A., Horvath T. B., Roth W. T., and Kopell B. S. (1979) Event-related potential changes in chronic alcoholics. *Electroencephalogr. Clin. Neurophysiol.* **47**, 637–647.

Picton T. W. (1986) Abnormal brainstem auditory evoked potentials: A tentative classification, in *Evoked potentials* (Cracco R. and Bodis-Wollner I., eds.), pp. 373–389. Arliss, New York.

Picton T. W. (1987) The recording and measurement of evoked potentials, in *A Textbook of Clinical Neurophysiology.* (Halliday A. M., Butler S. R., and Paul R., eds.) Wiley, New York, pp. 23–40.

Picton T. W. and Hillyard S. A. (1972) Cephalic skin potentials in electroencephalography. *Electroencephalogr. Clin. Neurophysiol.* **33**, 419–424.

Picton T. W. and Hillyard S. A. (1974) Human auditory evoked potentials. II Effects of attention. *Electroencephalogr. Clin. Neurophysiol.* **36**, 191–199.

Picton T. W. and Hink R. F. (1974) Evoked potentials: How? What? and Why? *Am. J. EEG Technol.* **14**, 9–44.

Picton T. W. and Stuss D. T. (1980) The component structure of the human event-related potentials. *Prog. Brain Res.* **54**, 17–49.

Picton T. W., Hillyard S. A., and Galambos R. (1976) Habituation and attention in the auditory system, in *Handbook of Sensory Physiology,* vol. 5, *Auditory system, Part 3* (Clinical and special topics), (Keidel W. D. and Neff W. D., eds.), pp. 343–389 Springer Verlag, Berlin.

Picton T. W., Hillyard S. A., Krausz H. I., and Galambos R. (1974) Human auditory evoked potentials. I. Evaluation of components. *Electroencephalogr. Clin. Neurophysiol.* **36**, 179–190.

Picton T. W., Hink R. F., Perez-Abalo M., Linden R. D., and Wiens A. S. (1984) Evoked potentials: How now? *J. Electrophysiol. Tech.,* **10**, 177–221.

Pieper C. F., Goldring S., Jenny A. B., and McMahon J. P. (1980) Comparative study of cerebral cortical potentials associated with voluntary movements in monkey and man. *Electroencephalogr. Clin. Neurophysiol.* **48**, 266–292.

Pirch J. H. (1980) Event related slow potentials in rat cortex during a reaction time task: cortical area differences. *Brain Res. Bull.* **5**, 199–201.

Pirch J. H., Corbus M. J., and Rigdon G. C. (1983) Single-unit and slow potential responses from rat frontal cortex during associative conditioning. *Exp. Neurol.* **82**, 118–130.

Pirch J. H., Corbus M. J., Rigdon G. C., and Lynes W. H. (1986) Generation of cortical event-related slow potentials in the rat involves nucleus basalis chrolinergic innervation. *Electroencephalogr. Clin. Neurophysiol.* **63,** 464–475.

Polich J. M., McCarthy G., Wang W. S., and Donchin E. (1983) When words collide: Orthographic and phonological interference during word processing. *Biol. Psychol.* **16,** 155–180.

Porjesz B., Begleiter H., and Samuelly I. (1980) Cognitive deficits in chronic alcholics and elderly subjects assessed by evoked brain potentials. *Acta Psychiatr. Scand. Suppl.* **286,** 62.

Pratt H. and Starr A. (1981) Mechanically and electrically evoked somatosensory potentials in humans: Scalp and neck distributions of short latency components. *Electroencephalogr. Clin. Neurophysiol.* **51,** 138–147.

Pratt H., Bleich N., and Berliner E. (1982) Short latency visual evoked potentials in man. *Electroencephalogr. Clin. Neurophysiol.* **54,** 55–62.

Prichep L. S., Sutton S., and Hakerem G. (1976) Evoked potentials in hyperkinetic and normal children under certainty and uncertainty: A placebo and methylphenidate study. *Psychophysiology* **13,** 419–428.

Prim M., Ojemann G., and Lettich E. (1983) Human cortical patterns of "P300" potentials to novel visual items. *Soc. Neurosci. Abstr.* **9,** 655.

Pritchard W. S. (1981) Psychophysiology of P300. *Psychol. Bull.* **89,** 506–540.

Pritchard W. S., Shappell S. A., and Brandt M. E. (1988) Psychophysiology of N200/N400: a review and classification scheme. In: *Advances in Psychophysiology* (Ackles P. K., Jennings J. R. and Coles M. G. H., eds.), JAI Press, Greenwich, CT, in press.

Purpura D. P. (1959) Nature of electrocortical potentials and synaptic organizations in cerebral and cerebellar cortex. *Int. Rev. Neurobiol.* **1,** 47–163.

Raeva S. (1986) Localization in human thalamus of units triggered during "verbal commands," voluntary movements and tremor. *Electroencephalogr. Clin. Neurophysiol.* **63,** 160–173.

Ranck J. B. Jr. (1973) Studies on single neurons in dorsal hippocampal formation and septum in unrestrained rates. Part 1: behavioral correlates and firing repertoires. *Exp. Neurol.* **41,** 462–531.

Rapin I., Schimmel H., and Cohen M. M. (1972) Reliability in detecting the auditory evoked response (AER) for audiometry in sleeping subjects. *Electroencephalogr. Clin. Neurophysiol.* **32,** 521–528.

Rebert C. S. (1972) Cortical and subcortical slow potentials in the monkey's brain during a preparatory interval. *Electroencephalogr. Clin. Neurophysiol.* **33,** 389–402.

Rebert C. S. (1973a) Slow potential correlates of neuronal population responses in the cat's lateral geniculate nucleus. *Electroencephalogr. Clin. Neurophysiol.* **35**, 511–515.

Rebert C. S. (1973b) Elements of a general cerebral system related to CNV genesis, in *Event-Related Slow Potentials of the Brain: Their Relations to Behavior* (McCallum W. C. and Knott J. R., eds.) *(Electroencephalogr. Clin. Neurophysiol.)*, pp. 63–67.

Rebert C. S. (1977) Intracerebral slow potentials changes in monkeys during the foreperiod of reaction time, in *Attention, Voluntary Contraction and Event-Related Cerebral Potentials* (Desmedt, J. E. ed.) *(Prog. Clin. Neurophysiol.*, vol. 1), Karger, Basel, pp. 242–253.

Rebert C. S. (1980) Neurobehavioral aspects of brain slow potentials, in *Motivation, Motor and Sensory Processes of the Brain* (Kornbuber H. H. and Deecke L., eds.) *(Prog. in Brain Res.*, vol. 54), Elsevier/North Holland, Amsterdam, pp. 381–402.

Regan D. (1972) *Evoked Potentials in Psychology, Sensory Physiology and Clinical Medicine* (Chapman and Hall, London).

Regan D. (1981) Evoked potential studies of visual perception. *Can. J. Psychol* **35**, 77–112.

Regan D. (1982) Comparison of transient and steady-state methods. *Ann. NY Acad. Sci.* **388**, 45–71.

Regan D. and Richards W. (1971) Independence of evoked potentials and apparent size. *Vision Res.* **11**, 679–684.

Remond A. (1956) Integration temporelle et integration spatiale a l'aide d'un meme appareil. *Rev. Neurol.* (Paris) **95**, 585–586.

Remond A. (1962) Correction des enregistrements elementaires en vue des presentations spatiotemporelles des EEG. *Rev. Neurol.* (Paris) **107**, 135–136.

Renault B. (1983) The visual emitted potentials: Clues for information processing, in *Tutorials in ERP Research: Endogenous Components* (Gaillard A. W. K. and Ritter W., eds.), Elsevier/North Holland, Amsterdam, p. 159.

Renault B. and Lesevre N. (1978) Topographical study of the emitted potential obtained after omission of an expected visual stimulus, in *Multidisciplinary Perspectives in Event-Related Brain Potential Research* (EPA 600/9-77-043) (D. A. Otto, ed.), US Govt. Printing Office, Washington, DC, p. 202–208.

Richer F., Barth D. S., and Beatty J. (1983) Neuromagnetic localization of two components of the transient visual evoked response to patterned stimulation. *Il Nuovo Cimento* **2**, 420–428.

Richer F., Johnson R. A., and Beatty J. (1983) Sources of late components of the brain magnetic response. *Neurosci. Abstr.* **9**, 656.

Rigdon G. C. and Pirch J. H. (1986) Nucleus basalis involvement in conditioned neuronal responses in the rat frontal cortex. *J. Neurosci.* **6,** 2535–2542.

Ritter W., Vaughan H. G., Jr., and Simson R. (1983) On relating event-related potential components to stages of information processing, in *Tutorials in ERP Research: Endogenous Components* (Gaillard A. W. K. and Ritter W., eds.), Elsevier/North Holland, Amsterdam, p. 143.

Ritter W., Simson R., Vaughan H. G., Jr., and Macht M. (1982) Manipulation of event-related potential manifestations of information processing stages. *Science* **218,** 909–911.

Ritter W., Ford J. M., Gaillard A. W. K., Harter M. R., Kutas M., Naatanen R., Polich J., Renault B., and Rohrbaugh J. (1984) Cognition and event-related potentials: The relation of negative potentials and cognitive processes, in *Brain and Information: Event-Related Potentials* (Karrer R., Cohen J., and Tueting P., eds), pp. 24–38.

Rockstroh B., Elbert T., Birbaumer N., and Lutzenberger W. (1982) *Slow Brain Potentials and Behavior* Urban and Schwartzenberg, Baltimore.

Rohrbaugh J. W., Synduldo K., and Lindsley D. B. (1976) Brain wave components of the contingent negative variation in humans. *Science* **191,** 1055–1057.

Rohrbaugh J. W., Syndulko K., and Lindsley D. B. (1978) Cortical slow negative waves following non-paired stimuli: Effects of task factors, *Electroencephalogr. Clin. Neurophysiol.* **45,** 551–567.

Rohrbaugh J. W., Syndulko K., Sanquist T. F., and Lindsley D. B. (1980) Synthesis of the contingent negative variation brain potential from noncontingent stimulus and motor elements. *Science* **208,** 1165–1168.

Roland P. E. (1985) Cortical organization of voluntary behavior in man. *Hum. Neurobiol.* **4,** 155–167.

Rolls E. T. (1983) The initiation of movements, in *Experimental Brain Research, Suppl. 7,* Springer-Verlag, Berlin, Heidelberg, pp. 97–113.

Romani G. L., Williamson S. J., Kaufman, L., and Brenner D. (1982) Characterization of the human auditory cortex by the neuromagnetic method. *Exp. Brain Res.* **47,** 381–393.

Rosenkilde C. E., Bauer R. H., and Fuster J. M. (1981) Single cell activity in ventral prefrontal cortex of behaving monkeys. *Brain Res.* **209,** 375–394.

Rosler F., Sutton S., Johnson R., Jr., Mulder G., Fabiani M., Plooij-Van Gorsel E., and Roth W. T. (1986) Endogeneous ERP components and cognitive components: a review, in *Cerebral Psychophysiology: Studies in Event-Related Potentials (EEG Suppl. 38)* (McCallum W. C., Zappoli R., Denoth F., eds.) Elsevier, Amsterdam, pp. 51–92.

Roth E. T., Pfefferbaum A., Horvath T. B., Berger P. A., and Kopell B. S. (1980) P3 reduction in auditory evoked potentials of schizophrenics. *Electroencephalogr. Clin. Neurophysiol.* **49**, 497–505.

Rowland V. (1968) Cortical steady potential in reinforcement and learning. *Prog. Physiol. Psychol.* **2**, 1–77.

Ruchkin D. S. and Sutton S. (1979) CNV and P300 relationships for emitted and for evoked cerebral potentials, in *Prog. Clin. Neurophysiol.*, vol. 6 (Desmedt J. E., ed.), Karger, Basel, pp. 119–131.

Rugg, M., Kok A., Barrett G., and Fischler I. (1986) ERPs associated with language and hemispheric specialization, in *Cerebral Psychophysiology: Studies in Event-Related Potentials (EEG Suppl. 38)* (McCallum W. C., Zappoli R., Denoth F., eds.) Elsevier, Amsterdam, pp. 273–300.

Rugg M. D. and Nagy M. E. (1987) Lexical contribution to non-word repetition effects: Evidence from event-related potentials. *Mem. Cognit.* **15**, 473–481.

Rugg M. D., Furda J., and Lorist M. (1988) The effects of task on the modulation of event-related potentials by word repetition. *Psychophysiology* **25**, 55–63.

Ruhm H., Walder E., and Flanigin H. (1967) Acoustically-evoked potentials in man: Mediation of early components. *Laryngoscope* **77**, 806–822.

Sakata H., Takoka Y., Kawarasaki A., and Shibutani H. (1973) Somatosensory properties of neurons in the superior parietal cortex (area 5) of the Rhesus monkey. *Brain Res.* **64**, 85–102.

Salamy A. and McKean C. M. (1977) Habituation and dishabituation of cortical and brainstem evoked potentials. *Int. J. Neurosci.* **7**, 175–182.

Sanquist T. F., Beatty J. T., and Lindsley D. B. (1981) Slow potential shifts of human brain during forewarned reaction. *Electroencephalogr. Clin. Neurophysiol.* **51**, 639–649.

Sanquist T. F., Rohrbaugh J. W., Syndulko K., and Lindsley D. B. (1980) Electrocortical signs of levels of processing: perceptual analysis and recognition memory. *Psychophysiology* **17**, 568–576.

Sano K., Miyake H., and Mayanagi Y. (1967) Steady potentials in various stress conditions in man. *Electroencephalogr. Clin. Neurophysiol., Suppl.* **25**, 264–275.

Sasaki K. (1976/1977) Electrophysiologic studies on the cerebellothalamo-cortical projections. *Appl. Neurophysiol.* **39**, 239–259.

Schafer E. W. P. (1967) Cortical activity preceding speech: Semantic specificity. *Nature* **216**, 1338–1339.

Schafer E. W. P., Amochaev A., and Russell M. J. (1981) Knowledge of stimulus timing attenuates human evoked cortical potentials. *Electroencephalogr. Clin. Neurophysiol.* **52**, 9–17.

Scherg M. (1984) Spatio-temporal modeling of early auditory evoked potentials. *Rev. Laryngol. Otol. Rhinol. (Bord),* **105,** 163–170.

Scherg M. and VonCramon D. (1985) Two bilateral sources of the late AEP as identified by a spatio-temporal dipole model. *Electroencephalogr. Clin. Neurophysiol.* **62,** 32–44.

Schimmel H. (1967) The ($\pm$) reference: accuracy of estimated mean components in average response studies. *Science* **164,** 92–94.

Schlag J. (1973) Generation of brain evoked potentials. *Bioelectric recording techniques, Part A,* Cellular processes and brain potentials, Academic, New York.

Schlag J. and Schlag-Rey M. (1987) Evidence for a supplementary eye field. *J. Neurophysiol.* **57,** 179–200.

Schneider M. R. (1974) Effect of inhomogeneities on surface signals coming from a cerebral current-dipole source. *IEEE Trans. Biomed. Eng.* **21,** 52–54.

Schreiber H., Land M., Lang W., Kornhuber A., Heise B., Keidel M., Deecke L., and Kornhuber H. H. (1983) Frontal hemispheric differences in the Bereitschaftspotential associated with writing and drawing. *Hum. Neurobiol.* **2,** 197–202.

Schwent V. L. and Hillyard S. A. (1975) Evoked potential correlates of selective attention with multi-channel auditory inputs. *Electroencephalogr. Clin. Neurophysiol.* **38,** 131–138.

Schwent V. L., Hillyard S. A., and Galambos R. (1976) Selective attention and the auditory vertex potential. I. Effects of stimulus delivery rate. *Electroencephalogr. Clin. Neurophysiol.* **40,** 604–614.

Seaba P. (1980) Electrical safety. *Am. J. EEG Technol.* **20,** 1–13.

Semlitsch H., Anderer P., Schuster P., and Presslich O. (1986) A solution for reliable and valid reduction of ocular artifacts, applied to the P300 ERP. *Psychophysiology* **23,** 695–703.

Sgro J. A. and Emerson R. G. (1985) Phase synchronized triggering: A method for coherent noise elimination in evoked potential recording. *Electroencephalogr. Clin. Neurophysiol.* **60,** 464–468.

Shibasaki H. (1975) Movement-associated cortical potentials in unilateral cerebral lesions. *J. Neurol.* **209,** 189–198.

Shibasaki H. and Kato M. (1975) Movement associated cortical potentials with unilateral and bilateral simultaneous hand movement. *J. Neurol.* **208,** 191–199.

Shibasaki H., Barrett G., Halliday E., and Halliday A. M. (1980a) Components of the movement-related cortical potential and their scalp topography. *Electroencephalogr. Clin. Neurophysiol.* **49,** 213–226.

Shibasaki H., Barrett G., Halliday E., and Halliday A. M. (1980b) Cortical potentials following voluntary and passive finger movements. *Electroencephalogr. Clin. Neurophysiol.* **50**, 201–213.

Shibasaki H., Barrett G., Halliday E., and Halliday A. M. (1981) Cortical potentials associated with voluntary foot movement in man. *Electroencephalogr. Clin. Neurophysiol.* **52**, 507–516.

Simson R., Vaughan H. G., Jr., and Ritter W. (1977a) The scalp topography of potentials in auditory and visual discrimination tasks. *Electroencephalogr. Clin. Neurophysiol.* **42**, 528–535.

Simson R., Vaughn H. G., Jr., and Ritter W. (1977b) The scalp topography of potentials in auditory and visual go/no go tasks. *Electroencephalogr. Clin. Neurophysiol.* **43**, 864–875.

Sindrup E., Thygesen N., Kristensen O., and Alving J. (1981) Zygomatic electrodes: Their use and value in complex partial epilepsy, in *Advances in Epileptology: XIIth Epilepsy International Symposium*, (Dam M., Gram L., and Penry J. K., eds.), Raven, New York.

Skinner J. E. (1971) Abolition of a conditioned, surface-negative, cortical potential during cryogenic blockade of the nonspecific thalamocortical system. *Electroencephalogr. Clin. Neurophysiol.* **31**, 197–209.

Skinner J. E. and King G. L. (1980) Contribution of neuron dendrites to extracellular sustained potential shifts. *Prog. Brain Res.* **54**, 89–102.

Skinner J. E. and Yingling C. D. (1976) Regulation of slow potential shifts in nucleus reticularis thalami by the mesencephalic reticular formation and the frontal granular cortex. *Electroencephalogr. Clin. Neurophysiol.* **40**, 288–296.

Skinner J. E. and Yingling C. D. (1977) Central gating mechanisms that regulate event-related potentials and behavior. A neural model for attention, in *Attention, Voluntary Contraction and Event-Related Cerebral Potentials* (Desmedt, J. E., ed.) *(Prog. Clin. Neurophysiol.*, vol. 1), Karger, Basel, pp. 28–68.

Skinner J. E., Reed J. C., Welch K. M. A., and Nell J. (1978) Cutaneous shock produces correlated shifts in slow potential amplitude and cyclic 3–5 adenosine monophosphate level in parietal cortex of the conscious rat. *J. Neurochem.* **30**, 699–704.

Skrandies W. amd Lehmann D. (1982) Spatial principal components of multichannel maps evoked by lateral visual half-field stimuli. *Electroencephalogr. Clin. Neurophysiol.* **54**, 297–305.

Slimp J. C., Tamas L. B., Stolov W. C., and Wyler A. R. (1986) Somatosensory evoked potentials after removal of somatosensory cortex in man. *Electroencephalogr. Clin. Neurophysiol.* **65**, 111–117.

Smith D. B., Sidman R. D., Henke J. S., Flanigin H., Labiner D., and Evans L. N. (1983) Scalp and depth recordings of induced deep cerebral potentials. *Electroencephalogr. Clin. Neurophysiol.* **55**, 145–150.

Smith M. E. and Halgren E. (1987a) Event-related potentials elicited by familiar and unfamiliar faces, in *Current Trends in Event-Related Potential Research* (Johnson R., Jr., Purasuraman R., and Rohrbaugh, J. W., eds.) *Electroencephalogr. Clin. Neurophysiol. Suppl. 40)*, Elsevier, Amsterdam, pp. 422–426.

Smith M. E. and Halgren E. (1987b) ERPs during lexical decision: Effects of repetition, word frequency, pronounceability, and concreteness, in *Current Trends in Event-Related Potential Research* (Johnson R., Jr., Purasuraman R., and Rohrbaugh J. W., eds.) *Electroencephalogr. Clin. Neurophysiol. Suppl. 40)*, Elsevier, Amsterdam, pp. 417–421.

Smith M. E. and Halgren E. (1989) Dissociation of recognition memory components following temporal lobe lesions. *J. Exp. Psychol. (Learn. Mem. Cogn.)* **15**, 50–60.

Smith M. E. and Halgren E. (1988) Attenuation of a sustained visual processing negativity after lesions that include the inferotemporal cortex. *Electroencephalogr. Clin. Neurophysiol.* (in press). **70**, 356–370.

Smith M. E., Halgren E., Sokolik M., Baudena P., Mussolino A., Liegeois-Chauvel C., and Chauvel P. Initial survey of the intracranial voltage distribution of endogenous potentials elicited during auditory discrimination (submitted).

Smith M. E., Stapleton J. M., and Halgren E. (1986) Human medial temporal lobe potentials evoked in memory and language tasks. *Electroencephalogr. Clin. Neurophysiol.* **63**, 145–159.

Smith M. E., Halgren E., Sokolik M., Baudena P., Mussolino A., Liegeois-Chauvel C., and Chauvel P. (1988) Intracranial distribution of human cognitive potentials. *Soc. Neurosci. Abstr.* **14**, 1014.

Somjen G. G. (1973) Electrogenesis of sustained potentials. *Prog. Neurobiol.* **1**, 199–237.

Somjen G. G. (1979) Extracellular potassium in the mammalian central nervous system. *Annu. Rev. Physiol.* **41**, 159–177.

Soso M. J. and Fetz E. E. (1980) Responses of identified cells in postcentral cortex of awake monkeys during comparable active and passive joint movements. *J. Neurophysiol.* **43**, 1090–1110.

Speckmann E. J. and Caspers H. (eds.) (1979) *Origin of Cerebral Field Potentials* (George Thieme: Stuttgart.)

Speckmann E. J., Caspers H., and Janzen R. W. C. (1978) Laminar distribution of cortical field potentials in relation to neuronal activities during seizure discharges, in *Architectonics of the Cerebral Cortex* (Brazier M. A. B. and Petsche H., eds.), Raven, New York, pp. 191–209.

Spehlmann R. (1985) *Evoked Potential Primer.* (Butterworth, Boston.)

Spekreijse J., Van der Tweel L. H., and Zuidema T. (1973) Contrast evoked responses in man. *Vision Res.* **13,** 1577–1601.

Spencer W. A. and Kandel E. R. (1962) Hippocampal neuron responses to selective activation of recurrent collaterals of hippocampofugal axons. *Exp Neurol.* **4,** 140–161.

Spencer W. A. and Kandel E. R. (1969) Synaptic inhibition in seizures, in *Basic Mechanisms of the Epilepsies* (Jasper H. H., Ward A. A., and Pope A., eds.), Little, Brown and Co., Boston. p. 575.

Sperling M. R. and Engel J., Jr. (1985) The EEG from the temporal lobes: A comparison of rear, anterior temporal, and nanopharyngeal electrodes *Ann. Neurol.* **17,** 510–513.

Sperling M. R. and Engel J., Jr. (1986) Sphenoidal electrodes. *J. Clin. Neurophysiol.* **3,** 67–63.

Spitz M. C., Emerson R. G., and Pedley T. A. (1986) Dissociation of frontal N100 from occipital P100 in pattern reversal visual evoked potentials. *Electroencephalogr. Clin. Neurophysiol.* **65,** 161–168.

Spydell J. D., Pattie G., and Goldie W. D. (1985) The 40 Hertz auditory event-related potential: normal values and effects of lesions. *Electroencephalogr. Clin. Neurophysiol.* **62,** 192–202.

Squire L. R. (1982) The neuropsychology of human memory. *Annu. Rev. Neurosci.* **5,** 241–273.

Squires N. K., Squires K. C., and Hillyard S. A. (1975) Two varieties of long-latency positive waves evoked by unpredictable auditory stimuli in man. *Electroencephalogr. Clin. Neurophysiol.* **83,** 387–401.

Squires N. K., Halgren E., Wilson C. L., and Crandall P. H. (1983) Human endogenous limbic potentials: cross-modality and depth/surface comparisons in epileptic subjects, in *Tutorials in ERP Research: Endogenous Components* (Gaillard A. W. K. and Ritter W., eds.), North Holland, Amsterdam, pp. 217–232.

Squires K. C., Chippendale T. J., Wrege K. S., Goodin D. S., and Starr A. (1980) Electrophysiological assessment of mental function in aging and dementia, in *Aging in the 1980's: Psychological Issues,* (Poon L. W., ed), American Psychological Association, Washington, DC, pp. 125–134.

Srebro R. (1985a) Localization of visually evoked cortical activity in humans. *J. Physiol. (London)* **360,** 233–246.

Srebro R. (1985b) Localization of cortical activity associated with visual recognition in humans. *J. Physiol. (London)* **360,** 247–259.

Stamm J. S. and Rosen S. C. (1972) Cortical steady potential shifts and anodal polarization during delayed response performance. *Acta Neurobiol. Exp (Warsz)* **32**, 193–209.

Stapleton J. M. and Halgren E. (1987) Endogenous potentials evoked in simple cognitive tasks: Depth components and task correlates. *Electroencephalogr. Clin. Neurophysiol.* **67**, 44–52.

Stapleton J. M., Halgren E., and Moreno K. A. (1987a) Endogenous potentials after anterior temporal lobectomy. *Neuropsychologia* **25**, 549–557.

Stapleton J. M., O'Reilly T., and Halgren E. (1987b) Endogenous potentials in simple cognitive tasks: Scalp topography. *Int. J. Neurosci.* **36**, 75–88.

Starr A. (1985) Auditory pathway origins of scalp-derived auditory brainstem responses, in *Evoked Potentials. Neurophysiological and Clinical Aspects* (Morocutti C. and Rizzo P. A., eds), Elsevier, Amsterdam, pp. 133–143.

Stephenson W. A. and Gibbs F. A. (1951) A balanced non-cephalic reference electrode. *Electroencephalogr. Clin. Neurophysiol.* **3**, 237–240.

Steriade M. and Deschenes M. (1984) The thalamus as a neuronal oscillator. *Brain Res.* **320**, 1–63.

Straschill M. and Takahashi H. (1980) Slow potentials in the human subthalamus associated with rapid arm movements, in *Motivation, Motor and Sensory Processes of the Brain: Electrical Potentials, Behavior and Clinical Use* (Kornhuber H. H. and Deecke L., eds.) (*Progress in Brain Research,* vol. 54) Elsevier/North Holland, Amsterdam p. 135.

Streletz L. J., Katz L., Hohenberger M., and Cracco R. Q. (1977) Scalp recorded auditory evoked potentials and sonomotor responses: An evaluation of components and recording techniques. *Electroencephalogr. Clin. Neurophysiol.* **43**, 192–206.

Streletz L. J., Bae S. H., Roeshman R. M., Schatz N. J., and Savino P. J. (1981) Visual evoked potentials in occipital lobe lesions. *Arch. Neurol.* **38**, 80–85.

Stuss D. T., Sarazin F. F., Leech E. E., and Picton T. W. (1983) Event-related potentials during naming and mental rotation. *Electroencephalogr. Clin. Neurophysiol.* **56**, 133–146.

Surwillo W. W. (1977) Cortical evoked response recovery functions: Physiological manifestations of the psychological refractory period? *Psychophysiology* **14**, 32–39.

Suzuki H. and Azuma M. (1977) Prefrontal neuronal activity during gazing at a light spot in the monkey. *Brain Res.* **126**, 497–508.

Suzuki I. and Mayanagi Y. (1984) Intracranial recording of short latency somatosensory evoked potentials in man: identification of origin of each component. *Electroencephalogr. Clin. Neurophysiol.* **59,** 286–296.

Syndulko K. and Lindsley D. B. (1977) Motor and sensory determinants of cortical slow potential shifts in man, in *Progress in Clinical Neurophysiology* (Desmedt J. E., ed.), Karger, Basel, pp. 97–131.

Syndulko K., Pettler-Jennings P., Cohen S. N., Cummings J., Halgren E., and Tourtellotte W. W. (1984) P300 in memory disorders of diverse etiology, in *Proceedings of the American Academy of Neurology, 36th Annual Meeting*, Abstract 298.

Syndulko K., Hansch M. A., Cohen S. N., Pearce J. W., Goldberg Z., Montan B., Tourtellotte W. W., and Potvin A. R. (1982) Long-latency event related potentials in normal aging and dementia, in *Advances in Neurology* vol. 32, (Courjon J., Maugiere F., and Revol M, eds.), Raven, New York, pp. 279–286.

Szirtes J., and Vaughan H. G., Jr. (1977) Characteristics of cranial and facial potentials associated with speech production. *Electroencephalogr. Clin. Neurophysiol.* **43,** 386–396.

Talairach J., Szikla G., Tournoux P., Prossalentis A., Bordas-Ferrer M., Covello L., Jacob M., and Mempel E. (1967) *Atlas d-Anatomie Stereotaxique du Telencephale.* (Masson et Cie, Paris).

Tamas L. B. and Shibasaki H. (1985) Cortical potentials associated with movement: A review. *J. Clin. Neurophysiol.* **2,** 157–171.

Tanji J. (1984) The neuronal activity in the supplementary motor area of primates. *Trends Neurosci.* **7,** 282–285.

Tanji J. and Kurata K. (1982) Comparison of movement-related activity in two cortical motor areas of primates. *J. Neurophysiol.* **48,** 633–653.

Tanji J., Taruguchi K., and Saga T. (1980) Supplementary motor area: neural response to motor instructions. *J. Neurophysiol.* **43,** 60–68.

Taylor M. (1978) Bereitschaftspotential during the acquisition of a skilled motor task. *Electroencephalogr. Clin. Neurophysiol.* **45,** 568–576.

Thatcher R. W., Krause P. J., and Hrybyk M. (1986) Cortico-cortical associations and EEG coherence: A two-compartmental model. *Electroencephalogr. Clin. Neurophysiol.,* **64,** 123–143.

Thickbroom G. W., Carroll W. M., and Mastaglia F. L. (1985a) Dipole source derivation. Application to the half-field pattern evoked potential. *Int. J. Biomed. Comput.,* **16,** 17–28.

Thickbroom G. W., Mastaglia F. L., Carroll W. M., and Davies H. D. (1985b) Cerebral potentials accompanying visually triggered finger movement in man. *Electroencephalogr. Clin. Neurophysiol.* **62,** 209–108.

Timsit-Berthier M., Gerono A., and Rousseau J. (1977) CNV variations of amplitude and duration during low level arousal: The "distraction-arousal" hypothesis reconsidered. *Electroencephalogr. Clin. Neurophysiol.* **43**, 471.

Tsubokawa T. and Moriyasu N. (1978) Motivational slow negative potential shift (CNV) related to thalamotomy. *Appl. Neurophysiol.* **41**, 202–208.

Tsubokawa T., Katayama T., Nishimoto H., Kotani A., and Moriyasu N. (1976/1977) Emotional slow negative potential shift (CNV) in the thalamus. *Appl. Neurophysiol.* **39**, 261–267.

Tsuji S., Shibasaki H., Kato M., Kuroiwa Y., and Shima F. (1984) Subcortical, thalamic and cortical somatosensory evoked potentials to median nerve stimulation. *Electroencephalogr. Clin. Neurophysiol.* **59**, 465–476.

Tukey J. W. (1978) A data analysts's comments on a variety of points and issues, in *Event-Related Brain Potentials in Man* (Callaway E., Tueting P., and Koslow S. H., eds.), Academic, New York, pp. 139–154.

Vanderwolf C. H. (1975) Neocortical and hippocampal activation in relation to behavior: effects of atropine, eserine, phenothiazines, and amphetamine. *J. Comp. Physiol. Psychol.* **88**, 300–323.

Vanderwolf C. H. and Baker G. B. (1986) Evidence that serotonin mediates noncholinergic neorcortical low voltage fast activity, noncholinergic hippocampal rhythmic slow activity, and contributes to behavior. *Brain Res.* **374**, 342–356.

Vanderwolf C. H., Kramis R., Gillespie L. A., and Bland B. H. (1975) Hippocampal rhythmical slow activity and neocortical low voltage fast activity: relation to behavior. In: *The Hippocampus: Neurophysiology and Behavior* (Isaacson R. L. and Pribram K. H., eds.), Plenum, New York, pp. 101–128.

Vanderwolf C. H., Leung L. W. S., and Stewart D. J. (1985) Two afferent pathways mediating hippocampal rhythmical slow activity, in *Electrical Activity of the Archicortex* (Buzsaki G. and Vanderwolf, C. H., eds.), Akademial Kiado, Budapest, pp. 47–66.

Van Hoesen G. W. (1982) The parahippocampal gyrus: New observations regarding its cortical connections in the monkey. *Trends Neurosci.* **5**, 345–350.

van Lith G. H. M., van Marle G. W., and Vijfvinkel-Bruinenga S. (1979) Two disadvantages of a television system as pattern stimulator for evoked potentials. *Doc. Ophthalmol.* 48, 261–266.

Vaughan, H. G. (1966) The perceptual and physiologic significance of visual evoked responses recorded from the scalp in man, in *Clinical Electroretinography* (Burian H. M. and Jacobson J. H., eds.), Oxford, Pergamon Press, pp. 203–223.

Vaughan H. G. (1969) The relationship of brain activity to scalp recordings of event related potentials, in *Average Evoked Potentials* (Donchin E. and Lindsley D. B., eds.), NASA, Washington, DC, pp. 45–75.

Vaughan H. G. (1974) The analysis of scalp-recorded potentials. in *Bioelectric Recording Techniques, Part B. Electroencephalography and human brain potentials* (Thompson R. F. and Patterson M. M., eds.), Academic, New York pp. 158–207.

Vaughan H. G. (1975) The motor potentials, in *Handbook of Electroencephalography and Clinical Neurophysiology*, vol. 8A Elsevier, Amsterdam, pp. 86–92.

Vaughan H.G., and Gross E. G. (1969) Cortical responses to light in unanesthetized monkeys and their alteration by visual system lesions. *Exp. Brain Res.* **8**, 19–36.

Vaughan H. G., Jr., (1969) The relationship of brain activity to scalp recordings of event-related potentials, in *Average Evoked Potentials* (Donchin E. and Lindsley D. B., eds.), NASA Sp-191, Washington DC, pp. 45–94.

Vaughan H. G., Jr. and Hull R. C. (1965) Functional relation between stimulus intensity and photically evoked cerebral responses in man. *Nature* **206**, 720–722.

Vaughan H. G., Jr. and Ritter W. (1970) The sources of auditory evoked responses recorded from the human scalp. *Electroencephalogr. Clin. Neurophysiol.* **28**, 360–367.

Vaughan H. G., Jr., Bossom J., and Gross E. G. (1970) Cortical motor potential in monkeys before and after upper limb deafferentation. *Exp. Neurol.* **26**, 253–262.

Vaughan H. G., Jr., Costa L. D., and Ritter W. (1968) Topography of the human motor potential. *Electroencephalogr. Clin. Neurophysiol.* **25**, 1–10.

Velasco F., Velasco M., Cepeda C., and Munoz H. (1980) Wakefulness-sleep modulation of cortical and subcortical somatic evoked potentials. *Electroencephalogr. Clin. Neurophysiol.* **48**, 64–72.

Velasco M., Velasco F., Romo R., and Alamanza S. (1984) Subcortical correlates of the auditory brain stem potentials in the monkey: Bipolar EEG and multiple unit activity responses. *Int. J. Neurosci.* **22**, 235–252.

Velasco M., Velasco R., Almanza X., and Coats A. C. (1982) Subcortical correlates of the auditory brain stem potentials in man: Bipolar EEG and multiple unit activity and electrical stimulation. *Electroencephalogr. Clin. Neurosphysiol.* **53**, 133–142.

Verleger R. (1988) Event-related potentials and memory: A critique of the context updating hypothesis and an alternative interpretation of P3. *Behav. Brain Sci.* **11,** 343–427.

Verleger R. and Cohen R. (1978) Effects of certainty, modality shift and guess outcome on evoked potentials and reaction times in chronic schizophrenics. *Psychol. Med.* **8,** 81–93.

Voorn F. J., Adamse H., Kop P. F. M., and Brunia C. H. M. (1987) Hippocampal potentials related to signal stimuli in unrestrained rats, in *Current Trends in Event-Related Potential Research* (Johnson R., Jr., Rohrbaugh J. W., and Parasuraman R., eds.) *(EEG Suppl. 40),* Elsevier, Amsterdam, pp. 493–498.

Walaas I. (1983) The hippocampus, in *Chemical Neuroanatomy* (Emson P. C., ed.), Raven, New York, pp. 337.

Walter D. O., Etevenon P., Pidoux B., Trotrat D., and Guillou S. (1984) Computerized topo-EEG spectral maps: difficulties and perspectives. *Neuropsychologia* **11,** 264–272.

Walter W. G. (1964) The convergence and interaction of visual, auditory and tactile responses in human nonspecific cortex. *Ann. NY Acad. Sci.* **112,** 320–361.

Walter W. G. (1965) Brain responses to semantic stimuli. *J. Psychosom. Res.* **9,** 51–61.

Walter W. G. (1975) Evoked response general, in *Handbook of Electroencephalography and Clinical Neurophysiology,* vol. 8A, Elsevier, Amsterdam, pp. 20–32.

Walter W. G., Cooper R., Aldridge V. J., McCallum W. C., and Winter A. L. (1964) Contingent negative variation: An electric sign of sensorimotor association and expectancy in the human brain. *Nature* **203,** 380–384.

Weinberg H. (1973) The contingent negative variation: its relation to feedback and expectant attention, in *Event-Related Slow Potentials of the Brain: Their Relations to Behavior* (McCallum W. D. and Knott J. R., eds.) *Electroencephalogr. Clin. Neurophysiol. Suppl. 33),* Elsevier, Amsterdam, pp. 219–228.

Weinberg H. and Brickett P. (1983) Slow magnetic fields of the brain preceding movements and speech. *Il Nuovo Cimento* **2,** 495–504.

Weinberg H., Michalewski H., and Koopman R. (1976) The influence of discriminations on the form of the contingent negative variation. *Neuropsychologia* **14,** 87–95.

Weinrich M., Wise S. P., and Mauritz K. H. (1984) A neurophysiological study of the premotor cortex in the rhesus monkey. *Brain* **107,** 385–414.

Whittaker S. G. and Siegfried J. B. (1983) Origin of wavelets in the visual evoked potential. *Electroencephalogr. Clin. Neurophysiol.* **55,** 91–101.

Wilder M. B., Farley G. R., and Starr A. (1981) Endogenous late positive component of the evoked potential in cats corresponding to P300 in humans. *Science* **211,** 605–607.

Wilke J. T. and Lansing R. W. (1973) Variations in the motor potential with force exerted during voluntary arm movements in man. *Electroencephalogr. Clin. Neurophysiol.* **35,** 259–265.

Williamson S. J. and Kaufman L. (1981) Biomagnetism. *J. Magnet. Mag. Mat.* **22,** 129–202.

Wise S. P. (1984) The nonprimary motor cortex and its role in the cerebral control of movement, in *The Nonprimary Motor Cortex and Its Role in the Cerebral Control of Movement* (Edelman G. M., Gall W. E., and Cowan W. M., eds.), Wiley, New York, pp. 524–555.

Wolpaw J. R. (1979) Single unit activity vs. amplitude of the epidural evoked potential in primary auditory cortex of awake cats. *Electroencephalogr. Clin. Neurophysiol.* **47,** 372–376.

Wolpaw J. R. and Penry J. K. (1975) A temporal component of the auditory evoked response. *Electroencephalogr. Clin. Neurophysiol.* **39,** 609–620.

Wood C. C. (1982) Application of dipole localization methods to human evoked potentials. *Ann. NY Acad. Sci.* **388,** 139–159.

Wood C. C. (1987) Generators of event-related potentials, in *A. Textbook of Clinical Neurophysiology* (Halliday A. M., Butler S. R., Paul R., eds.), Wiley, New York, pp. 535–568.

Wood C. C. and McCarthy G. (1984) Principal component analysis of event-related potentials: Simulation studies demonstrate misallocation of variance across components. *Electroencephalogr. Clin. Neurophysiol.* **59,** 249–260.

Wood C. C., and McCarthy G. (1985) A possible frontal lobe contribution to scalp P300. *Soc. Neurosci. Abstr.* **11,** 879.

Wood C. C. and Wolpaw J. R. (1982) Scalp distribution of human auditory evoked potentials. II. Evidence for over-lapping sources and involvement of auditory cortex. *Electroencephalogr. Clin. Neurophysiol.* **54,** 25–38.

Wood C. C., Cohen D., Cuffin B. N., Yarita M., and Allison T. (1985) Electrical sources in human somatosensory cortex: Identification by combined magnetic and potential recordings. *Science* **227,** 1051–1053.

Wood C. C., McCarthy G., Allison T., Goff W. R., Williamson P. D., and Spencer D. D. (1982) Endogenous event-related potentials following temporal lobe excisions in humans. *Soc. Neurosci. Abstr.* **8,** 976.

Wood C. C., McCarthy G., Kim J. H., Spencer D. D., and Williamson P. D. (1988) Abnormalities in temporal lobe event-related potentials predict hippocampal cell loss in temporal lobe epilepsy. *Society for Neuroscience Abstracts* **14,** 5 (Abstract).

Wood C. C., McCarthy G., Squires N. K., Vaughan H. G., Woods D. L., and McCallum W. C. (1981) Anatomical and physiological substrates of event related potentials: Two case studies. Papers presented at the Sixth Int. Conf. on Event-Related Potentials, Lake Forest, Illinois.

Wood C. C., Spencer D. D., Allison T., McCarthy G., Williamson P. D., and Goff W. R. (1988) Localization of human sensorimotor cortex during surgery by cortical surface recording of somatosensory evoked potentials. *J. Neurosurg.* **68,** 99–111.

Woodbury J. W. (1960) Potentials in a volume conductor, in *Medical Physiology and Biophysics* (Ruch T. C. and Fulton J. F., eds.), Saunders, Philadelphia, pp. 83–91.

Woody C. D. (1967) Characterization of an adaptive filter for the analysis of variable latency neuroelectric signals. *Med. Biol. Eng.,* **5,** 539–553.

Yabe H., Mita M., Aoki N., and Mimatsu Y. (1981) Temporal depression of EMG activity prior to a rapid voluntary movement in man. *Electroencephalogr. Clin. Neurophysiol. (Suppl)* **52,** S64.

Yagi A. (1981) Averaged cortical potentials (lambda responses) time-locked to onset and offset of saccades. *Physiol. Psychol.* **9,** 318–320.

Yamada T., Kimura J., Wilkinson J. T., and Kayamori R. (1983) Short- and long-latency median somatosensory evoked potentials. *Arch. Neurol.* **40,** 215–220.

Yiannikas D. and Walsh J. C. (1983) The variation of the pattern shift visual evoked response with the size of the stimulus field. *Electroencephalogr. Clin. Neurophysiol.* **55,** 427–435.

Yingling C. D. and Hosobuchi Y. (1984) A subcortical correlate of P300 in man. *Electroencephalogr. Clin. Neurophysiol.* **59,** 72–76.

Zappoli R., Papini M., Briani S., Benvenutti P., and Pasquinelli A. (1975) CNV in patients with known frontal lobe lesion. *Electroencephalogr. Clin. Neurophysiol.* **39,** 216.

Zappoli R., Papini M., Briani S., Benvenuti P., and Pasquinelli A. (1976) CNV in patients with frontal lobe lesions and mental disturbances, in *The Responsive Brain* (McCallum W. C. and Knott J. R., eds.), Wright, Bristol, pp. 158–163.

Zemon V., Kaplan E., and Ratliff F. (1986) The role of GABA-mediated intracortical inhibition in the generation of visual evoked potentials, in *Evoked Potentials* (Cracco R. and Bodis-Wollner I., eds.), AR Liss, New York, pp. 287–295.

Zimmermann G. N. and Knott J. R. (1974) Slow potentials of the brain related to speech processing in normal speakers and stutterers *Electroencephalogr. Clin. Neurophysiol.* **37,** 599–607.

From: *Neuromethods, Vol. 15: Neurophysiological Techniques: Applications to Neural Systems* Edited by: A. A. Boulton, G. B. Baker, and C. H. Vanderwolf Copyright © 1990 The Humana Press Inc., Clifton, NJ

Field Potentials in the Central Nervous System

Recording, Analysis, and Modeling

Lai-Wo Stan Leung

1. Introduction

In contrast to unit action potentials recorded from discrete neurons, field potentials, as the name implies, are not restricted to the spatial domain of a neuron or of the brain. As a result of the volume-conducting properties of the brain, field potentials reflect activity of a population of neurons. They are often used, therefore, as a monitor of the gross brain state during sleep, behavioral activation, and epilepsy.

In addition to serving as a gross monitor of brain states, field potentials yield important physiological information that is not otherwise available. Postsynaptic potentials in a population of neurons manifest themselves in the field, and such potentials may be difficult to record intracellularly, especially in a behaving animal. Field potentials also yield spatiotemporal data that can be used for the study of parallel neuronal interactions in a neuronal population (Freeman, 1975; Freeman and Skarda, 1985). The data recorded and analyzed are macroscopic (at a level larger than the size of a neuron) rather than microscopic. However, in cortical structures where neurons are aligned in parallel, the current-source-density (CSD) analysis of the field potentials may elucidate the sites of synaptic action, which otherwise may be obtained only with such difficult techniques as dendritic impalements.

The subject of field potentials has been reviewed and described in various depths (Freeman, 1975; Hubbard et al., 1969; Lorente de Nó, 1947a,b; Nicholson and Freeman, 1975; Mitzdorf, 1985). The purpose of this chapter is not to review the literature exhaustively. Rather, the purpose is to present a brief and self-contained treatment of field potentials, with emphasis on a better intuitive understanding of the subject, and to describe the techniques used in field-potential recording and analysis, including current-source-density analysis and synthesis (modeling) of field potentials. Some equations are included, but those who are not quantitatively inclined may skip those sections.

2. Field Potential Theory

2.1. General

The electromotive forces (emf) for intra- and extracellular current lie in the membrane. Conductance changes at the membrane, whether the results of action or synaptic potentials, cause local depolarization or hyperpolarization. The difference in potential within the neuronal core conductor causes spatial current flows that tranverse both the intra- and extracellular media. The passive electrotonic potentials are important in conducting between the dendritic synapse (or receptors) and the action-potential trigger zone (axon hillock or first node of Ranvier). They are also important for the passive depolarization of the membrane during propagation of an action potential.

Extracellular potentials in a conducting medium are a consequence of the membrane emf. It can be imagined that currents are injected into the extracellular medium (source) or removed from it (sink) at discrete locations. The field potential may be derived theoretically if the sources and sinks are known. At any location, the field potential depends on the linear sum of potentials from each of the current sources and sinks, weighted according to distance and the extracellular conductivity. The dependence on the conductivity may be complex, since the conductivity may be neither uniform (homogeneous) nor isotropic (the same in all directions). At a microscopic level, the neuropil may look extremely inhomogeneous. However, at a macroscopic level (i.e., larger than the domain of a single neuron), the conductivity may often be assumed to be isotropic or homogeneous, at least to a first approximation. Conductivity of tissues outside of the active area of the brain, e.g. ventricles, skull, and scalp, also enters into the calculation of field potentials, as so-called boundary conditions.

2.2. Principles of Current Flow

There are two main principles to current flow in the brain: (1) the currents are mainly resistive or ohmic, except through the cell membrane, and (2) the currents flow in a closed loop. Conventionally, a current is a flow of positive charges or ions from a high to a low potential.

Capacitative current flow through the extracellular medium has been shown to be negligible in the brain at physiological frequencies of 1 KHz or lower (Ranck, 1963; Plonsey, 1969). In addition, the absence of magnetic materials imply a lack of inductive effects. As a consequence, potential fields in the brain are quasi-static, and depend only on resistive or ohmic current flows (Plonsey, 1969).

The emf for all currents in the brain reside in the membrane. However, the currents spread through the conductive intra- and extracellular media. These currents flow in closed loops, with many loops traversing both the intra- and extracellular media. For example, during the peak of an action potential (Fig. 1A), the voltage-dependent ion channels open at the membrane and sodium currents enter the axon (at point A). The conservation of charges at any point in the brain (Kirchoff's second law) dictates that the current inflow equals the current outflow. Thus, the accumulation of positive (Na^+) charges inside the membrane will directly lead to outflow of current (positive charges) from that location. The current outflow will cause charge accumulation elsewhere in the intracellular medium, which will create another current flow, until the current flow has closed a loop. To complete this loop, at some location (point B in Fig. 1A), the current has to exit from the intracellular medium. This outgoing current deposits positive charges at the inner side of the membrane and causes depolarization (decrease in charge across the membrane) at point B. Initially, this depolarization at point B is totally passive, i.e., driven by the emf at point A. However, with sufficient depolarization, voltage-dependent Na^+ channels at point B will regenerate the action potential, and the sequence of events repeats itself. Thus, the passive spread of current or the creation of the current loop is essential for the propogation of the action potential.

Synaptic currents also flow in a closed loop, and these currents loops are important for synaptic transmission. Let us assume that

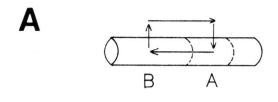

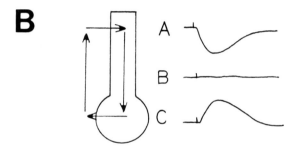

Fig. 1. (A) Current flows in a closed loop when an action potential begins at point A (with inward sodium currents). Passive currents exit at point B. (B) Synaptic excitation at the distal dendrites drives a current loop that flows from positive (point C) to negative potentials (point A) in the extracellular medium. Response transients, positive upward.

excitation at the distal dendrites causes distal dendritic depolarization (Fig. 1B). This makes the intracellular potential at distal dendrites more positive than at other parts of the membrane. As a consequence, an intracellular current flows from high to low membrane-potential, away from the distal dendrites. Using the current loop principle, the intracellular current has to complete an extracellular loop. This assumption requires that the main extracellular current flow in a direction opposite to the intracellular current. The extracellular potential at point C (Fig. 1B) will be positive (since a small current may flow from this point to a far-away point at zero potential), whereas that at a point A will be negative. Somewhere between points A and C, at point B, a zero potential point may be encountered (where no currents will flow to a distal reference point). Therefore, in the extracellular medium, there exist both positive and negative potentials (in other words, a dipole field).

At a snapshot, the field potentials from an action or synaptic current are not much different. If the distal dendrities can generate an action potential, then Fig. 1B, drawn for dendritic synaptic excitation, will essentially describe the main current flows during the peak of this action potential. The main differences between action and synaptic currents are in their regenerative nature and time course. The synaptic currents do not move if the same synapses are activated; their extracellular field may be regarded as standing. On the other hand, action currents propagate, generating a moving field (Nicholson and Llinas, 1971). Another difference is that the fast sequence of source–sinks of an action potential (high temporal frequency) will cause more capacitative currents to flow through the membrane locally and will result in a faster spatial decay in the neuronal cable (Lux, 1967).

An important issue on field potential interpretation is that field potentials depend primarily on current sources and sinks (or current flows), rather than on the level of depolarization. The following two examples illustrate this point (*see also* section 2.5.): (1) During an action potential (Fig. 1A) or a synaptic potential (Fig. 1B), depolarization is seen at all points intracellularly, yet, extracellularly, either positive or negative field potentials are encountered. (2) Simultaneous and uniform depolarization of all parts of the neuronal membrane will result in no spatial or extracellular currents.

2.3. Equations for Current Flow

This section presents the basic equations describing intra- and extracellular current flows. In general, the intra- and extracellular compartments may be treated as independent compartments. Thus, we may explain the generation of field potentials in two discrete steps. First, the intracellular potentials are established by equations describing capacitative and resistive flow through the cable representation of the neuron; this is the cable equation. Second, extracellular potentials are generated by the current-source-density, i.e., membrane currents that flow out of (sources) or into (sinks) the intracellular medium; the essential equation is a Poisson equation that describes current flow in a volume conductor. (Readers not quantitatively oriented may skip this section.)

2.3.1. Electrical Model of the Membrane

The electrical properties of the membrane are represented by a capacitance and a resistance in parallel (Cole, 1968; Jack et al., 1983). The current I_m is therefore

$$I_m = C_m \frac{dV}{dt} + \frac{V}{R_m} \tag{1}$$

Injection of a current step I_o through the membrane will slowly charge up the membrane (Fig. 2), and

$$V(t) = I_o R_m \left[1 - \exp(-t/\tau)\right] \tag{2}$$

where t = time
$\tau = R_m C_m$ = time constant
R_m = membrane resistance [ohm cm^2]
C_m = membrane capacitance [F/cm^2]

When I_o is removed, voltage decays as

$$V(t') = I_o R_m \exp(-t'/\tau) \tag{3}$$

where t' = time from the instant I_o is changed back to zero.

2.3.2. Continuous Cable Representation

The geometry of the intracellular medium can be complicated. Often, however, it may be represented by a core-conductor of the shape of a cylindrical cable (cf Jack et al., 1983; Rall, 1977). Rall (1959, 1964) has used cables for the simulation of somas, dendrites, and axons. In a simple cylindrical cable, radial currents are assumed negligible, and the main current is longitudinal. The extracellular potentials are often negligible in the determination of intracellular current flow, so that the transmembrane potential may be approximated as the intracellular potential $V(x,t)$. The longitudinal current i_l is given by

$$i_l = -\frac{1}{r_l} \frac{\partial V}{\partial x} \tag{4}$$

when r_l = longitudinal resistance [ohm/cm].
The membrane current is given by the loss of the longitudinal current, or

$$i_m = -\frac{\partial i_l}{\partial x} = \frac{1}{r_l} \frac{\partial^2 V}{\partial x^2} \tag{5}$$

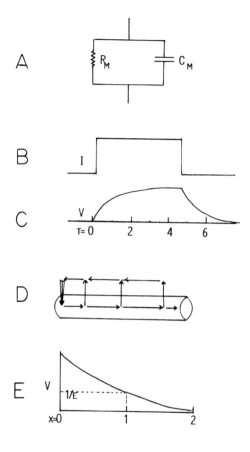

Fig. 2. (A–C) Electrical model of a passive membrane is a resistance (R_m) and a capacitance (C_m) in parallel. Injection of a current square wave (B) causes voltage response across the membrane (C). The rise and fall of the voltage are determined by the time constant $\tau = R_m C_m$ (*see* text). Time (T) in units of τ. (D–E) Injection of a constant current at the end of an axon or dendrite results in decremental current and voltage drop-off away from the injection site. The steady-state voltage (membrane potential) falls off exponentially with the space constant λ. Distance (x) in units of λ.

This membrane current is identical to that flowing across the leaky capacitance (Eq. 1)

$$i_m = \frac{1}{r_l}\frac{\partial^2 V}{\partial x^2} = c_m\frac{\partial V}{\partial t} + \frac{V}{r_m} \tag{6}$$

where (Eq. 1) is rewritten with the partial derivative in time and c_m and r_m are expressed as per unit length of the cable, where

$$r_l = R_i/\pi a^2 \tag{7a}$$

$$r_m = R_m/2\pi a \tag{7b}$$

$$c_m = C_m 2\pi a \tag{7c}$$

a = radius of the cylindrical cable
R_i = intracellular resistivity [ohm cm]

Thus,

$$\frac{aR_m}{R_i}\frac{\partial^2 V}{\partial x^2} = C_m R_m\frac{\partial V}{\partial t} + V \tag{8}$$

Define space constant

$$\lambda = (aR_m/R_i)^{1/2} \tag{8a}$$

and, as before

$$\tau = C_m R_m \tag{8b}$$

Then

$$\lambda^2\frac{\partial^2 V}{\partial x^2} = \tau\frac{\partial V}{\partial t} + V \tag{9}$$

which is the cable equation.

The space constant determines the decay of the potential with distance. If a steady current is injected at $x = 0$ of an infinite cable (Fig. 2D), the steady-state voltage distribution (Fig. 2E) is

$$V(x) = V_0 e^{-(x/\lambda)}, \; x > 0 \tag{10}$$

where V_0 = intracellular potential at $x = 0$.

In other words, the voltage decays exponentially with distance as determined by the space constant λ. A large space constant means that current will flow for considerable distances longitudinally with no membrane current loss when R_m is large and/or R_i is small.

Similarly, a large space constant is found for cables with a large radius (a). Thus, large axons have large space constants and require "boosting" only at relatively long distances. The approximate value of λ in neuronal processes varies from about 100 μm (for $a = 0.1$ μm) to 3 mm ($a = 100$ μm), assuming $(R_m/R_i) \simeq 40$. Therefore electrotonic spread occurs over large distances (>100 μm), and the distribution of current sources and sinks is also spatially extensive.

2.3.3. Volume Conduction

The previous section describes the membrane current for a single neuronal cable. The current-source-density (CSD) is the sum of the membrane currents for all the neurons in a local volume. CSD is a descriptor for the current accumulation (formally equivalent to charge) per volume of the extracellular medium, thus the term "density". It has been noted that there is no net charge accumulation anywhere in the brain if both intra- and extracellular media are included. However, in the generation of field potentials, we may assume that the extracellular medium is impressed with CSD and use standard electric field equations to describe the resulting extracellular current ($\bar{J}$), electric ($\bar{E}$) or potential (ϕ) fields. The fields are essentially described in three equations (*see* an introductory physics text, such as Halliday and Resnick, 1962 for reference):

$$\bar{E} = -\bar{\nabla}\phi \tag{11}$$

$$\bar{J} = \sigma\bar{E} = -\sigma\bar{\nabla}\phi \tag{12}$$

and

$$\bar{\nabla} \cdot \bar{J} = -I_v \tag{13}$$

where σ = conductivity tensor

$$\bar{\nabla} = \frac{\partial}{\partial x}\,\hat{\imath} + \frac{\partial}{\partial y}\,\hat{\jmath} + \frac{\partial}{\partial z}\,\hat{k} \text{ gradient operator}$$

and

$$\bar{\nabla} = \left(\frac{\partial}{\partial x}\,\hat{\imath} + \frac{\partial}{\partial y}\,\hat{\jmath} + \frac{\partial}{\partial z}\,\hat{k}\right) \cdot \text{ divergence operator}$$

Equation 11 describes the conservation of energy in an electric field, and the existence of a scalar potential as a function of space (but not of path or history). Equation 12 describes the relation between the two vectors, $\bar{J}$ and $\bar{E}$. The most general case is when the conductivity is a tensor (or a 2-dimensional matrix relating the various components of $\bar{J}$ and $\bar{E}$). Equation 13 describes the conservation of charges, stating that the increase in current in a local volume is caused by the impressed volume CSD I_v.

Combination of Eqs. 11–13 results in

$$\bar{\nabla} \cdot (\sigma \bar{\nabla} \phi) = -I_v \tag{14}$$

This is the Poisson equation. In a region without I_v, $\bar{\nabla}(\sigma \bar{\nabla} \phi) = 0$ is known as the Laplace equation. If σ is dependent on direction (anisotropic), but is homogeneous in one direction, then

$$\sigma_x \frac{\partial^2}{\partial x^2} \phi + \sigma_y \frac{\partial^2}{\partial y^2} \phi + \sigma_z \frac{\partial^2}{\partial z^2} \phi = -I_v \tag{15}$$

where σ_x, σ_y and σ_z = conductivity in x, y, and z directions. Given that a discrete current I_0 is injected at the center of a polar coordinate system ($r = 0$), i.e.,

$$I_v = -I_0\, \delta(r) \tag{16}$$

with Dirac delta function $\delta(r) = 1$ at $r = 0$
                        and $\delta(r) = 0$ at $r \neq 0$

then, for an anisotropic but homogeneous medium,

$$\phi(x, y, z) = [I_0/4\pi(\sigma_y\sigma_z x^2 + \sigma_x\sigma_z y^2 + \sigma_x\sigma_y z^2)] \tag{17}$$

With the assumption of an isotropic and homogeneous medium, i.e.,

$$\sigma_x = \sigma_y = \sigma_z = \sigma \tag{18a}$$

and

$$x^2 + y^2 + z^2 = r^2, \tag{18b}$$

the relation between ϕ and I_v is given by

$$\frac{\partial^2 \phi}{\partial x^2} + \frac{\partial^2 \phi}{\partial y^2} + \frac{\partial^2 \phi}{\partial z^2} = -\frac{I_v}{\sigma} \tag{19}$$

and a discrete $I_v = -I_0\delta(r)$ current will give

$$\phi(r) = \frac{I_0}{4\pi\sigma r} \tag{20}$$

Equation 20 describes the potential field of a monopole in an infinite homogeneous medium, with a decay of r^{-1} with distance.

Since the equation relating ϕ and CSD (I_v) is linear, the potential at any point is a linear sum of a series of discrete CSDs. A complex distribution of CSDs may be approximated by a series of discrete CSDs, and the potential at any point is caused by the sum of that caused by each discrete CSD.

In a local volume, different neurons may generate membrane currents of various magnitudes or polarities. The differences may be caused by differences in synaptic actions (e.g., excitation vs inhibition) or by a spatial dispersion of neuronal elements (dendrites excited in some neurons vs somas in the others). Cancellation of positive and negative membrane currents will occur in the CSD. This underscores the fact that CSD is a macroscopic (field) rather than a microscopic (single neuronal) descriptor.

2.4. Qualitative Properties of Field Potentials

2.4.1. Main Characteristics

In a series of detailed studies, Lorente de Nó analyzed and discussed the main characteristics of action and synaptic potential fields. We shall discuss selectively the results of these papers, emphasizing those relevant to this chapter. For details, the readers are referred to the original papers (Lorente de Nó, 1947a,b).

In one study (Lorente de Nó, 1947a), the extracellular potential field generated by a compound action potential in the frog's sciatic nerve was systematically mapped. The following results were established

1. The magnitude, duration, and waveform of the extracellular potential were different from the intracellular potential. The extracellular field near the nerve trunk could be described mainly as a positive–negative–positive transient. This reflects the dependence of the extracellular potential on current sources and sinks, or membrane currents that flow between intra- and extracellular media (*see* Eq. 6 above). In a cable representation, the sources and sinks are dependent on the second-order derivative of the transmembrane potential ($\frac{\partial^2 V}{\partial x^2}$ in Eq. 6). In

a traveling wave (action potential) described by a function $V(x - kt)$, $\dfrac{\partial^2 V}{\partial x^2} = \dfrac{1}{k^2}\dfrac{\partial^2 V}{\partial t^2}$; i.e., the wave-shape of the space derivative is similar to that of the time derivative. A second-order time derivative of an (intracellularly recorded) action potential yields a triphasic time course.

2. At a snapshot, the extracellular potentials were distributed widely in the volume conductor. There was a general decline of field amplitude away from the nerve trunk. In general, the field potential at any particular location depends on the current sources and sinks at all other sites, though the dependence on the nearest sink or source is strongest.

3. The propagating compound action potential resulted in a propagating field associated with two zones of positive potentials surrounding a negative zone.

In another study, Lorente de Nó (1947b) described the concept of closed vs open fields. A closed field has a radial symmetry (Fig. 3B). It may result either from radially symmetric activation of a single cell or from activation of a nuclear structure, resulting in a radially symmetric extracellular current flow. In ideal closed fields, no extracellular current flows outside of the domain of the cell or nucleus that is activated. The field has the same polarity everywhere, and this polarity depends on the sign of the centrally located current-source-density. If the centrally located current density is a source, e.g., hyperpolarization of the cell body of a cell with spherically symmetric dendrities, then the field is everywhere positive. This closed field is thus called a monopole field. However, the field is NOT generated by a "monopole" current-source-density, but by radially opposing sources and sinks (Fig. 3B).

In contrast, an open field is characterized by an extensive extracellular current and potential field (Fig. 3A). This type of field results from activation of laminated structures like the cortex and cerebellum, where palisades of cells are aligned parallel to each other. The existence of long dendritic trees in the cortex and the predominance of synaptic inputs on the dendrites enhance the flow of extracellular currents along the long axis of the cell. For a given active synaptic site, dipole or tripole fields (classified by polarity of the potential field) may result.

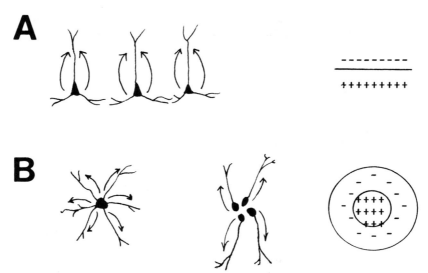

Fig. 3. (A) Excitation of the distal apical dendrites of pyramidal cells gives rise to mainly axial currents; the electrostatic model is a dipole layer that gives an open field. (B) Excitation of the distal dendrites of a single stellate cell or excitation of the periperal dendrites of cells in a nuclear structure gives rise to radial currents; the electrostatic model is one of concentric layers of charges that generate a closed field.

The realistic situation most likely involves fields that are intermediate between ideal open and closed fields, termed open–closed fields by Lorente de Nó (1947b). A uniform activation of the olfactory bulb is an example of such a field (Klee and Rall, 1977).

2.4.2. Contribution of Action and Synaptic Currents to the Electrocorticogram

It has been recognized for some time that the electrocorticogram and extracellularly recorded evoked responses are mainly generated by postsynaptic potentials, not by action potentials (*see* review by Purpura, 1959). The relative lack of contribution of the action potential may be the result of several factors:

1. Somatic action potentials are brief (<2 ms duration), and the action potentials among a population of neurons seldom fire synchronously in the

spontaneous condition. In contrast, postsynaptic potentials typically have durations of 10 ms or longer.

2. An action potential consists of fast, high-frequency changes in conductances. As a result, action currents (Na^+ or K^+) flow preferentially through the membrane capacitance at or near the active locus. The latter results in a relatively small physical separation between sink and source(s). The extracellular field at a distance is proportional to the distance between the source and sink (or the dipole moment). Thus, a closely clustered source–sink pair will result in a smaller extracellular field at large distances (Humphrey, 1968).

3. When different neurons are considered, and these neurons are dispersed in space or depth, source and sink cancellation will occur easily for action potentials, since their source–sink separation is small (Humphrey, 1968).

4. Action potentials at the soma will likely generate a source–sink–source CSD configuration, formally a quadrupole "charge" formation. The potential field of the quadrupole "charge" decays quickly with distance as $1/r^3$, as compared to $1/r$ for the monopole "charge", and $1/r^2$ for the dipole "charge" (Halliday and Resnick, 1962). As described above (e.g., Figs. 1B and 3A), distal dendritic synapses may generate a predominantly dipole field that decays with $1/r^2$.

It has sometimes been stated that the extracellular medium behaves like a low-pass filter (cf Elul, 1972). This is used to account for the small contribution of unitary action potentials to the spontaneous field potential. The statement is technically incorrect, since impedance measurement of cortex has not revealed a significant capacitative component at less than 5 KHz (Ranck, 1963; Nicholson and Freeman, 1975).

Glial cells may contribute to the electrocorticogram if they have the necessary geometrical alignment and if they are depolarized preferentially at one end of their axial processes. The currents of glial cells may only account for the dc or slow (<1 Hz) component of the electrocorticogram. For example, the Müller (glial) cells in the retina are known to generate the slow b-wave of the electroretinogram (Newman and Odette, 1984).

The reader is referred to the reviews by Creutzfeldt (1974), Elul (1972), and Mitzdorf (1985) for the neuronal mechanism underlying various components of the neocortical electrocorticogram. Generation of EEG by the olfactory cortex and hippocampus has been reviewed, respectively, by Freeman (1975) and Leung (1984).

2.5. Simulation of Field Potentials

The simulation of field potentials serves both theoretical and empirical purposes. It is sometimes necessary to distinguish between different hypotheses of neuronal activation. For example, Nicholson and Llinas (1971) found that the experimental field profiles were not similar to theoretical profiles generated by synaptic activation of passive Purkinje cells in the alligator cerebellum. Instead, the experimental profiles matched those caused by a propagating dendritic spike that was subsequently verified by intracellular recording (Llinas and Nicholson, 1971). The concept of mitral cells exciting granule cells through dendrodendritic synapses is reinforced and extended by the theoretical reconstruction of the high-amplitude field potential generated by granule cells in the olfactory bulb (Rall and Shepherd, 1968). However, despite the success of these outstanding contributions, the simulation of field potentials remains underused (*see,* however, Humphrey, 1968; Nicholson, 1973; Newman and Odette, 1984). Theoretical reconstruction is important for the interpretation of the local fields. In all scientific attempts, an inductive, synthetic (modeling) approach should complement an analytical one (below).

We advocate a three-step process in the modeling of the generation of field potential (Leung, 1984).

1. The first step is the generation of intracellular potentials by means of dendritic cable models (Rall, 1959, 1964). The compartment cable model of Rall (1964) is especially useful for computer simulation. The structure of the neuronal processes and certain biophysical properties of the membrane (e.g., time constant, space constant) are needed for this simulation.

2. The second step is the generation of CSDs from the intracellular potentials. This involves the calculation of membrane current for each neuronal cable (Eq. 6), and summing the membrane currents for all (or part of) the neurons in the local volume (to give CSD); a certain density or geometry of neuronal packing has to be assumed.

3. The third step is the simulation of field potentials by means of Poisson equation, given the imposed CSDs (Eq. 15 or 19). The location of the CSDs, the conductivity, and the boundary conditions enter into the field potential generation.

The main rationale for using the three-step approach is clarity and correspondence to available experimental data. Intracellular potentials, field profiles, and CSD profiles can all be recorded in the same preparation. The use of Rall's discrete compartment formulation is ideal for digital computation, and avoids the use of lengthy analytical formulae and Laplace transforms. The generation of field potentials from CSDs is theoretically rigorous, and the use of a "potential-divider" (Rall and Shepherd, 1968) that contains arbitrary constants is avoided. The latter is a derived, rather than a first principle (Nicholson and Llinas, 1971; Klee and Rall, 1977).

Figure 4 illustrates the simulation process for a 9-compartment representation of a neuron with dendritic processes. It is assumed that the ends of the cable represents the basal and apical dendrites, respectively, and that the cell body is at compartment 3. Synaptic excitation given at compartment 1 is described by a time function (S transient in Fig. 4B)

$$S(t) = te^{-10t} \tag{21}$$

The peak of this function is at $t = 0.1$ units of the time constant; i.e., with $\tau = 10$ ms, the peak of the activation is at 1 ms. Differential equations were solved by Runge-Kutta formulae of orders 5 and 6, at $t = 0.05$ steps. The intracellular potentials V for compartments 1–9 demonstrate the properties of cable electrotonus (Fig. 4A). At the synapse (compartment 1), the EPSP is fast and large, whereas compartments more distal to the excitation show smaller and slower responses. The early decay at the synapse reflects both the dendritic electrotonus and the brief excitation function, but the final decay at the membrane decay constant (reciprocal of time

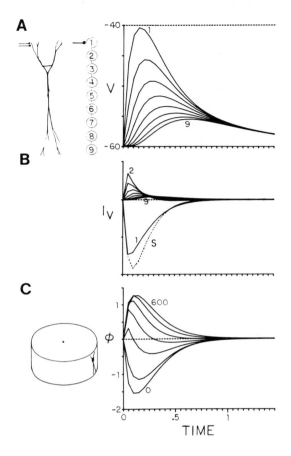

Fig. 4. (A) Basal dendritic excitation of a hippocampal pyramidal cell is modeled by a 9-compartment cable with sealed ends. Right, the peak of the intracellular transient responses (*V*) declines gradually, with delays, from compartment 1 (top, with excitation) to compartment 9 (bottom). Note that responses in all compartments decay ultimately at the same rate. (B) The membrane current flow (proportional to current-source-density I_v) at each of the 9 compartments. Compartment 1 has a current influx activated by the excitatory time function (S), and compartments 2–9 have current outflow, decreasing from compartment 2 to compartment 9. (C) The excited pyramidal cells are assumed to occupy a cylinder of 1-mm radius. Assuming uniform excitation and an infinite, homogeneous, and isotropic medium, the extracellular responses at the center of the cylinder, in 100-μm depth intervals from 0 μm (level of distal basal dendrites) to 600 μm, are shown; note an approximate reversal of potentials, i.e., a dipole field (*see* text).

constant) is the same for all compartments. Membrane currents and CSDs (Fig. 4B) generally show sinks at the synapse, and sources elsewhere. For field generation, it is assumed that the neuronal population activated is contained within a cylinder, and that the extracellular medium is isotropic, homogeneous, and infinite (Eq. 19). The extracellular field potential at different depths in a track through the center of the active neuronal population is shown in Fig. 4C. The dipole field is negative at the synapse, and positive at the cell body. This dipole field shows a distal–proximal shift of the zero isopotential during the first 0.1 time units, corresponding to the spread of the sink. The extracellular field transients are shorter than the intracellular ones. At one time unit, the field has decayed to zero, and the intracellular profiles in all compartments are almost identical. This is a demonstration that the field is generated by spatial differences in intracellular potentials, and not by depolarization alone.

3. Techniques in Field Potential Recording and Analysis

3.1. Field Potential Mapping (Laminar Analysis)

We have discussed the theoretical issues concerning the generation of field potentials. The characteristics of the field depends very much on the nature and geometry of activation of a population of neurons, as confirmed by computer simulation of field potentials. In the experimental situation, we have to solve the inverse problem, i.e., how can meaningful physiological information be obtained from a given distribution of field potentials?

Experimentally, the spatial distribution of the potential is determined by mapping. The design of mapping protocol is facilitated by relevant anatomical information. If fibers are stimulated, the projection of these fibers to the region of interest will determine the initial spatial spread of the field potentials. The spatial extent of the mapping region should encompass the structure(s) of interest. Anatomical data are also important for the interpretation of the field potentials, as discussed later.

Mapping is usually conducted in planes, i.e., in rectangular coordinates. This is partly determined by the design of the conventional micromanipulator, which is typically most accurate in Cartesian coordinates. Mapping may be performed by fixed electrode arrays or by sequential recording by a single microelectrode, typically using a reference electrode far away from the active region (such that the reference is effectively at zero potential).

Fixed electrode arrays are of two types: surface or depth electrode arrays (Appendix). The main advantage of using arrays lies in the possibility of recording from multiple electrodes at the same time. Theoretically, a potential field is generated instantaneously, and multiple electrodes may capture this instantaneous picture. This may be essential for the mapping of spontaneous events in the EEG (e.g., interictal spikes) that may not be the same at another time. However, the hardware required for amplification, filtering, and sampling of multiple (typically <100) electrodes is not trivial. Technical problems may also preclude or jeopardize the use of electrode arrays. For example, surface arrays are usually restricted to cortical structures where a clear anatomical surface can be defined. Depth electrode arrays typically have a fairly large shaft diameter and may do severe damage to the brain tissue (*see also* discussion in Kostopoulos et al., 1982).

If sequential mapping is done by a single electrode, as is common in mapping evoked responses, consideration must be given to maintaining the stability or stationarity of the response. One control is by use of a stationary recording electrode for monitoring the responses during the mapping procedure. this stationary electrode is best situated downstream of the afferent input to the region of mapping, so that tissue damage may be easily detected. An additional control is recording the responses several times before, during, and at the end of a mapping procedure. The number of mapping sites (i.e., the spatial extent and interval of mapping) and the number of averages of the response at each site both may be subjected to the constraint of the time duration in which stationarity can be maintained, and the damage the tissue can sustain. Typically, 1–3 planes and 5–10 tracks may be mapped in one preparation (cf Freeman, 1975). Automated electrode stepping will improve the accuracy and speed of mapping.

At the end of a mapping procedure, the location of the brain tissue corresponding to a salient field event (e.g., maximum or reversal) should be marked histologically. This can be accomplished by passing dyes out of a micropipet or driving metallic ions (ferric or tungsten) out of a metal microelectrode.

Two types of displays are commonly used in the mapping of field potentials. First, the time transients are plotted at the different sites of recording. This usually constitutes the raw data. Second, at sequential time instants, spatial maps of the field are plotted (Fig. 5). The spatial maps can be formed by linking points with the same potential, i.e., by means of isopotentials, and thus resemble a contour map. The plot of potential at one time instant is essential for the interpretation of field potential. As discussed above, each potential field is an instantaneous event. Thus, considerations should be given to ensure that the same time instant is sampled for each of the sequential records. For example, temporal variation of the instant of the sampling should be minimized.

3.2. Measurements of Conductivity

The conductivity of a particular part of the brain (approximate range 0.8–10 mmho/cm) depends on multiple factors, such as the direction of fiber tracts or dendrites, the constitution of the neuropil and its packing density, and in part, the distribution of blood vessels. It has been found that white matter typically has a lower conductivity than grey matter (Van Harreveld et al., 1963), and that the conductivity is lower in a direction transverse rather than parallel to the main direction of a fiber tract (Nicholson, 1965; Ranck and Bement, 1965; Nicholson and Freeman, 1975).

The measurement of tissue conductivity is usually based on simplifying assumptions. Current sources and/or sinks are imposed on the (extracellular) brain tissue, and the potentials at different points are measured. Typically, homogeneity is assumed, and boundary conditions between inhomogeneous layers or regions are ignored. Anisotropy may be estimated, typically in Cartesian coordinates. Variations in the techniques of conductivity measurement are in (1) the type of electrode used to impose currents, (2) the frequency or waveform of the applied current, and (3) the detailed equation used in deriving conductivity.

Some studies are large parallel plates for imposing extracellular currents (cf Haberly and Shepherd, 1973). Potentials are then mapped along an axis perpendicular to, and at the middle of, the electrode plates. Since currents flow only perpendicularly to the plates, the conductivity of a single direction can be determined. The problem with this approach is the difficulty in positioning large parallel plates of electrodes in vivo without damage to the brain.

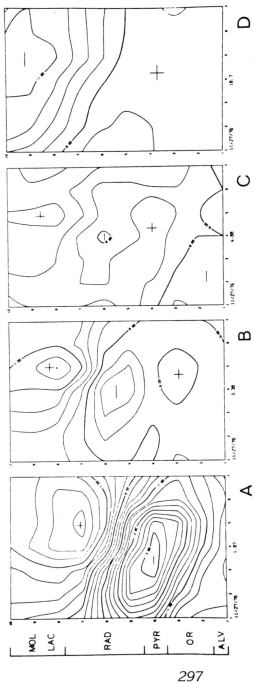

Fig. 5. Contour map of the average evoked potential (AEP) at (A) 1.87, (B) 3.38, (C) 4.88, and (D) 18.7 ms following an alvear tract stimulation. The AEP ($N = 50$) was mapped sequentially at each of the 70 grid points (600 μm mediolateral × 900 μm deep) in hippocampal CA1 region in a coronal plane. Ventrolateral is at the upper left. ALV, alveus, layer of the alvear tract; OR, Stratum oriens, basal dendritic layer; PYR, pyramidal cell layer; RAD, stratum radiatum, mid-apical-dendritic layer; MOL-LAC, stratum molecularelacunosum, distal apical-dendritic layer. See Fig. 10 for schematic of neuronal arrangement. Contour interval is 15 μV (from Leung, 1979b).

A more flexible approach uses a single electrode to impose an extracellular current (and potential) field. Assume that the source current is I_o at the origin $x = 0$, $y = 0$, $z = 0$ or $(0, 0, 0)$, and the potential is recorded at the three points, V_x at $x = a$, $y = 0$, $z = 0$ $(a, 0, 0)$, V_y at $(0, a, 0)$ and V_z at $(0, 0, a)$. Then, for an anisotropic medium of conductivity σ_x, σ_y, and σ_z along the x, y, and z axes, the potentials are given by using equation 17, i. e.,

$$V_x = I_o/4\pi\sqrt{\sigma_y\sigma_z} \tag{22a}$$

$$V_y = I_o/4\pi\sqrt{\sigma_x\sigma_z} \tag{22b}$$

$$V_z = I_o/4\pi\sqrt{\sigma_x\sigma_y} \tag{22c}$$

and

$$\sigma_x = I_oV_x/4\pi V_yV_z \tag{23a}$$

$$\sigma_y = I_oV_y/4\pi V_xV_z \tag{23b}$$

$$\sigma_z = I_oV_z/4\pi V_xV_y \tag{23c}$$

The dependence of the potential recorded along one axis on the conductivity of the two other axes, e.g., V_x dependence on σ_y and σ_z, but not on σ_x, should be noted.

Readers are referred to the papers of Ranck and Bement (1965), Nicholson and Freeman (1975), Yedlin et al. (1974), and Plonsey 1969 p. 358) for the modifications and refinements used by the different researchers.

Mapping of the field resulting from imposed currents may reveal whether the assumptions of isotropicity along the direction of the axis and homogeneity are justified. Sinusoidal currents of different frequencies may be used to test the frequency dependence of the conductivity. In general, the conductivity is not strongly dependent on frequency within the physiological range (cf Ranck, 1963; Nicholson and Freeman, 1975). Thus square wave current pulses will give similar results as sinusoidal currents.

3.3. The Current Field

The extracellular current $\bar{J}$ is related to the extracellular electric field $\bar{E}$ and the conductivity tensor σ. In isotropic medium, $\bar{J}$ and $\bar{E}$ are proportional, and $\bar{E}$ can be derived readily as the voltage gradient. Although a number of investigators prefer to derive and interpret CSD profiles without the intermediate step of deriving voltage gradients, estimation and display of the current flow field facilitate data interpretation, because of the prime importance of current flow in neurophysiology.

Current flow is derived from the relation.

$$\bar{J} = -\sigma\bar{\nabla}\phi \qquad (12)$$

In an homogenous but anisotropic medium,

$$\bar{J} = J_x\hat{i} + J_y\hat{j} + J_z\hat{k}$$

$$= -\sigma_x \frac{\partial\phi}{\partial x}\hat{i} - \sigma_y \frac{\partial\phi}{\partial y}\hat{j} - \sigma_z \frac{\partial\phi}{\partial z}\hat{k} \qquad (24)$$

In practice, if sampling of the potential is at regular spatial intervals of Δl, the differentiation is approximated by differencing, e.g.

$$J_x = -\sigma_x[\phi(x + \Delta l, y, z) - \phi(x, y, z)]/\Delta l \qquad (25)$$

This $\bar{J}$ estimate derived is formally at position $(x + \Delta l/2, y + \Delta l/2, z + \Delta l/2)$. The $\bar{J}$ vector derived may be plotted in a plane (Fatt, 1957; Leung, 1979b; Fig. 6). These $\bar{J}$ maps give an important picture as to where are the main currents and their direction of flow. For a quantitative estimation of the location and strength of sources and sinks, CSD is preferred over $\bar{J}$ field.

3.4. Current-Source-Density Analysis

CSD analysis theoretically gives the location and time course of changes in membrane currents. Volume conductor effects are eliminated, and CSD describes the local macroscopic membrane currents. A source occurs when currents enter the extracellular medium (from the intracellular one), and a sink occurs when currents exit the extracellular medium.

The equation for CSD is given as

$$I_v = -\bar{\nabla}(\sigma\bar{\nabla}\phi) \qquad (14)$$

In an anisotropic homogenous medium

$$I_v = -\sigma_x \frac{\partial^2\phi}{\partial x^2} - \sigma_y \frac{\partial^2\phi}{\partial y^2} - \sigma_z \frac{\partial^2\phi}{\partial z^2} \qquad (15)$$

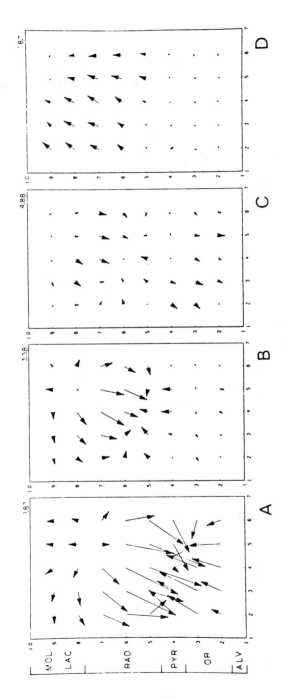

Fig. 6. Electric field or current-flow field (assuming homogeneity and isotropy) at (A) 1.87, (B) 3.38, (C) 4.88, and (D) 18.7 ms following alvear tract stimulation. Calibration: length of base of grid = 2.2 mV/mm (from Leung, 1979b).

Practically, potential can be sampled only at discrete intervals, and CSDs are determined by differencing instead of differentiation. The simplest approximation is

$$\frac{\partial^2 \phi}{\partial x^2} \simeq \frac{1}{\Delta x} \left[\frac{\phi(x + \Delta x, y, z) - \phi(x, y, z)}{\Delta x} - \frac{\phi(x, y, z) - \phi(x - \Delta x, y, z)}{\Delta x} \right]$$

$$\simeq \frac{1}{(\Delta x)^2} [\phi(x + \Delta x, y, z) - \phi(x - \Delta x, y, z) - 2\phi(x, y, z)] \quad (26)$$

Note that electric field E_x is approximated by

$$E_x = -\frac{\partial \phi}{\partial x} = \frac{\phi(x, y, z) - \phi(x + \Delta x, y, z)}{\Delta x} \quad (27)$$

The following are some practical concerns in applying CSD analysis:

1. Dimensionality: Many applications use one-dimension CSD analysis without providing an empirical justification that currents flow essentially in one direction. Establishing the latter fact requires mapping in two or three dimensions. The $\bar{J}$ maps (Fig. 6) will graphically illustrate the presence or absence of unidirectional flow.

2. Spatial interval of mapping: The sampling theorem dictates that the sampling frequency must be at least twice the maximal frequency in the signal. Otherwise, (spatial) aliasing may occur (Leung, this volume). In order to determine the spatial frequency of the event in question, the spatial variation of the potential of the event (using a very small sampling interval) and a spatial power spectrum should be determined. The power spectrum will indicate the maximum spatial frequency contained in the signal (Freeman and Nicholson, 1975). In general, the relatively large space constant of the neuronal processes, 100 µm–1 mm (corresponding 0.1–10 µm diameter, *see above*), will effectively smooth the extracellular potential. Intervals of 25–200 µm have been used by different researchers.

3. Smoothing and differencing formulae: Equation 26 above for the CSD represents the simplest

approximation to the second-order differentiation. Other differentiation formulae (*see* Freeman and Nicholson, 1975) assume fitting a polynomial through three points or more and finding the second-order derivative from the best-fitted curve. An implicit smoothing and then differentiation (differencing) is implied. It is interesting to note that if the potential (in one direction) is spatially smoothed by

$$\phi'(x) = \phi(x + \Delta x) + 2\phi(x) + \phi(x - \Delta x) \qquad (28)$$

and

$$\text{CSD}_x = \frac{\partial^2 \phi}{\partial x^2} \simeq \phi'(x + \Delta x) + \phi'(x - \Delta x) - 2\phi'(x) \qquad (29)$$

Then effectively,

$$\text{CSDx} = \phi(x + 2\Delta x) + \phi(x - 2\Delta x) - \phi(x) \qquad (30)$$

or an effective $2\Delta x$ interval is now used in the differencing approximation (though the sampling is at Δx intervals). The effectiveness of different smoothing and differencing formulae can only be evaluated with actual data. Freeman and Nicholson (1975) found that the simple smoothing and differencing procedure described above (Eqs. 28–30) gives CSDs with reasonable signal-to-noise ratios, equivalent or superior to more sophisticated procedures.

4. Accuracy in time and space: Sampling accuracy is extremely important in CSD analysis, because the differencing procedure amplifies noise. Stability of a preparation is essential for a sequential mapping procedure, and averaging of individual responses may reduce random sporadic noise. The accuracy of the micromanipulator is important, since CSD error is heavily dependent on the error in the spatial interval through the $(\Delta x)^2$ term.

CSDs are typically displayed in two ways: (1) plotting a CSD map or CSD strength at different depths (Fig. 7), and (2) plotting the time transients of CSD at each location (Fig. 9).

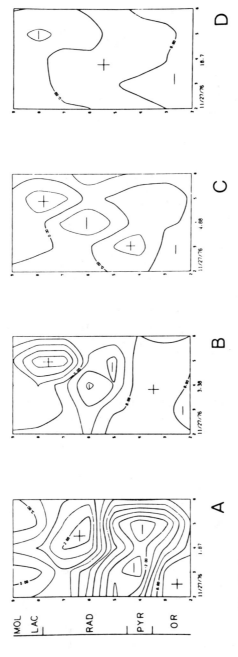

Fig. 7. Current-source-density map at (A) 1.87, (B) 3.38, (C) 4.88, and (D) 18.7 ms following alvear tract stimulation. Contour interval = 3 mV/mm² (from Leung, 1979b).

303

4. Interpretation of Field Potentials

4.1. General Principles

Given a set of field potentials, volume conduction makes the exact delineation of active vs inactive regions impossible. However, since the potential decays with distance away from the current source, the maximum or minimum of the surface potentials can usually be considered as approximately the epicenter of activity. Although the location of a potential maximum (or minimum) does correspond to the location of a source (or a sink), it may not correspond to the location of the largest source or sink. Only CSD analysis (of the correct dimensionality) will give the correct profile of sources and sinks.

It is difficult to interpret cellular processes with only field or CSD profiles. A positive CSD (source) may imply an active local membrane hyperpolarization, or passive local *depolarization* driven by more depolarized emf elsewhere (e.g., EPSP at a distant synapse). Furthermore, CSD or field analysis reveals only the global picture of current flow. A population of neurons undergoing sequential synaptic activation (e.g., EPSP–IPSP sequence) or two populations of neurons receiving different synaptic inputs may give rise to complex potential or CSD fields that may cancel each other or be difficult to decompose. Thus, additional neuroanatomical and unit physiological information should be utilized. The location and branching patterns of the axon and dendrites of different cells (neurons and glia) would suggest the likelihood of their participation in a field event. For example, stellate cells would tend to give closed fields, whereas pyramidal cells would tend to give open fields (Fig. 3). The extent of extracellular current sources and sinks should correspond to the spatial extent of the particular cell population that generates the sources and sinks. In terms of physiological data, intracellular recording in different cell populations will be the most useful, since it will reveal cellular polarization. Lacking intracellular impalements, increase or decrease in unit firing may be interpreted, with some degree of uncertainty, as caused by underlying EPSPs or IPSPs.

Some researchers consider EPSPs, rather than IPSPs, as the prime source of synaptic currents (Mitzdorf, 1985). It is true that for many CNS neurons at the resting potential, IPSPs are typically slower and of lower amplitude than EPSPs. Thus, capacitative and resistive flows during an IPSP may be smaller than those during an EPSP. However, there are conditions under which the IPSP fields are large, e.g., when IPSPs are highly synchronous among cells (this may be facilitated by an IPSP duration longer than that of an EPSP) or when membrane potentials are tonically depolarized. Thus, the contributions of EPSPs and IPSPs may vary in different conditions.

The interpretation of CSD or field potentials is a deductive as well as an inductive one. For each cell population, it may be asked whether a particular type of depolarization/hyperpolarization caused by an intrinsic or a synaptic process may give rise to the particular profile of field potentials or CSD. Geometrical and morphological data, such as the dendritic branching of the type of cell and the distribution of cells through the region, will be factors that determine the characteristics of the extracellular field. Whereas qualitative aspects of the field may be envisioned using first principles, quantitative aspects of the field potentials can be obtained only by biophysical models, such as the one proposed above. A model should incorporate branching and biophysical properties of a single neuron and geometry of the neuronal population, and generate CSDs and extracellular potential fields. A mismatch between the model-generated and the actual fields will necessitate reevaluating the interpretation of the field potentials.

4.2. Examples

The scheme in Fig. 8 was proposed by Mitzdorf and Singer (1978) to explain the sequence of activation of area 18 of the visual cortex following optic radiation stimulation (Fig. 9). The initial event (peak 1, not labeled) was the presynaptic volley, which yielded only small CSDs. Peak 3 was interpreted as the monosynaptic excitation (sink) on the proximal apical dendrites at layer IV of the pyramidal cells. The monosynaptic activity generated by the small stellate calls, where most optic afferents terminate, was not represented in the field potentials or CSDs. This may not be unexpected, because of the closed field generated by the stellate cells. The existence of concurrent sources in layer III and V is incompatible with the small stellate cells that extend few dendritic processes outside of layer IV. Peaks 4 and 5 were interpreted as mainly caused by di- and trisynaptic activity generated by excitatory synapses at layer III and II, respectively. The inverse

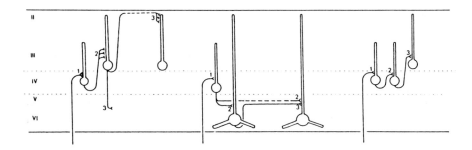

Fig. 8. Schematic diagram of the three main pathways in area 18 that give rise to the main current-source-densities following optic radiation stimulation (*see* Fig. 9). 1, 2, and 3 correspond to mono-, di- and trisynaptic synapses (from Mitzdorf and Singer, 1978).

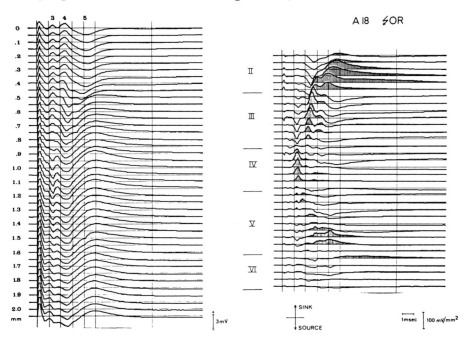

Fig. 9. Left, average evoked potentials and right, current-source-densities along a track through area A18 of the cat following electrical stimulation of the optic radiation. The sinks, interpreted as active EPSP currents, are hatched vertically. Cortical layers are indicated on the left. Kindly provided by U. Mitzdorf (unpublished).

polarity of peak 5 as compared to earlier peaks is consistent with the distal vs the proximal excitation.

The scheme in Fig. 10 was used for the interpretation of the local responses following alvear tract stimulation (Leung, 1979b; Richardson et al., 1987). A compound action potential (antidromic) was conveyed by (horizontal) alvear fibers that invaded the cell bodies and then the dendrites. At 3 ms latency, the excitation at the superficial stratum oriens was observed, followed by a long-latency, long-duration inhibition of the soma and proximal dendrites. All the events were generated mainly by pyramidal cells, though interneuronal participation was possible.

The interpretation of the field and CSD events following alvear stimulation was supported by other electrophysiological data:

1. The antidromic spike was also recorded extra- or intracellularly at 1.5–2.5 ms latency following alvear stimulation, and it followed up to 100 Hz stimulation with fixed latency (Leung, 1979a).
2. Excitation of pyramidal cells at 2.5–5 ms latency was observed.
3. The intracellularly recorded IPSP, suppression of PSTH activity, and the long-latency field event had similar physiological properties:
   a. they all have late onset latency and long duration of >50 ms,
   b. they saturated at low stimulus intensities,
   c. they did not follow stimulus frequency of >10 Hz, and
   d. they could be evoked by stimulation of various input pathways (Leung, 1979c). Neuroanatomical data indicated that basket cells, presumably inhibitory, form a plexus around the somata of pyramidal cells. Inhibitory synapses at the somata and proximal dendrites would generate the long-duration field event (also cf Andersen et al., 1964).

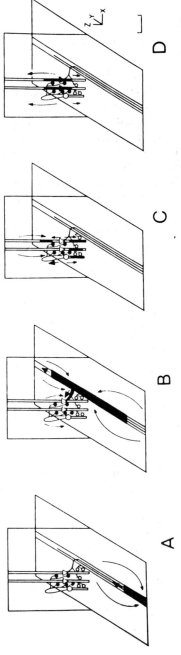

Fig. 10. Model of events in CAl following an alvear tract stimulus. Long elements, pyramidal cells with basal dendrites (short cylinder) and apical dendrites (long cylinder); short element with spherical soma, basket cell. Same layout as in Figs. 5–7. (A) Compound action potential moving in direction of thick arrow; currents (curved arrows) mostly in a horizontal plane. (B) Action potentials invaded the cell bodies (1.87 ms) and then (C) the proximal dendrites (3.38, 4.88 ms) as synaptic excitation of pyramidal cells and basket cells increased. (D) Basket cells activated inhibitory synapses on pyramidal cells in strata pyramidale and radiatum (18.7 ms) for more than 100 ms.

Appendix

Multiple Electrode Arrays

Multiple electrode arrays consist of individually fabricated types, such as assembly of a bundle of wires into vertical arrays (Barna et al., 1981; Karmos et al., 1982) or surface arrays (Eastman, 1974). Printed circuit arrays, which are smaller and allow more precise separation between electrodes, have also been used for field recording (Kuperstein and Eichenbaum, 1985; Prohaska et al., 1979; Pochay et al., 1979). Horizontal arrays can also be used to record from tissue culture or brain slices in vitro (cf. Novak and Wheeler, 1986).

At present, there are at least two commercial vendors for printed circuit electrodes:

1. Otto Sensors Corporation (cf Prohaska et al., 1979), 1100 Cedar Ave., Cleveland, OH 44106 (216) 229-3068. Thin-film, chamber-type, multisensor electronic probes are made for the recording of extracellular potential, oxygen, temperature, and ions (including pH).
2. Micro Probe Inc. (cf Kuperstein and Eichenbaum, 1985), P.O. Box 87, Clarksburg, MD 20871 (301) 972–7100. Distributed printed-circuit, 24-channel microelectrode.

Both vendors also make matching amplifier and other interface accessories.

References

Andersen P., Eccles J. C., and Løyning Y. (1964) Location of postsynaptic inhibitory synapses on hippocampal pyramids. *J. Neurophysiol.* **27,** 592–607.

Barna J. S., Arezzo J. C., and Vaughan H. G., Jr. (1981) A new multielectrode array for the simultaneous recording of field potentials and unit activity. *Electroencephalogr. Clin. Neurophysiol.* **52,** 494–496.

Cole K. S. (1968) Membranes, Ions and Impulses. (University of California Press, Berkeley), 569 pp.

Creutzfeldt O. (1974) The neuronal generation of the EEG, in *Handbook of Electroencephalography and Clinical Neurophysiology* vol 2(c) (Creutzfeldt O., ed.) Elsevier, Amsterdam, pp. 1–157.

Eastman C. (1974) Construction of miniature electrode arrays for recording cortical surface potentials. *J. Electrophysiol. Tech.* **5**, 28–30.

Elul R. (1972) The genesis of the EEG. *Int. Rev. Neurobiol.* **15**, 227–272.

Fatt P. (1957) Electric potentials occurring around a neuron during its antidromic activation. *J. Neurophysiol.* **20**, 27–60.

Freeman J. A. and Nicholson C. (1975) Experimental optimization of current source-density technique for Anuran cerebellum. *J. Neurophysiol.* **38**, 369–382.

Freeman W. J. (1975) *Mass Action in the Nervous System* (Academic, New York).

Freeman W. J. and Skarda C. A. (1985) Spatial EEG patterns, non-linear dynamics and perception: the eno-Sherringtonian view, *Brain Res. Rev.* **10**, 147–175.

Haberly, L. B. and Shepherd, G. M. (1973) Current-density analysis of summed evoked potentials in opossum prepyriform cortex. *J. Neurophysiol.* **36**, 789–802.

Halliday D. and Resnick R. (1962). *Physics, Part II.* (Wiley, New York).

Hubbard J. I., Llinas R. and Quastelo M. J. (1969) *Electrophysiological Analysis of Synaptic Transmission* (Williams & Williams, Baltimore).

Humphrey D. R. (1968) Re-analysis of the antidromic cortical response II. On the contribution of cell discharge and PSPS to the evoked potentials. *Electroencephalogr. Clin. Neurophysiol.* **25**, 421–442.

Jack J. J. B., Noble D. and Tsien R. W. (1983) *Electric Current Flow in Excitable Cells* (Clarendon, Oxford).

Karmos G., Molnar M., and Csépe V. (1982) A new multielectrode for chronic recording of intracranial field potentials in the cat. *Physiol. Behav.* **29**, 567–571.

Klee M. and Rall W. (1977) Computed potentials of cortically arranged populations of neurons. *J. Neurophysiol.* **40**, 647–666.

Kostopoulous G., Avoli M., Pelligrini A., and Gloor P. (1982) Laminar analysis of spindles and of spike of the spike and ware discharge of feline generalized penicillin epilepsy. *Electroencephalogr. Clin. Neurophysiol.* **53**, 1–13.

Kuperstein M. and Eichenbaum H. (1985) Unit activity, evoked potentials and slow waves in the rat hippocampus and olfactory bulb recorded with a 24-channel microelectrode. *Neuroscience* **15**, 703–712.

Leung L. S. (1979a) Potentials evoked by alvear tract in hippocampal CAl region of rats. I. Topographical projection, component analysis, and correlation with unit activities. *J. Neurophysiol.* **42**, 1557–1570.

Leung L. S. (1979b) Potentials evoked by alvear tract in hippocampal CA1 region of rats. II. Spatial field analysis. *J. Neurophysiol.* **42,** 1571–1589.

Leung L. S. (1979c) Orthodromic activation of hippocampal CA1 region of the rat. *Brain Res.* **176,** 49–63.

Leung L. S. (1984) Model of gradual phase shift of the theta rhythm in the rat. *J. Neurophysiol.* **52,** 1051–1065.

Leung L. S. (1990) Computer techniques in neurophysiology, this vol.

Llinas L. and Nicholson C. (1971) Electrophysiological properties of dendrites and somata in alligator Purkinje cells. *J. Neurophysiol.* **34,** 532–551.

Lorente de Nó R. (1947a) Analysis of the distribution of the action currents of nerve in volume conductors. *Stud. Rockefeller Inst. Med. Res.* **132,** 384–477.

Lorente de Nó R. (1947b) Action potential of the motoneurons of the hypoglossus nucleus. *J. Cell. Comp. Physiol.* **29,** 207–287.

Lux H. D. (1967) Eigenschaften eines neuron-modells mit dendriten begrenzter lange. *Pflugers Arch.* **297,** 238–255.

Mitzdorf U. (1985) Current source-density method and application in cat cerebral cortex: Investigation of evoked potentials and EEG phenomena. *Physiol. Rev.* **65,** 37–100.

Mitzdorf U. and Singer W. (1978) Prominent excitatory pathways in the cat visual cortex (A17 and A18): A current source density analysis of electrically evoked potentials. *Exp. Brain Res.* **33,** 371–394.

Newman E. A. and Odette L. L. (1984) Model of electroretinogram b-wave generation: a test of the K^+ hypothesis. *J. Neurophysiol.* **51,** 164–182.

Nicholson C. (1973) Theoretical analysis of field potential in anisotropic ensembles of neuronal elements. *IEEE Trans. Biomed. Eng.* **BME-20,** 278–288.

Nicholson C. and Freeman J. A. (1975) Theory of current source-density analysis and determination of conductivity tensor for anuran cerebellum. *J. Neurophysiol.* **38,** 356–368.

Nicholson C. and Llinas R. (1971) Field potentials in the alligator cerebellum and theory of their relationship to Purkinje dendritic spikes. *J. Neurophysiol.* **36,** 509–531.

Nicholson P. W. (1965) Specific impedance of cerebral white matter. *Exp. Neurol.* **13,** 386–401.

Novak J. L. and Wheeler B. C. (1986) Recording from the Aplysia abdominal ganglion with a planer microelectrode array. *IEEE Trans. Biomed. Eng.* **BME-33,** 196–202.

Plonsey R. (1969) *Bioelectric Phenomenon* (McGraw Hill, New York).

Pochay P., Wise K. D., Allard L. F., and Rutledge L. T. (1979) A multi-channel depth probe fabricated using electron-beam lithography. *IEEE. Trans. Biomed. Eng.* **BME-26,** 199–206.

Prohaska O., Pacha F., Pfundner P., and Petsche H. (1979) A 16-fold semi-microelectrode for intracortical recording of field potentials. *Electroencephalogr. Clin. Neurophysiol.* **47,** 629–631.

Purpura D. P. (1959) Nature of electrocortical potentials and synaptic organizations in cerebral and cerebellar cortex. *Int. Rev. Neurobiol.* **1,** 47–163.

Rall W. (1959) Branching dendritic trees and motoneuron membrane resistivity. *Exp. Neurol.* **1,** 491–527.

Rall W. (1964) Theoretical significance of dendritic trees for neuronal input-output relations, in: *Neural Theory and Modeling* (Reiss R. F., ed.), (Standford U. Press, Stanford). pp. 73–97.

Rall W. (1977) Core conductor theory and cable properties of neurons, in *Handbook of Physiology, The Nervous System I* (Am. Physiol. Soc., Bethesda, Maryland) pp. 39–97.

Rall W. and Shepherd G. M. (1968) Theoretical reconstruction of field potentials and dendrodendritic synaptic interaction in Olfactory bulb. *J. Neurophysiol.* **31,** 884–915.

Ranck J. B., Jr. (1963) Specific impedance of rabbit cerebral cortex. *Exp. Neurol.* **7,** 144–152.

Ranck J. B., Jr. and Bement S. L. (1965) The specific impedance of the dorsal columns of cat: an anisotropic medium. *Exp. Neurol.* **11,** 451–463.

Richardson T. L., Turner R. W., and Miller J. J. (1987) Action-potential discharges in hippocampal CAl pyramidal neurons: Current source-density analysis. *J. Neurophysiol.* **58,** 981–996.

Van Harreveld A., Murphy T., and Noble K. W. (1963) Specific impedance of rabbit's cortical tissue. *Am. J. Physiol.* **205,** 203–207.

Yedlin M., Kwan H., Murphy J. T., Nguyen-Hun H., and Wong Y. C. (1974) Electrical conductivity in cat cerebellar cortex. *Exp. Neurol.* **43,** 555–569.

From: *Neuromethods, Vol. 15: Neurophysiological Techniques: Applications to Neural Systems* Edited by: A. A. Boulton, G. B. Baker, and C. H. Vanderwolf Copyright © 1990 The Humana Press Inc., Clifton, NJ

Computer Techniques in Neurophysiology

Lai-Wo Stan Leung

1. Introduction

1.1. General Introduction

Many advances in neurophysiology depend on prior advances in technology and physical sciences. Neural signals are small electrical and chemical events, and sophisticated equipment is required to record and analyze these events. Many technological advances like the mirror galvanometer, the vacuum tube, the transistor, and the integrated circuit (IC) have been used to explore the human and the animal brain. Currently, the microprocessor promises to revolutionize the neurophysiological laboratory.

The microprocessor is a tiny chip of many ICs that controls and performs computations. The first commercially available microprocessor-based digital computer was built in about 1976. Twelve years later, a microprocessor now retails at $1–1000 and a microcomputer at $100–6000, easily within the budget of a modest research grant. In addition, today's microcomputer exceeds the performance of minicomputers built 10 years ago. In contrast to earlier machines, the microcomputer is cheap and affordable, yet extremely versatile and powerful. Its size is small enough to fit on the bench top or equipment rack. Other than a small, low-noise fan at the back, it does not require external air conditioning. The electronic components are quite reliable, and regular maintenance and servicing are minimal. When components do break down, the problem can usually be traced to a particular board or IC that can be replaced readily.

There seem to be two main impediments to the realization of the full potential of a microcomputer in an electrophysiological laboratory. First, there is a certain degree of computer phobia among technicians and scientists not previously exposed to computers. This group has to realize that microcomputers are in the laboratory to stay. A microcomputer can only do what it is instructed to do, and is no more intelligent in this way than any other piece of equipment. In order to use a piece of equipment effectively, you must know its capability and how to operate it. To use a microcomputer does not require that you become a programmer or a system analyst. Many of us can use electronic equipment adequately without knowing much about circuit design. Second, among those willing or enthusiastic souls, scientific software may be hard to come by. The time and effort required for the development of appropriate programs are formidable. The relatively small market for scientific software keeps the number of commercial products small and their prices high. This problem can be alleviated by increasing the pool of computer-enthusiastic scientists.

This chapter attempts to provide basic information on data acquisition and some common analysis techniques in neurophysiology that can readily be used on a microcomputer. This should extend and supplement the current literature on microcomputer use in the laboratory (Kerkut, 1985; Mize, 1985). In addition, previous literature on laboratory minicomputers (e.g. Brown, 1976; Bureš et al., 1982) may also provide useful information on the capabilities of current microcomputers. The knowledge of computer hardware and programming is too vast to be dealt with adequately, and the reader is referred to books on microcomputer basics (e.g., Osborne, 1979, and Zaks, 1980). A brief introduction and a glossary are provided for those unfamiliar with computer terminology, but only selected topics relevant to scientific computing are included.

With the appropriate hardware and programs, a microcomputer may function as a digital oscilloscope, digital recorder, analog-delay line, averager (both average evoked potential and poststimulus time histograms), digital filter, frequency analyzer, animal activity monitor, digital programming device (for behavioral experiments), timer, and counter. There are many functions that a microcomputer can perform, by virtue of its programming flexibility, that are not easily done by specialized equipment. Many analysis routines, e.g., cross-spectral analysis and waveform analysis, can be performed economically by a microcomputer.

1.2. A Microcomputer System

1.2.1. Basic Concepts

A digital computer deals with binary numbers, or numbers that contain either 0 or 1. A binary digit (0 or 1) is known as a bit. In the real world, we ordinarily use numbers with base (or radix) 10. Therefore, it is necessary to know the interconversion between decimal and binary numbers. Hexadecimal (or base 16) numbers are also commonly used in a computer. A hexadecimal contains 4 bits ($2^4 = 16$). In microcomputer usage, a byte is regarded as 8 bits. A word is typically the basic unit of a microprocessor, generally 8–32 bits.

The operations in a digital computer are on the binary digits 0 and 1. Addition and subtraction of binary numbers are equivalent to a combination of logical functions, such as AND, OR, and NOT (inversion). Multiplication and division can be reduced to multiple steps of addition and subtraction. Therefore, Boolean algebra, or the algebra of logical operations, is the key to computer operation.

In a computer, logical operations are done by electronic circuits. There may be many types of technology available (e.g., CMOS, TTL, and so forth), but the essential elements of computing are the same. There must be circuits to perform logical and arithmetical operations (processing unit), and there must be places to store information (memory locations). The basic memory is a logic gate that can be either open or closed (0 or 1; true or false).

Notwithstanding its ability to perform operations at greater than 1,000,000 ×/s, the real power of a computer lies in its versatility in being programmable. The outcome of the computer operations depends on the program being run. Thus, the term software is used to describe programs, which are flexible and adaptable as compared to hardware, which is the electronic circuitry that is hardwired and fixed.

1.2.2. Hardware: Processor, Peripherals, and Interface

1.2.2.1. PROCESSORS.   Continuing advances are made in computer design. Pioneering designs make use of parallel processing and multiple processors. In this section, we shall focus only on the serial-processing, single-processor microcomputer.

A general computer usually consists of three major components: processor, memory, and input/output (Fig. 1). A processor is the central core of a computer that interprets and executes

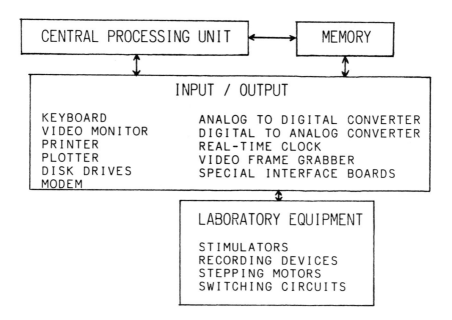

Fig. 1. Computer organization in the neurophysiological laboratory, with emphasis on the input/output interface.

instructions. It usually has a number of temporary storage locations, called registers. The instructions may involve reading and writing of a specific memory location or reading and writing of an input and output port, i.e., receiving data and transmitting signals to the external world. Instructions may also involve computations (addition, subtraction, logical operations). Processing of information is synchronized by a clock. The clock rate of microcomputers is approximately 1–20 MHz, and some operations require more than one clock cycle. Therefore, the current microcomputer performs about 1,000,000–20,000,000 operations/s.

A microprocessor is a processor on a single IC chip; some examples are given in Table 1. The older ones process 8-bit data (i.e., with each datum having 2^8 [256] discrete values) and can directly address 64K (64 × 1024 = 65,536) memory locations; the newer ones normally process 16- or 32-bit data and can address up to 16M (16,777,216) memory locations. Some microprocessors can be coordinated with a coprocessor that facilitates multiplication and division (floating-point processing, glossary).

Table 1
Some Popular Microprocessors

Microprocessor	Data bus, bit	Address bus, bit	Clock rate, MHz	Microcomputer
MOSTEK 6502	8	16	2	Apple II
Zilog Z80A	8	16	4	Cromemco II
Intel 8080	8	20	4.77	IBM-PC, -XT
Intel 80286	16	24	6–8	IBC-AT and compatibles
Intel 80386	32	32	16–20	Compaq, AST
Motorola 68000	16	24	8–10	Amiga, Macintosh

The memory is the part of the computer where programs and data are stored. There are different levels of memory in the computer. The main memory consists of semiconductor gates that are accessible in 10–2000 ns. Each memory location in the main memory is identified by an address and is accessible without interrogating another memory location (RAM, or random access memory). Secondary memory on hard disk or floppy disk may require access times of a few to many ms. Disk storage is usually divided into tracks and sectors (glossary). Storage and retrieval on magnetic cassette (or reel-to-reel) tapes require long sequential access times, and are usually used only for backing up programs and data. There is also read-only memory (ROM), which may be erasable and programmable (EPROM). Memory may be static or dynamic. The latter is volatile and is refreshed periodically; it disappears when the power is turned off.

Different parts of a microcomputer are interconnected through "bus lines". Input/output ports and memory are connected through an address bus. The loading of an address on this bus will enable a particular memory location or input/output port. Data from and to peripherals are communicated through a data bus line.

1.2.2.2. PERIPHERALS.   The instructions, data, and results of computation must be communicated to and from the external environment. For these purposes, there are many input and output devices (called peripherals), some of them used specifically in a

Table 2
Microcomputer Peripherals in the Laboratory

Keyboard for typing characters and numbers
Video for the display of graphic and text data
Printer for the printing of lines of text or for the dot printing of graphic
  data
Plotter for graphics of better quality than that given by the printer
MODEM (modulator-demodulator) for transfer of information through
  telephone lines
Floppy and hard disk drives
Tape backup devices more specific to the laboratory
Real-time clock to give exact times
Analog-to-digital converters that convert analog data to the digital format
  of the micrcomputer
Digital-to-analog converters that convert digital computer data to analog
  format
Digitizer tablets (x–y graphics input)
Relays and digital switches that interface with actual laboratory equip-
  ment

---

laboratory (Fig. 1; Table 2). Each peripheral is connected to the microcomputer through a port or an addressable connection that may provide temporary data storage (buffer).

A keyboard is a fairly standard device that codes characters (numbers and symbols) as 7- or 8-bit ASCII codes (glossary) and sends them to the computer. Choice of a keyboard usually lies in its ergonomics, e.g., whether the keyboard is detachable, the layout of symbols outside of the alphabet, the location of the function keys or number pad, and the touch of the keys.

A video monitor may be color or monochrome, and different degrees of resolution are available. Color is a combination of red, green, and blue, and monochrome may appear green, amber, or gray. Both color and monochrome monitors may have different intensity coding. The resolution of a monitor is described by the number of pixels (picture elements) in the horizontal and vertical dimensions. For example, a 768×240 resolution means that 768 elements in the horizontal axis and 240 in the vertical axis can be individually manipulated. The pixel resolution usually is relevant only for graphic display. Fully formed characters are usually generated and displayed as arrays of 5 × 7 or 7 × 9 dots (a dot matrix). Depending on the horizontal resolution, there may be 40, 80, or more characters per line of text. Some video monitors communicate by separate wires, each specifying the horizontal location, vertical location, and intensity and color of each pixel. Other monitors use the standard television cable (e.g., RS 170) and transmit a composite signal through a coaxial cable. For the color composite signal, the transmission format depends on the different systems used in different parts of the world.

A printer may print characters on paper as dot matrices or as fully formed characters. It communicates with a computer either by a serial or by a parallel interface *(see below)*. Many dot matrix printers can also be used for graphical display. The resolution of a lasar printer may even be better than some plotters. A high-speed printer (>100 characters per second) would facilitate large volumes of printing. A printer buffer may be part of the printer or the computer, or can be added on as a separate device. A print buffer stores the data directed to the printer, allowing use of the computer for other tasks.

A digital plotter is indispensible for making high-quality hard copies of graphic data. A plotter may use one or many (color) pens. Resolution of the pen is usually given in number of steps per inch or centimeter. For large volumes of plotting, automatic feeding or scrolling of paper is preferred. Since plotters are intelligent devices using their own unique command codes, consideration should be given to the availability of software to drive the plotter. Graphics data represented by a map or a tracing, or a projected film image may be entered into the computer by an x–y digitizer. Eight digitizers have been reviewed recently (Hearn 1986).

A disk drive is an essential part of a microcomputer. Information is stored on either a hard disk or a floppy disk. A hard disk may store 10–100 Mbytes using a magnetic metallic medium. Many hard disks are not removable from the computer, but there are also some removable hard disks. A floppy disk (diskette) stores approximately 0.1–1 Mbytes on a magnetic-coated plastic medium. Floppy disks come in 3-, 5 ¼-, and 8-in diameter, and they may be of single, double, or quad-density recording medium. Since electrophysiological data acquisition may generate many Kbytes in a second, adequate external memory storage is needed. Data may also be stored on digital magnetic tape. However, retrieval from magnetic tape is slow, and its only common use is for backing up data.

Storage of data on cassette tape recorders is extremely slow and is not recommended.

Communication between computers or terminals may take place through a telephone line. In order to modulate and de-modulate signals for telephone transmission, a modem is needed at both the sending and the receiving ends. Commercially available modems transmit at 300–2400 bits/s, and are not meant for massive data transfer. High-speed (Megabits/s) transfer can be achieved using fixed coaxial or fiber optics cables.

Some peripherals are more specifically used in the laboratory (Fig. 1). An analog-to-digital converter is essential for the digitizing of continuous current and voltage values. The digitizing timing should be provided by a real-time clock. A digital-to-analog con-verter may be needed for the microcomputer to display data or control equipment. A video-frame-grabber board is used to digitize video images, and may be needed in behavioral analysis. Digital input and output for the microcomputer may involve commercial and homemade interface or driver circuits, e.g., in detecting switch closure or in driving stepping motors, stimulators, and recording devices.

1.2.2.3. COMMON INTERFACES.   The interface is the connection between microcomputers and peripherals. It may be serial or paral-lel. A serial interface transmits data in one direction and through a single wire, each character coded with a temporal sequence of on and off voltages. A second wire transmits data in the opposite direction, and other wires indicate whether data are available for receiving or transmitting. A common serial interface standard is the EIA RS232C (Table 3). It typically sends by means of ASCII codes, a data communications standard. A parallel interface trans-mits data through many wires at the same time (e.g., 8-bit data through 8 separate lines). A strobe pulse is needed to synchronize the sending and receiving ends. Other pulses may be used for handshaking (glossary) or to indicate whether data are ready for sending or receiving (Table 3). The speed of communication is specified in baud rate (bits/s). The IEEE488 bus, a special instru-ment interface sometimes known as the HPIB (Hewlett-Packard interface bus), can be used to talk, to listen, or to control up to 15 pieces of compatible equipment.

1.2.2.4. INTERRUPTS.   Direct memory access. Many peripherals do not need attention most of the time. Rather than polling these peripherals constantly, most microcomputers have an interrupt

Table 3
Standard Interfaces

RS-232C serial interface (DB25 connector typically)
  pin 2 transmitted data
  pin 3 received data
  pin 7 ground
Parallel Interface basics
  pin 1 data strobe
  pin 2–9 data bit 1–8, respectively
  pin 10 acknowledge
IEEE-488 digital interface
  pin 1–4 data lines (D101–D104, respectively)
  pin 5 EOI (End or identify)
  pin 6 DAV (Data valid)
  pin 7 NRFD (Not ready for data)
  pin 8 NDAC (not data accepted)
  pin 9 IFC (Interface cleared)
  pin 10 SRQ (Service request)
  pin 11 ATN (Attention)
  pin 12 shield
  pin 13–16 data lines (D105–D108, respectively)
  pin 17 REN (Remote enable)
  pin 18–23 ground
  pin 24 logic ground

---

mode that is used to service a peripheral when needed. The latter device sends an interrupt request to the computer, which then determines the calling device and performs the servicing (data transfer) before returning to the main program. Interrupts may be prioritized so that urgent calls will be serviced first. Unnecessary interrupts may be masked or denied access to the computer.

Direct memory access (DMA) is a rapid way of data transfer that can take place without the participation of the central processor. Instead, the peripheral device takes control of the address and data bus, and directly transfers data to and from memory.

1.2.3. Software Support

A disk-operating system (DOS) is available from the microcomputer vendor to go with a particular system. The DOS is used to manipulate information (usually organized as files) and to perform routine printing or disk functions. File manipulations include copy, delete (erase), rename, directory, and so on. An editor program, for storing strings of characters in data or program files, is also important. Some common utility programs (e.g., disk formatting, printing) are usually provided with the DOS.

Computer language is classified as high- or low-level, depending on how closely it resembles the binary codes (machine language) for microcomputer operation. ASSEMBLY language is a low-level symbolic language that is very close to machine codes, and therefore is identified with a particular microprocessor. Other (high-level) languages, e.g., BASIC, FORTRAN, FORTH, PASCAL, and C, have to be compiled by a special program called a compiler in order to translate them into ASSEMBLY or machine codes. In addition, BASIC can be run in the interpreter mode, in which the computer interprets and executes a program source line by line. The programmer will then have immediate results of simple operations, and the feasibility of a small program can readily be tested. When a program consists of several modules or subroutines, a link/load program is run after compilation of individual subroutines. A recent language, like PASCAL, has powerful capability, e.g., it favors structured programming or gives better control of the flow of the program. New versions of BASIC and FORTRAN may also have additional, more powerful features than old versions. Each language has its strength: BASIC is easy to learn, C is relatively portable across microcomputers, FORTRAN has a long history of scientific use and is still popular, and ASSEMBLY is sometimes crucial in real-time control applications.

Consideration for software must take into account its compatibility with other peripherals. A data acquisition board may come with software functions (like data acquisition, subroutines, or graphics packages) written in a particular language. In starting a new system, it is preferable to use software that is familiar to people around you, so that you can benefit from their experience. A combination of FORTRAN and ASSEMBLY can usually handle all the chores of a neurophysiological laboratory. There are probably more scientific programs and subroutines written in FORTRAN than in any other language. FORTRAN subroutines or subprograms can be compiled and linked together with ASSEMBLY subroutines. The latter is relatively difficult to write, and may be reserved only for input/output manipulations in which speed is important. Direct manipulation of memory and input/output ports using a high-level language is not usually efficient in real time.

In addition to being a scientific tool, a microcomputer is useful for writing manuscripts (wordprocessing), using a spreadsheet, organizing data bases (e.g., references to papers) drawing figures (graphics), searching references over the telephone line, and as a terminal to a larger computer system. Many programs for statistical and mathematical analyses (e.g., ANOVA, IMSL subroutines) are now available on the microcomputer.

1.2.4. Single and Multiple-User Systems and Networks

Local area network is a linkage of microcomputers in order that they can communicate with each other and with other peripherals. It may be a useful solution to share expensive devices like high-speed printers, plotters, or software. During data acquisition, there is little time left for the microcomputer to deal with other input, and a single-user system is preferred for this reason.

1.2.5. Getting a Laboratory Microcomputer System*

There are many microcomputers available today. Even a slower one (like the 8-bit Apple II) can be a valuable asset in the scientific laboratory. However, if you (or a colleague you can count on for help) have no previous experience on other machines, the IMB PC, PC-XT or PC-AT, or compatible models are probably the best choice for two main reasons: economy and popularity. There are inexpensive IBM-compatible machines (at one-half or one-third of the IBM prices) that will support almost all of the software and hardware made for the real IBM microcomputers. Because of their popularity and market competition, the prices of these models are very low, and the hardware (board level) and software support is very wide. There are probably more boards and devices (for memory, analog-to-digital conversions, and so on) for the IBM PC-compatible models than for any other models. One important caution is that IBM-compatibility is a graded, but not an all-or-none attribute, especially with reference to scientific software. There-

*Every effort has been made to present accurate and up-to-date information. However, because of space limitation and perhaps lack of information, not all vendors and their products are described or listed. The information is meant to be useful to the neuroscientific community and does not constitute an endorsement of the product. The author assumes no responsibility or liability for the products presented.

fore, the compatibility of the essential software and hardware must be confirmed before purchase. For the user requiring more speed and memory, an IBM PC-AT is recommended. Poler et al. (1985) and Moreton (1985) have written reviews on the selection of hardware and software for a microcomputer in the neurobiology laboratory.

2. The Computer in a Neurophysiological Laboratory

2.1. *Recording of Neurophysiological Signals*

2.1.1. *Neural Signals*

Neural signals are electrochemical events. Sensory signals are transduced into a graded receptor potential, which then triggers an all-or-none action potential propagating down the nerve fiber. At the synapse, depolarization of the presynaptic terminal causes the release of neurotransmitters, which then interact with postsynaptic receptors, generating an excitatory (or inhibitory) postsynaptic potential. The latter may increase or decrease the firing of action potentials in the postsynaptic neuron.

Different types of electrodes, large (macroelectrodes), small (microelectrodes), or ion-sensitive (to potassium, calcium, sodium, and so on) may be placed in different parts of the brain. Recording may be intracellular or extracellular. Two main types of neural signal can be classified: pulse (action potentials) and wave (graded potentials) (cf Vanderwold and Leung, 1985). Action potentials are all-or-none events with brief time courses of usually less than 2 ms; they are often treated statistically as point processes that occur at an instant of time. The frequency, and perhaps the temporal pattern, of action potentials are behaviorally significant. Graded potentials (wave) consist of postsynaptic potentials (PSPs) measured intra- or extracellularly. In stratified structures, such as the cortex, many PSPs occur at the dendrites (dendritic potential), and extracellular (field) potentials are of high amplitude (up to approximately 10 mV) and can be recorded outside of the active region (e.g., electroencephalogram on the scalp).

In this section, microcomputer registration of electric events will be described. The use of microcomputers in functional mapping of the brain (cf Hopt et al., this volume) is described in Mize (1985) and will not be considered here. Some aspects of data acquisition have been described by Park (1985), Teyler et al. (1985) and Bagust (1985).

2.1.2. Wave Registration

Digitization of a time-varying wave signal is equivalent to imposing the signal on a rectangular grid and approximating it by a staircase. The digitization of the signal strength (vertical axis) is commonly known as quantization, and the digitization on the horizontal time axis as sampling.

2.1.2.1. SAMPLING THEOREM. The most important rule concerning digitization of an analog (wave) signal is the sampling theorem. This theorem specifies that in order to sample (digitize) an analog signal of frequency f, the sampling rate must be at least $2f$ (twice the signal frequency). Other than not being able to include the higher signal frequency, a sampling frequency (f_s) less than $2f$ will actually cause misrepresentation of the signal frequency contents. Signal frequency above $f_s/2$ will be represented as frequency ($f–f_s$) or ($f_s–f$).

An intuitive understanding of the sampling theorem can be obtained from a simple exercise (Fig. 2). If we assume a sine wave of 5 Hz (period 200 ms) as the signal, sampling at 10 Hz is adequate to get the peaks and valleys of the signal. The sampled signal has the correct frequency. However, a sampling rate of 4 Hz (every 250 ms) will generate sampling at the open squares (Fig. 2). The sampled data points have a period of 1000 ms (1 Hz). Interestingly, sampling at 6 Hz (every 166.7 ms) generates a different set of points (triangles in Fig. 2), but the period is also 1 Hz. The power spectra in Fig. 2 illustrates that the signal frequency of 5 Hz is represented at (5–4) = 1 Hz with 4 Hz sampling, or as (6–5) Hz with a mirror image (folding) at f_s = 6 Hz. The mispresentation of signal frequencies as a consequence of an inadequate sampling rate is therefore also known as aliasing (or Faltung/folding). Without a priori knowledge, the data generated after inadequate sampling cannot be used to reconstruct the real signal frequency. A 7-Hz as well as a 5-Hz signal will appear as a 1-Hz wave when sampled at 6 Hz.

Neural signals usually have a rather wide bandwidth. In order to satisfy the sampling theorem, the sampling frequency must be twice the maximal frequency of the neural signal. To find the frequency contents of a signal, it is desirable to sample at a high sampling rate (>10 KHz) and then construct a power spectrum of

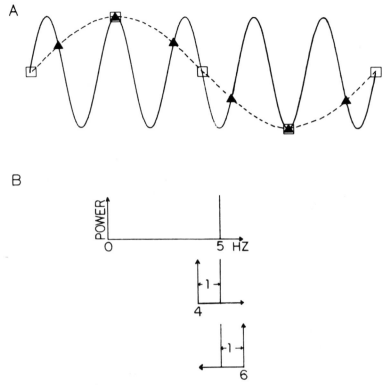

Fig. 2. (A) A signal of 5 Hz (continuous line) is sampled every 250 ms (4 Hz, open squares) or every 166.67 ms (6 Hz, triangles). At a 10-Hz sampling rate (e.g., at peaks and valleys of the wave), the period of the signal is represented correctly. At 4- or 6-Hz sampling, the sampled points fall on a sine wave of 1-Hz frequency (dotted line). (B) A power spectrum of the signal, adequately sampled, shows a single peak at 5 Hz. At a sampling frequency at f_s Hz($<$10 Hz), the vertical axis can be considered to shift to f_s Hz, such that the apparent frequency of the signal is [$f_s -$ 5] Hz, i.e., an apparent 1 Hz for both 4-Hz and 6-Hz sampling.

the signal. Practically, the maximal frequency of a signal may be considered as that beyond which there is a rapid drop-off of the power (or amplitude). Alternatively, a low-pass filter with preferably >12 dB decade roll-off should be used *before* digital sampling. Filtering may be regarded as a time-saving data reduction, but it may also give a limited view of the data.

2.1.2.2. QUANTIZATION.   Quantization is the transformation of the continuous amplitude of a signal into one of discrete, uniformly spaced steps. The procedure of quantization *per se* adds noise to the digitized signal. The mean value of the quantization error is half the least significant bit (LSB) or the quantization step. The variance of the error is $(LSB)^2/12$. If a histogram of the amplitude distribution of the signal can be constructed (by means of a high-resolution converter), the quantization step may be chosen as half the width of the narrowest peak in this amplitude histogram (Glaser and Ruchkin, 1976). This quantization step is equivalent to the sampling interval (inverse sampling frequency) discussed in the last section.

2.1.2.3. HARDWARE.   Analog-to-digital converters (ADC) operate with different methods (Artwick, 1980). Successive approximation methods may use a comparator to determine if a converter-generated signal exceeds the input voltage. Fast successive approximation starts with the most significant bit (MSB). If input voltage exceeds the MSB, the bit is left on, and the next bit is tried. A total number of n successive trials is needed for all n bits of the ADC. A cheaper ADC may generate a staircase for comparison (counter method). In this case, 2^n comparisons are needed. The dual-slope integration method integrates an input signal over a constant time and charges up a capacitor. The time for the capacitor to discharge is proportional to the built-up charges and the input voltage. The fastest and most expensive ADC operates by the simultaneous parallel conversion (flash) method. This requires 2^n number of comparators, each of which outputs a 0 or a 1, depending on whether the input signal exceeds the reference level of an individual comparator. A decoder then decodes the bit values and generates a binary code for output.

Some important features of an ADC are discussed in the following:

1. Quantization Resolution. The resolution of ADCs may be 8, 10, 12, 14, or 16 bits. An 8-bit ADC gives resolution of 0.39% of the maximal voltage, while 10-bit and 12-bit ADCs give 0.098% and 0.024%, respectively. If both high- and low-amplitude signals, of more than $10 \times$ difference in magnitude, require precise digitization, a 12-bit (or better) ADC is preferred. For example, when action potentials

occur with 100-mV peaks in an intracellular record, a 12-bit and 8-bit ADC will allow quantizing steps of 0.024 mV and 0.39 mV, respectively. If miniature postsynaptic potentials occur with 0.2–0.5 mV amplitude, the 12-bit ADC that gives 8–40 quantal steps may be considered adequate, but not the 8-bit ADC.

2. Input Voltage Range. The actual voltage that the ADC can receive may vary bipolarly from –2.5 V to 2.5 V ($\pm$ 2.5 V), $\pm$5 V, $\pm$10 V, or unipolarly from 0 to 5 or 10V. In order to obtain maximal sensitivity from the ADC, the largest signal should be close to the maximal input voltage. Therefore, it is not optimal to have an amplifier signal of $\pm$5 V feeding into an ADC with an input range of 0–10 V. First, the negative signals are neglected, and second, the positive signals will never reach 10 V, and the MSB of the ADC is never used. Fortunately, many ADCs can be configured for either unipolar or bipolar inputs. Signals smaller than the ADC input maximum can be amplified, and signals larger than the input maximum can be attenuated, e.g., by use of voltage dividers. A useful feature in some ADCs is a programmable gain, commonly 1, 2, 4, 8, and sometimes up to 1000 $\times$. Software can then be implemented to increase or decrease the input signals to obtain the maximal quantization sensitivity. Digital formats after conversion may be binary (possibly with an offset) or two's complement (glossary). The actual input voltage can be calculated from each of these codes, but the calculation is different in each case.

3. Number of Channels and Configuration. Typically ADCs have 1–16 channels. Some are expandable by daisy-chain to 64 or 256 channels. The input may be single-ended (SE) or differential (DI). An SE signal is one referred to ground, whereas a DI is one referred to another signal. The latter offers better noise immunity, which is also partially provided by a pseudodifferential configuration using a return ground wire for each single-ended input. Many

ADCs may be connected with jumper cables for either SE or DI operation. For multiple channel acquisition, the signals are usually multiplexed to a single converter, and software strobes, or automatic channel advances, are needed to switch the converter to the multiple inputs.

4. Clock. Many ADCs allow both internal and external clock sources. It is desirable to trigger conversions from external pulses. The maximal sampling or throughput rate must match the laboratory requirement. Usually, this indicates only a maximal processing rate through the ADC, and the actual acquisition rate depends on the software. Therefore, in multiple-channel recording, the sampling rate at each channel is, at best, the quoted throughput rate divided by the number of channels. For data acquisition systems sold with software, the limits of the acquisition rate of the software may prevail, whether in single- or multiple-channel application (*see also* section 2.1.4., below).

5. Other Features. Data from the ADC may be memory- or I/O- (input/output) mapped, i.e., directed to a memory or input port location. Direct memory access provides quick block transfer of ADC data to the memory without processor intervention. It may be an important feature despite its higher cost.

A list of some commonly available ADC boards for the IBM-PCT, XT, and AT is given in Table 4, together with some of their features. Boards with their own microprocessors are typically capable of high sampling rates (especially when writing to the board memory), more expensive, and supported by specific software through the same vendor. The less expensive boards may be supported by general software provided by other vendors (Tables 4 and 5).

2.1.2.4. SOFTWARE. A simple flow chart for sampling a single signal channel is shown in Fig. 3A. The clock is a real-time clock that may be internal or external to the computer. Timing by software loops is imprecise and inadequate for most neurophysiological acquisitions. The flow chart can be implemented by polling the firing status of the clock pulse, without necessarily using interrupts

Table 4
Data Acquisition and Control Boards[1]

With no on-board processor

Name	ADC[2]	Bits	Maximum sampling rate	Programmable clocks	Digital inputs/ outputs	DAC	Remarks
Cyborg[3] ISAAC 91	16S 8D	12	10 KHz	0	16/16	4	
Data Translation[3] 2801A	16S	12	27.5 KHz	1	8/8	2	with DMA
IBM-DACA	4D	12	15 KHz	1	16/16	2	
(Tecmar)[3] Labmaster	16S 8D	12	40 KHz	5	24/24	2	

With separate processor (and memory)

CED 1401 Lab Interface	16	12	67 KHz	64K	4	16/16	4
Coulbourn Signamax	2	8,12	100 KHz	16K	–	1	–
MI² M100 & M202	8	12	333 KHz	24K	3	8/8	Modular design
RC Electron. Computerscope	16S	12	1 MHz	64K	?	?/2	(1?)

[1] Information in this table was obtained from brochures supplied by the vendor. While every effort has been made to be accurate, the author assumes no responsibility for missing or wrong information.
[2] S = single-ended; D = differential.
[3] Other models are available from the same vendor.

331

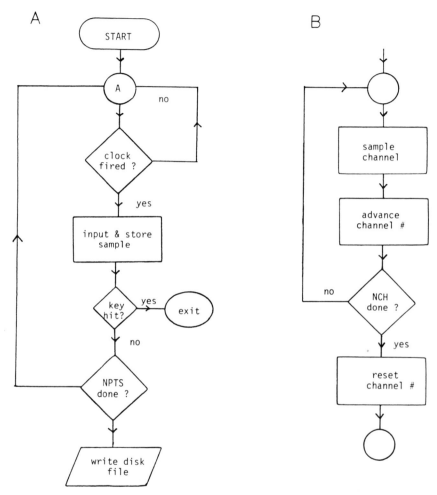

Fig. 3. (A) Flow chart for sampling on a clock pulse. (B) Multiple-channel sampling block (to replace input and store sample block in A).

to the processor. The sample and store operations should be sufficiently few that the program can return to point A (Fig. 3A) *before* another clock pulse occurs. Otherwise, clock pulses will be missed, and the sampling will not be uniform in time, i.e., some sampling intervals will be longer than others. The sampling is completed when a specified number of data points (NPTS) are done. This may be interrupted by the user (e.g., by hitting a key on the keyboard, Fig. 3A).

Some simple tests can be performed to test a sampling program. First, a steady dc signal can be used as an input, and the varying dc level should give different sampled values. If this fails, the connection and the (computer) address of the ADC must be checked. Second, in order to check precise counting of clock pulses, a fixed number of internal or external pulses can be sent to trigger ADC. The program must exit when the correct number of pulses are counted, no more and no less. If this fails, all software relating to the test of the presence of a clock pulse must be scrutinized, including an estimation of the real time required for the longest software loop (must be less than the sampling interval). Finally, a segment of a simple waveform should be sampled. The best waveforms are a linearly rising ramp, a triangular wave and a sinusoidal wave. The digitized data should be printed to see if they conform to the expected trend. Pure sinusoids can be analyzed to see if they correspond to a single symmetric peak in a power spectrum. Some of the above tests should also be applied to test commercially developed software.

2.1.3. Multiple-Channel Wave Acquisition

Many channels of analog (wave) data are usually multiplexed to a single ADC. Software commands may be needed to advance the multiplexer and sample the next channel (Fig. 3B). If the number of channels (NCH) is variable, channel advance must be provided by software (except when it is incorporated in hardware). The most rigorous multiple-channel ADC uses a sample-and-hold circuit for each channel. At one time instant, accurately provided by an internal/external clock, all circuits start sampling their individual channels, and the sampled data are held until the ADC can digitize it through the multiplexer. In this case, the sampled signals from the multiple channels are simultaneous.

Since the costs of a multiple-channel sample-and-hold ADC are quite high, alternative methods may be considered. With the current technology, near-simultaneous samples of some neurophysiological data cannot practically be distinguished from precisely simultaneous samples. Many common ADCs have a minimum of 25 KHz throughput rate, and adjacent channels can be accessed within 40 μs or better. Therefore, even if no simultaneous sample-and-hold circuits are incorporated in the ADC used in the

Table 5
Vendors

Data acquisition and control boards (cf Table 2)
  CED (Cambridge Electronic Design Ltd.), Science Park, Milton Rd.,
    Cambridge CB4 4FE, U.K. (0223) 316186
  Coulbourn Instruments, Box 2551, LeHigh Valley, PA 18001
    (215) 395–3771
  Cyborg, 55 Chapel St., Newton, MA 02158 (617) 964-9020
  Data Translation, Inc., 100 Locke Dr., Marlboro, MA 01752
    (617) 481-7300
  MI^2 (Modular Instruments Inc.) P.O. Box 447, Southeastern, PA 19399
    (215) 337-4507
  RC Electronics, 5386 Hollister Ave., Santa Barbara, CA 93111
    (805) 964-6708
  Scientific Solutions (formerly TECMAR), Inc., 6225 Cochran Rd.,
    Solon, OH 44139 (216) 349-4030

Stepping motor and accessories supplies
  Stepping motors (selected suppliers)
    AIRPAX   Japanese Products Corp.
    North American Philips Con-   7 Westchester Plaza
      trols Corp.
    Cheshire Division   Elmsford, NY 105 23
    Cheshire Industrial Park   (914) 592-8880
    Cheshire, CT 06410
    (203) 272-0301   Superior Electric Company
                                        383 Middle Street
    Sigma Instruments Inc.   Bristol, CT 06010
    Braintree, MA 02184   (203) 582-0682
    (617)843-5000

  Interface boards
    Rogers Labs (4 axis stepper   Big Stepper (external driver)
      driver)
    2727 #E. So Croddy Way   Centroid
    Santa Ana, CA 92704   P.O. Box 739
    (714) 751-0442   State College, PA 16801
                                        (814) 237-4535
    Scientific Solutions (stepper motor controller)
    (address above)

Video boards/equipment
  DT2803 (PC), DT2851 (AT) frame grabbers, Data Translation (above)
  Video tracking system, HVS, Ltd, sold by San Diego Instruments, 8148-A Ronson Rd., San Diego, CA 92111 (619) 560-7800
  Movement analysis systems, Motion Analysis Corp. 93 Stony Cir., Santa Rosa, CA 95401 (707) 579-6511

  Software for data acquisition and analysis
  ASYST, MacMillan Software Company, 866 3rd Ave., New York, NY 10022 (212) 702–3241
  LABPAC, sold by Scientific Solutions (above)
  LABSOFT, sold by Cyborg (above)
  PCLAB, ATLAB, sold by Data Translation (above)
Programs for EEG analysis
  Stellate Systems, 616 Belmont Ave., Westmount, Quebec, Canada H3Y2V9. (514) 486-1306
Programs for patch-clamp, voltage-clamp, and other experiments
  Axon Instruments Inc., 1101 Chess Drive, Foster City, CA 94404. (415) 571-9400
Programs for patch-clamp and other experiments
  Indec Systems, 128-A Mtn. View/Alviso Rd., Sunnyvale, CA. 94089. (408) 745-1842
Programs for unit, multiunit, and other analysis
  Brain Wave Systems, 3400 Industrial Lane, Suite 3, Broomfield, CO 80020. (303) 466-6190.
Programs for unit and EEG analysis, CED, and RC electronics
  (addresses above)

---

sampling flow chart of Fig. 3B, the acquisition of the second channel will follow that of the first within 40 μs. In many applications, <40 μs delay can be considered as practically simultaneous. In Fourier analysis, 40 μs causes 0.72° phase delay of a 50 Hz EEG rhythm, which is probably tolerable. However, the time and phase delay increase with the number of channels, and a 10.8° phase delay between the first and sixteenth channels may not be tolerable.

In some applications, multichannel sampling may be facilitated by using a burst of NCH (= number of channels) with a fixed burst interval (Fig. 4B; *see* section 2.1.5.). Each clock pulse is used

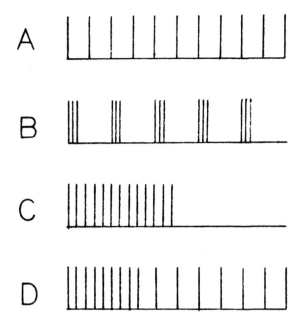

Fig. 4. Possible pulse trains generated by a timing program (*see* TIMET program, Leung, 1985). (A) Continuous pulses at a fixed interval. (B) Burst of pulses at fixed burst interval, number in each burst = NCH. (C) Triggered train of pulses at fixed interpulse interval. (D) Triggered train of pulses at high followed by low frequency.

for one sample, and the group of NCH pulses is meant for the sampling of NCH channels. Therefore, three channels are sampled during each burst in Fig. 4B. The interchannel sampling time should be as short as the ADC can allow. In our experience, we found two occasions in which a bursting pattern of clock pulses is useful. First, the sampling loop is simplified and sampling speed improved, since the test of whether NCH channels are completed (Fig. 3B) is no longer needed. Second, in some software (e.g., PC-LAB used with Data Translation 2801), it may be difficult to do interchannel sampling and sampling rate/channel at different rates, but an external source with bursts of pulses can solve this problem.

Multiple-channel acquisitions should be tested by passing identical signals of a simple waveform to all the channels. The actual time delays, if using a sequential sampling paradigm, can be assessed. Channels that are not used should be grounded to prevent cross-talk of noise into adjacent channels. The implemented program should be tested for its maximal sampling rate, which may vary with the number of channels used.

2.1.4. Timing Pulses for Spontaneous and Evoked Responses

The timing pulses (Fig. 4) can be supplied by an internal timer/counter board or by external oscillators/stimulators. Some scientific solution boards (LabMaster, LabTender, AD212) have 5 counters/timers that can be programmed to generate the different patterns of timing pulses in Fig. 4 (Leung 1985). The pattern in Fig. 4A can be used for spontaneous ongoing wave/pulse sampling; those in Figs. 4B, C, and D are triggered pulse trains used for sampling evoked or event-related responses.

Evoked responses are transient responses that follow a stimulus. In this chapter, we shall consider only responses to an impulse (a brief stimulus), e.g., an electrical shock, a light flash, or an auditory click. This stimulus is associated with a pulse trigger preceding or simultaneous to the stimulus. If sampling is done by means of a free-running internal clock, the trigger is first detected and the first clock pulse then initiates the first sample. On the average, therefore, the clock pulse is half a clock cycle delayed from the trigger. When multiple sweeps are averaged, there will be a jitter caused by the lack of absolute synchrony between trigger and free-running clock pulses. When the clock frequency is high, the jitter is negligible. This jitter is also minimized if a train of sampling pulses can be triggered with a precise, unvarying delay (Fig. 4C; Leung, 1985). A train of quick pulses followed by slow pulses (Fig. 4D) may be useful in studying the early and late periods of an evoked response (*see* section 2.2.2.).

Random or pseudorandom pulses may be generated by separating pulses by a random interval (e.g., Poisson, exponential, uniform statistics) previously stored in the computer memory. These pulses may be used to present random stimulations (e.g., by triggering a stimulation or visual display unit).

2.1.5. Pulse Registration.

2.1.5.1. WAVEFORM DETECTION. Action potentials may be recorded extracellularly by different types of microelectrodes (for review, *see* Vanderwolf and Leung, 1985). Partly dependent on the characteristics of the microelectrodes and on the recording conditions, single or multiple units (from single or multiple neurons, respectively) may be registered. Multiple-unit recording may be the unavoidable situation in a behaving animal or human. The presence of multiple units at a single electrode may even be regarded as advantageous, since it gives a better representation of the local neural activity.

Single neuronal firing may be teased out from multiple-unit recording by classifying certain characteristics (parameters) of the action potential (spike) waveform, which is presumably unique for a single neuron or axon (unit). The type of waveform classification algorithm can vary from simple (and quick) to complex (and time-consuming). The simplest method is to discriminate the peak (or peak-to-peak) amplitude of the spike, as done in the typical hardware window discriminator. The amplitude distribution of a single recorded unit typically had a Gaussian distribution. Different Gaussian distributions, each corresponding to a single unit, may be resolved from the amplitude spectrum of a multiple-unit record (Schwarz et al., 1976). The most complex software methods of unit classification require the digitization of the complete waveform of an action potential (*see* review by Schmidt, 1984), and then use template or feature-matching procedures. Many of these procedures are time-consuming and require an extremely fast processor or off-line analysis. Specific-function preprocessors may be developed to speed up the analysis (e.g., Gerstein et al., 1983). The most effective unit-classification algorithms probably lie somewhere between the time-consuming template matching and the simple amplitude discrimination. Usually, only a few parameters of the spike waveform are used for classification, e.g., the first peak of the filtered signal (V_{max}), the second peak (V_{min}), and the separation between peaks (t_m) (Fig. 5C; Vibert and Costa, 1979). More parameters, such as slopes of the signal or duration of its positive and negative phases, may give redundant and unnecessary information (Vibert and Costa, 1979). A close cluster around a particular triplicate coordinate of V_{max}, V_{min}, and t_m may be regarded as a single unit, which can be statistically discriminated from other single units.

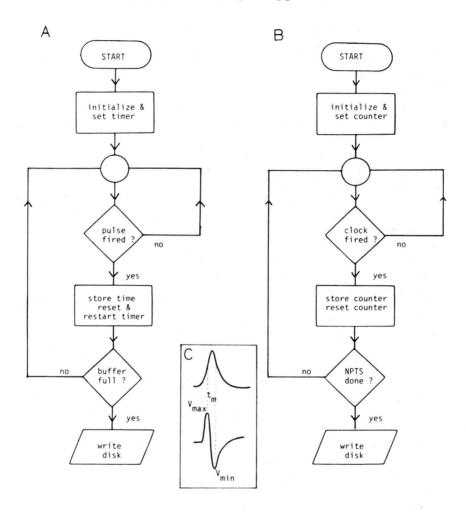

Fig. 5. (A) Flow chart for recording pulse intervals. (B) Flow chart for poststimulus time histogram (pulses/bin). (C) Unfiltered (top) and filtered (bottom) waveform of an action potential. V_{max} and V_{min} are the amplitudes of the peak and valley of the filtered signal, separated by interval t_m.

There are exceptions to the principle that each single unit has a unique waveform. For example, there could be changes in initial segment-somatic dendritic (IS-SD or AB) components of the action potential, depending on membrane polarization or firing rate. Also, neurons that fire in a burst of action potentials may have decremental heights in the action potentials, presumably because of cathodal block. Discrimination of decremental bursting units may be achieved by recording through two adjacent electrodes (stereotrode). The amplitude ratio of the action potentials recorded through the two electrodes may be used as an additional parameter for single-unit discrimination (McNaughton et al., 1983).

2.1.5.2. SAMPLING OF PULSES.   Once detected, most analyses on action potentials regard them as point processes occurring at an instant of time. The time interval between spikes can best be estimated by a timer that is started by a spike. With the occurrence of the next spike, the time elapsed is stored (to 1 ms or 0.1 ms accuracy), and the timer is then reset and restarted (Fig. 5A). Time reference to stimulus (or behavioral event) can also be maintained if the interval between the stimulus (or event) to the first pulse is stored and then all subsequent adjacent interpulse intervals are stored. A peristimulus time histogram (PSTH) can be reconstructed from the intervals, and interval histograms are readily generated.

If the precise intervals between spikes are not needed, it is possible to count pulses within a fixed time bin (of, for instance, 1 ms width). A clock source (or 1 KHz for 1 ms bin width) provides the time for reading and storing a pulse counter, which is then reset and restarted (Fig. 5B). Multiple counters may be used for multiple pulse channels distinguished by different electrodes or a preADC specialized circuit. By means of a triggered train of clock pulses (Fig. 4C, 4D), multiple sweeps of evoked spike response data can be acquired and summed to give the PSTH *(see below)*.

An alternate method to construct a PSTH is to convert the pulse data to an analog waveform.* This may be useful for users who do not have a software-addressable digital counter. A single pulse occurrence is converted to a voltage that is held for a fixed period of time equivalent to the PSTH bin width. The ADC then

---

*This strategy has been implemented by Dr. C. Y. Yim (Dept. Physiology, University of Western Ontario) using a specially built sample-and-hold circuit, a multiplexer, Data Translation 2801A, and locally developed programs using DMA.

samples the analog voltage, which codes for the presence or absence of a pulse. Multiple units can be multiplexed, each generating a distinct voltage step corresponding to a single bit of the ADC (e.g., 1, 2, 4, 8). If each neuronal unit is assumed not to fire twice within a time bin, individual unit firings can be decoded from the multiplexed voltage and individual PSTHs generated.

2.1.6. Simultaneous Pulse and Wave Recording

In order to study the relation between unit and wave, it is necessary to record both processes at the same time. An example is provided by the UNWAVE program implemented for the analysis of the relation between spontaneous wave and units (Fig. 6, Leung and Buzsaki, 1983). A single channel of pulse and NCH channels of wave (EEG) are recorded for NPTS number of samples. The sampling clock rate is separately set by a TIMET program generating a series of recurring pulses at fixed intervals of, for instance, 5 ms (Fig. 4A). At each pulse, the interpulse interval is read and a timer/counter is reset. The time interval of the first pulse in relation to the start of EEG sampling is registered, as are all subsequent interpulse intervals. A sequential polling method is used to check whether the EEG should be sampled (clock status high) or the unit has fired (pulse counter out high). Sampling is completed when NPTS wave samples have been performed. This allows a reconstruction of the complete pulse train, as well as its temporal relation to the EEG wave (Fig. 6). Subsequent analysis of the unit and wave data is presented in section 2.2.

If exact interpulse intervals are not required, both EEG and pulse-per-bin sampling may be initiated from a single clock pulse (Fig. 7). This method is a direct extension of previous wave or pulse sampling, and may be applied to multiple channels or evoked responses.

2.1.7. Recording of Events Past

Not all neural events can be studied as a response to a stimulus, or an effect of a cause. Many events occur spontaneously, and the preceding neural activities need to be investigated. An example is voluntary movement that is preceded by a slow negative wave in the frontal scalp EEG (motor prepotentials of Kornhuber or contingent negative variation of Walter). Another example is the spontaneous interictal spike observed in the EEG of epileptic patients or animals. Neural activities preceding the interictal spike

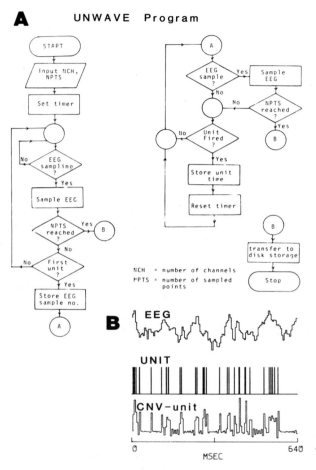

Fig. 6. (A) Sampling of unit and EEG uses a sequence of two programs. The first program, TIMET (not shown), sets the external pulses
that triggered analog-to-digital conversion (ADC). These pulses may be
continuously free-running or triggered (Fig. 4). The UNWAVE (UNit-
WAVE) program samples NCH channels of EEG at NPTS points (separated by the sampling interval set in TIMET). The time instants of unit
firing (after window discrimination) are stored as the time after the
previous unit or after the EEG sample number (for the first unit). These
programs are implemented on a Cromemco System 3 microcomputer
with a TECMAR AD212 timer/ADC board. The unitary data are further
convoluted in time by another program (MAKUNA), and spectrally an-

may indicate that other brain areas are active before the recorded spike. A simple technique to record precedent activities is the continuous storage of all relevant data, until an event occurs. This approach is both time-consuming and impractical, especially when the events are infrequent. One variant of this technique is to record the data on magnetic tape and play the tape back in the reverse direction, if the tape recorder has such a function. Another technique, described below, is to use a microcomputer for backsampling.

Obviously, no device can actually record activities *before* a particular event (trigger) in time. The paradigm of backsampling involves continuous recording, but the computer "remembers" only those samples preceding the particular event. A cyclic memory buffer that is continually storing data is used (Fig. 8A). If the particular event trigger occurs, the preceding samples (NCH channels each of N1 points in Fig. 8A) are stored. Posttrigger samples (N2 points) are also stored. If the trigger occurs too frequently, insufficient samples preceding (<N1) or following (<N2) the trigger may generate incomplete sweeps. Since all triggers occur at a fixed bin in each sampled sweep, the data can be readily averaged (back averaging). The computer technique is superior to the reverse tape playback technique, since both forward- and backsampling are achieved in one sweep (run).

2.2. Manipulation and Analysis of Data

Signal analysis using a digital computer has been used for more than 20 years. Only techniques that are commonly used and within the domain of microcomputers are presented here. For more detailed and elaborate neural signal analysis, readers may consult Glaser and Ruchkin (1976) and the references cited below.

---

alyzed by fast Fourier transform (SPECU). (B) Illustration of sampling program. Top trace: raw single-channel EEG sampled at 5-ms interval. Middle trace: units as standard pulses plotted from the stored occurrence times. Bottom trace: convoluted unit train sampled at 5-ms intervals (result of MAKUNA program) (reproduced with permission from Leung and Buzsaki, 1983).

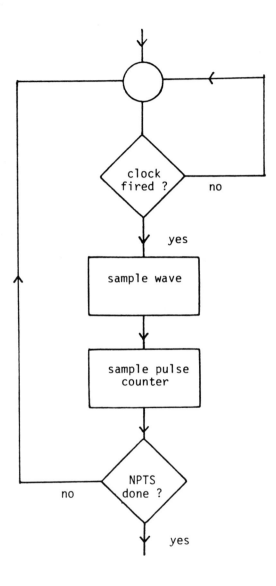

Fig. 7. Subroutine flow chart for sampling wave amplitude and pulse counts/bin at each clock pulse, for NPTS bins.

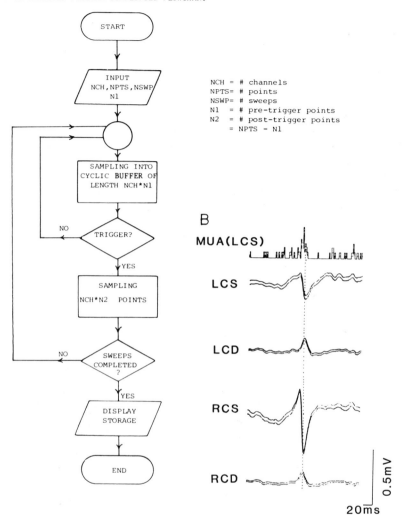

START

INPUT
NCH,NPTS,NSWP,
N1

NCH = # channels
NPTS= # points
NSWP= # sweeps
N1 = # pre-trigger points
N2 = # post-trigger points
    = NPTS - N1

SAMPLING INTO
CYCLIC BUFFER OF
LENGTH NCH*N1

NO

TRIGGER?

YES

SAMPLING
NCH*N2   POINTS

NO

SWEEPS
COMPLETED
?

YES

DISPLAY
STORAGE

END

B

MUA(LCS)

LCS

LCD

RCS

RCD

0.5mV

20ms

Fig. 8. (A) Backsampling program flow chart. (B) An example of
backsampling. An average EEG-spike (transient) recorded across the cell
layers (III/IV) of the left (LCS, LCD) and right (RCS, RCD) posterior
cingulate cortex. Multiple unit activity (MUA) was discriminated at LCS
and acquired simultaneously with the waves as a peri-"event" time histogram. The "event" was the sharp rising slope of the EEG transient at LCS
(reproduced with permission from Leung and Borst, 1987).

345

2.2.1. Averaging (AEP and PSTH)

The main assumption underlying averaging is that there is an invariable signal time-locked to the stimulus. This signal sums linearly, but does not interact with the random noise, which may be intrinsic (electronic or spontaneous neural activity) or extrinsic (e.g., power line). This latter assumption on averaging may be violated if evoked responses are different at various phases (e.g., during the positive vs the negative peak of a rhythmic wave) of the spontaneous slow waves (e.g., Rudell et al., 1980). Distinction between signal and noise is difficult when the stimulus reorganizes the phase of the ongoing spontaneous activity (Sayers et al., 1974).

Mathematically, the main assumption is

$$r_i(t) = s(t) + n_i(t) \tag{1}$$

where $r_i(t)$ = recorded waveform for the ith trial
$s(t)$ = signal
$n_i(t)$ = noise for the ith trial

The average $\bar{r}(t)$ is the sum of all N trials divided by N, i.e.,

$$\bar{r}(t) = \frac{1}{N} \sum_{i=1}^{N} r_i(t) = s(t) + \frac{1}{N} \sum_{i=1}^{N} n_i(t) \tag{2}$$

If the noise is random and independent for each trial, the expected value of the noise term is zero, and the SEM is $\sigma/(N)^{1/2}$ where σ = standard deviation of the noise, assumed to be time-independent. Thus, the error decreases as $1/(N)^{1/2}$.

The stimulus repetition rate in the evoked response should be chosen with the following considerations: First, with a fast rate, a larger N may be achieved in a fixed time, perhaps within a stationary behavioral state. (However, some neural systems may not respond linearly at fast rates; e.g., frequency potentiation may occur, or a stimulus may occur during the response to the previous stimulus.) Second, in order to avoid averaging spontaneous intrinsic rhythms, a random rather than a regular stimulus interval is preferred (see section 2.1.4.).

If an SEM has been estimated, comparison between AEPs may be made using the t-test. The Satterthwaite's t-test, which reduces the degrees of freedom according to the inhomogeneity of variances between the two responses, is used for Fig. 9 (Leung et al., 1982a). Groups of average responses may be compared using

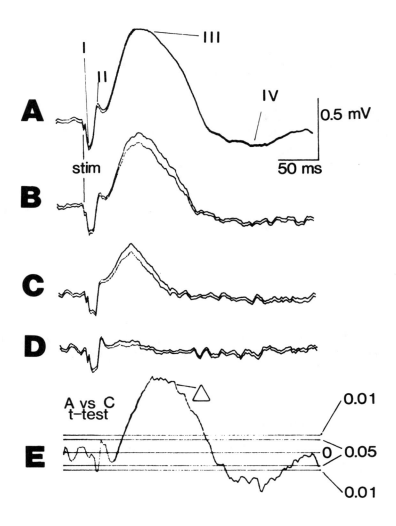

Fig. 9. Interhemispheric transcallosal evoked responses (IHRs) for four different behaviors: waking immobility (A), head-turn (B), walk (C) and struggle (D). Each consists of a prestimulus baseline and four components (I-IV), as labeled. The SEM is plotted on top of the average response. The number of averaging sweeps are 98 for A and 16 each for B, C, and D. In E, the t-values for the immobile-IHR and the walking-IHR (△, not calibrated) is drawn with the Satterthwaite's t of $P = 0.01$ and $P = 0.05$. Differences beyond the boundaries of a pair of P lines of a particular value are significant at that P value (reproduced with permission from Leung et al., 1982a).

nonparametric statistics that do not assume a normal distribution of values.

The above analysis of evoked response applies to both AEPs and PSTHs. It also applies to back or forward averaging. Fig. 8B is an illustration of unit perievent time histogram acquired simultaneously with analog waveforms (all averages with SEM) triggered by a sharp EEG-spike in the cingulate cortex.

2.2.2. Digital Filtering

Similar to analog filters, digital filters consist of low-pass, high-pass, band-pass and band-reject types. In addition, interpolation between digitized points is effectively a low-pass filter. The general operation of a digital filter, on a time series u_i, to give the output series y_n is written as

$$y_n = \sum_{k=-N}^{N} c_k u_{n-k} \tag{3}$$

where c_k, $k = -N$ to N is the filter spanning $(2N+1)$ digitized points.

The equation is the equivalent of the temporal convolution in the continuous time domain, where

$$y(t) = \int_{-\infty}^{\infty} c(\tau)u(t - \tau)d\tau \tag{4}$$

and in the frequency domain,

$$Y(f) = C(f)\, U(f) \tag{5}$$

where $y(t)$ = continuous output of filter
$\quad\quad\quad u(t)$ = continuous input of filter
$\quad\quad\quad c(t)$ = analog filter
$\quad\quad\quad Y(f)$ = $F[y(t)]$
$\quad\quad\quad C(f)$ = $F[c(t)]$
$\quad\quad\quad U(f)$ = $F[u(t)]$
and F = Fourier transform operator

The type of filter, smoothing (low pass) or differentiation (high pass) depends on the coefficients c_k in the digital filter series. Smoothing filters remove high frequencies and consist of a symmetric series of positive c_k. For example, a 3-point smoothing filter gives

$$Y(n) = (u_{n-1})/4 + (u_n)/2 + (u_{n+1})/4 \tag{6}$$

where $c_0 = 1/2$ and $c_{-1} = c_1 = 1/4$.

For a detailed description of filter designs, the reader should consult Hamming (1983).

2.2.3. Interval and Correlation Analysis of Spike Trains

For many purposes, the action potential from a single or multiple neuron (axons, cell bodies) is considered as an event that occurs at an instant of time. The actual waveform of the action potential is useful in its isolation, but often neglected in the analysis. In other words, the action potential and its apparently random pulse train is considered as a stochastic point process whose realizations consist of a series of point events instantaneous and indistinguishable (except in terms of position in time) (Perkel et al., 1967a).

The last section describes methods to store the interval time between pulses or spikes. The interval histogram, a plot of the number of occurrence of each interval (grouped into bins), is readily constructed from the sampled intervals. The usual statistics (mean, standard deviation, and kurtosis) can be calculated. Segmenting these intervals into earlier and later periods may reveal trends in the interval distribution. Such trends will reveal nonstationarity, i.e., departure from a fixed statistic, perhaps because of deterioration or state changes in the cell or preparation. Orderly changes of intervals may also be estimated by spectral analysis of intervals (Cox and Lewis, 1966, pp. 67). In addition, the order-dependence of interpulse intervals may be estimated from the serial correlation coefficients of interval lengths (Perkel et al., 1967a). One example is the joint interval histogram, in which the value of the interpulse interval (y-variable) is plotted against the value of the previous interval (x-variable). The deviation of the scatter diagram from a flat line will indicate the lack of dependence between adjacent intervals. For example, if a neuron tends to fire occasionally in a burst of high frequency, then the firing may be order-dependent, as short intervals tend to be followed by short ones only, whereas long intervals are followed by either short or long ones.

A common technique in order-dependent statistics is to estimate the autocorrelation function (ACF) of a spike train. The ACF is also known as the autocorreleogram or renewal density function, and it measures the probability that a unit will fire at time t, given that it had fired at time zero. A rough estimate of this function can be acquired on-line by constructing a PSTH triggered from a spike.

Since spikes within a sweep are not used as triggers, the resulting PSTH is not a true spike autocorrelation, which is the PSTH constructed by using all of the spikes as triggers. Effectively, the calculation is one of the convolution of a time series with itself, i.e.,

$$\phi_{xx}(t) = \int_{-\infty}^{\infty} x(\tau)x(\tau - t)d\tau \tag{7}$$

The autocorrelation function can be used to reveal the refractory period after a spike, or the periodicity in a rhythmic cell.

The correlation of one pulse train to itself can be extended to that between two pulse trains $x(t)$ and $y(t)$ (Perkel et al., 1967b). The cross-correlation function (CCF) or cross-correleogram is given by

$$\phi_{xy}(t) = \int_{-\infty}^{\infty} x(\tau)y(\tau - t)d\tau \tag{8}$$

The algorithm for the estimation of the CCF of two spike trains is similar to the autocorrelation function: select each and every pulse of one train and use it as a trigger to make a PSTH from the other train. The interpretation of the CCF is similar to the ACF; it is the probability that unit two will fire at time t, given that unit one had fired at time zero.

Cross-correlation techniques may be used to determine if two spike trains are dependent on each other. Independence between two trains is indicated by a flat CCF. However, satisfactory statistical tests of the null hypothesis of independent firings have not yet been fully developed (cf Perkel et al., 1967b). Cross-correlation techniques have been employed to study interactions between a pair of neurons (cf Toyama et al., 1981). CCF may be derived from firings of neuronal pairs during spontaneous (no stimulation) conditions or during stimulation. Periodic stimulations, e.g. auditory or visual (Perkel et al., 1967b; Toyama et al., 1981), are often used. During stimulation, the firing rate of each of the two neurons may change from the spontaneous condition, and each unit may fire in response to the stimulus (as revealed by their individual PSTHs). The CCF during stimulus-on conditions is thus different from that during stimulus-off, but may be attributed to a linear sum of a shared-input effect and a neuronal-interaction effect (if the stimulus does not change the neuronal interactions). This neuronal-related cross correlogram has been estimated for different neuronal pairs in the auditory and visual cortex. For example, Toyama et al. (1981) observed mutual excitation, delayed excitation (Fig. 10), and

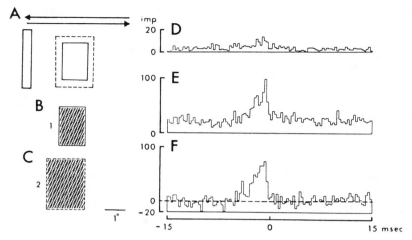

Fig. 10. Two complex cells in the cat's visual cortex, with overlapping receptive fields, were stimulated by a moving slit of light (A). B and C show coextensive on- and off-response areas in the receptive fields of cell 1 and cell 2. (D) Cross-correleogram with no stimulus. (E) Similar to D, but with iontophoretic injection of glutamate ions at the multibarrel electrode recording cell 2, thus increasing the spike rates of cell 2 and cell 1. (F) Neural-related correleogram derived from subtracting the stimulus-rated correleogram from the cross-correleogram during stimulation with the moving light slit *(see text)*. Note the firing of cell 2 before cell 1 (negative time on time axis, about –0.6 ms) (reproduced with permission from Toyama et al., 1981).

delayed inhibition between pairs of neurons in the cat's visual cortex during visual-field or glutamate-iontophoretic stimulations. The sensitivity of the CCF for the detection of inhibition may be lower than that for the detection of excitation (Aertsen and Gerstein, 1985).

The correlation functions are best used for estimates of time-delay or for estimates (phase, frequency) of a single dominant frequency. If more than one frequency is present in the time-series, frequency domain analysis is probably more revealing. Mathematically, the autocorrelation function is the time domain equivalent of the autopower spectrum and the cross-correlation function that of the crosspower spectrum. Therefore, all information in the time domain is contained in the frequency domain, and vice versa. In practice, time estimates (e.g., delay time) are better estimated in the time domain and frequency estimates (e.g., dominant frequency, bandwidth) in the frequency domain.

2.2.4. Fourier (Frequency Domain) Analysis

Frequency analysis has a long history in physical and engineering sciences, and many books have been written on the subject. The computation of the Fourier coefficients by digital computers is greatly facilitated by the Fast Fourier Transformer (FFT) algorithm (cf Jenkins and Watts, 1968). This algorithm reduces the number of computations from N^2 to $N\log N$ for a number N of digital samples.

A simple illustration of the Fourier transform for one signal is given in Fig. 11. A pure sine wave gives a power spectrum of a single peak (Fig. 11A). A higher-frequency sine wave gives a peak at a higher frequency (Fig. 11C). A linear sum of two (or more) frequencies is resolved into two (or more) peaks (Fig. 11D). The signal with two harmonics (a harmonic is an integral multiple of a fundamental frequency) is resolved into two peaks (Fig. 11B), as is a mixture of low and high frequency (Fig. 11D). Fig. 11E illustrates the addition of white noise to the signal in Fig. 11D. White noise gives a flat spectrum.

Theoretically, the sharp power peaks in Fig. 11 apply only to a signal of infinite duration, whereas all signals are time-limited in the real world. The shorter the time segment T, the broader is the frequency peak(s). This is the quintessence of the Heisenberg uncertainty principle in quantum mechanics, where the momentum and location (or energy and time) of a particle cannot both be determined with infinitesimal accuracy. Instead of a sharp impulse (Dirac delta) function, the power spectrum of a time-limited truncated sine wave is a broad peak with side lobes (leakage). Also, the frequency resolution for the segment of duration is $f_R = 1/T$. This frequency resolution is directly related to the width of the leakage side-lobes.

In a practical application of Fourier analysis, the uncertainty principle dictates that the frequency resolution must be traded off to achieve statistical reliability (confidence limits) of the measure and vice versa. A very long time segment T (within the limits of biological stationarity) gives a sharp frequency resolution, but the spectral estimate will have a large error (or a low reliability) because of a small degree of freedom (df). Averaging across N power spectra, each estimated from T/N time segments, increases df (by N

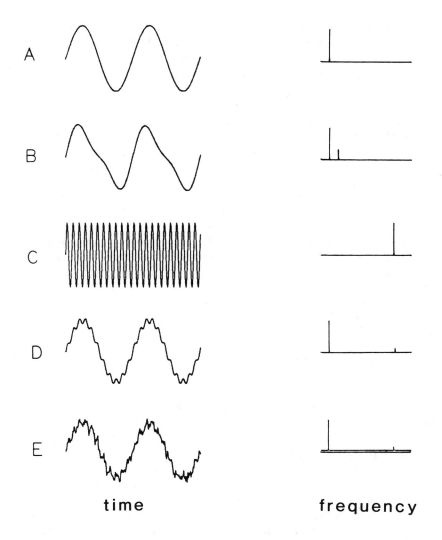

time   **frequency**

Fig. 11. Illustration of time and frequency domain of a signal (*see text* for explanation).

times) and the reliability of the spectral estimate, but decreases frequency resolution. Similarly, smoothing across adjacent points in a power spectrum will also increase df (Jenkins and Watts, 1968; Otnes and Enochson, 1972). The decision on an optimal segment size T and df depends on the biological application. Lopes da Silva (1982) suggested df to be greater than 60 for the power spectrum. The confidence limits or the error of the phase and coherence estimates (below) are even more sensitive than the power spectrum to low df, and an even larger df is recommended.

A cross-spectrum estimates the linear statistical relation between two signals (Fig. 12). Typically, this is displayed as the phase and coherence estimates, each as a function of frequency. The phase is an estimate of the phase lead or lag at a particular frequency. The square coherency estimates the degree of linear statistical correlation at a particular frequency. The coherence value is similar to the (absolute value of the) correlation coefficient, except it is frequency-dependent. It is also commonly reported as a coherence z-transform ($z = \ln[(1+c)/(1-c)]/2$ where $c =$ linear coherence), since the latter estimate is approximately normally distributed if the signal consists of Gaussian white noise (Otnes and Enochson, 1972).

2.3. Control and Output Functions

2.3.1. General

In industrial applications, microprocessors may be used in automatic process control, manufacturing, and robotics. Other than operating in harsh and hostile environments (a situation perhaps not applicable to most physiological laboratories), the microcomputer can assume routine procedures that may be too boring or too elaborate for the operator. It may also achieve a precision and a speed that is not attained manually. In a sophisticated laboratory with many pieces of equipment, it is convenient to have an ultimate control center in the microcomputer. Often, the result of the action is fed back into the computer by sensors or transducers, completing a feedback loop. Thus, the computer may become the sensory and motor system as well as the "brain" behind the actions.

The internal signal within a microcomputer is in digital format. The microcomputer output is also digital. Various ways of communication between a microcomputer and another external device,

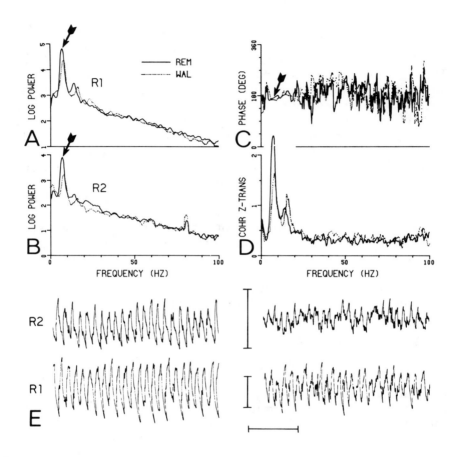

Fig. 12. Overlaid spectra for dorsal hippocampal EEG at electrodes above (R2) and below (R1) the CA1 cell layer, during rapid-eye-movement sleep (REM) and walking (WAL). A and B are power spectra at R1 and R2, respectively. The logarithmic power units [in $(\mu V)^2/Hz$] are not calibrated, but the calibration factor was constant across behavioral states. C and D are the phase and z-transform coherence spectra of R2 vs R1, which together constitute the cross-spectrum. Note the high Θ rhythm peak (at about 7 c/s) for both REM and WAL. The signals at R2 and R1 share a common coherent Θ frequency, with about 180° phase shift (arrow) from each other. E shows the raw EEG data during REM (left) and during WAL (right). Calibration 1 mV, 1 s (reproduced with permission from Leung et al. 1982b).

e.g., a piece of equipment, have been designed. Some modern neurophysiological equipment may be equipped with a standard serial (e.g., RS232C) or parallel interface, or an IEE488 interface. Through this standard interface, serial or parallel pulses representing commands may be passed on to the equipment. Other equipment may not need sophisticated control by a set of commands. Instead, a single digital pulse may be sufficient to trigger certain actions, like switching a relay or turning an instrument on or off.

Computer interface boards may be commercially available, or in special applications, may need to be homemade. One important function of the interface board is to provide a matching between computer output and driven devices, e.g., in boosting the power or current. Another is to isolate the computer circuits from the external world, usually through optical or inductive (magnetic) means. Such an isolation is important to protect the computer from high power surges that may occur in the external circuit. Some common interfaces, the serial (RS232C) and parallel interfaces, have been described in section 1.2.2.3. In the following sections, examples of the use of digital and analog control devices will be given.

2.3.2. Digital Control (Switching)

The ultimate microcomputer output signal is a digital pulse, usually TTL-compatible. A driver circuit is recommended, even if this output pulse may directly drive external circuits. This will limit the load driven by the computer as well as offer some protection to the computer circuitry. For other applications that involve driving high power loads, protection may be provided by optical or magnetic isolation. In the former, the input causes a light-emitting diode to emit photons that are detected by a phototransistor, resulting in an output current. Thus, the input and output circuits are coupled only by light, not electrically. Magnetic relays also offer input–output isolation.

Logical switching by TTL signals may control stimulus delivery (flash, click, electrical shock), or reward/punishment (food/water feeder, foot shock) in a behavioral experiment. In a recording situation, the stimulator may be controlled by one or a series of pulses, and a tape recorder (video recorder) may be turned on or off during the recording.

In order to switch on a high current or voltage, special devices are needed. High ac voltage (e.g., 115 V) are switched on by thyristors or silicon-controlled rectifiers (SCRs). As implied by its name, SCRs only pass half of the ac wave. A triac gives the complete ac wave, basically by coupling two SCRs. Mechanical (magnetic, reed) relays may also achieve ac switching. Modern devices include the VFET (V-shaped channel MOS-field effect transistor) and solid state relays. These devices may need only 5 V and a small input current (<20 mA) for turning on outputs up to 115 V (ac) and several amperes.

2.3.3. Analog (Continuous) Control

2.3.3.1. DIGITAL-TO-ANALOG CONVERTER   (DAC). As the reverse case of digitization involving on ADC, DAC converts a digital train of signals to an analog staircase. After bandpass filtering (at below twice the conversion rate), the signal will appear rather smooth. Any kind of waveform may therefore be output by the microcomputer as a smooth function of time, provided that the function frequency does not exceed half the DAC conversion rate (the inverse of the sampling theorum). Sinusoids, triangles, square waves, ramps, or various duty cycles can be output in order to drive microelectrodes or external mechanical devices. A driver circuit, e.g., an operational amplifier, may be needed to boost the power of the DAC output.

2.3.3.2. STEPPING MOTOR.   Among the output devices, the stepping motor deserves a brief description. This is a motor that can be digitally controlled and can make very precise and reproducible steps. The motor consists of a gear-like inner permanent magnetic rotor surrounded by two or more stator coils. The coils are activated in a time sequence that energizes alternatively north or south magnetic fields, which causes the rotor to rotate clockwise or counter-clockwise. Typically, the torque (or turning power) given by stepping motors decreases with increased step rate. A high step rate (steps/s) means a large rotational speed (revolutions/s). Step angles of less than 1° and stepping rate more than 200/s are available.

There are various ways to drive a stepping motor. ICs (e.g., AIRPAX SAA 1027) are available to convert single pulses into the actual time sequence of activating the motors. This is probably the most economical, and possibly the most flexible, interface if the experimenter is willing to do the programming. Complete interface boards are available (Table 5) that may be accompanied by software. There are also independent devices that may have manual controls, but can be brought under computer control via standard (e.g. serial RS232) interfaces.

2.3.4. Examples of Equipment Control

Stepping motors are useful for placing electrodes in neurophysiological experiments. Micromanipulators that are moved by turning a knob may be gear-connected to a rotating stepping motor. Three-dimensional electrode placements can be achieved by using three motors, each driving one direction. Such a system has been implemented by W. J. Wadman at the University of Amsterdam. The system could be used for automatic placement of a microelectrode at a precise location in the brain or brain slice. Automated recording and mapping of extracellular field potentials could be achieved. Alternatively, only one direction (depth) may be manipulated. Brown and Flaming (1977) described the use of a stepping motor to step an intracellular microelectrode at 1-μm steps with a Kopf hydraulic drive. The motor is stopped when a cell is impaled, as indicated by a negative dc shift. Some micromanipulators (e.g., Burleigh inch-worm, but not the Narishige SM21) are equipped with a microcomputer interface.

Another use of equipment control is given by Mullikan and Davis (1985). These authors used an IBM-XT microcomputer to drive an optical bench through interfaces made by MI². By means of DACs and digital outputs driving stepping motors, it is possible to control the position, velocity, orientation, length, and width of a bar presented in the visual field of a subject.

3. Behavioral Analysis Using a Microcomputer

3.1. General

Rapid progress in behavioral analysis may be expected in the near future. The main discussion here will be focused on the monochrome video signal, which may contain information concerning the location of an animal (and its various parts of the body) in space. The video format is popular (making cameras and recorders affordable), and it is amenable to digital analysis. In a later section, some alternate movement analysis systems are considered briefly.

3.2. The Video Signal

This signal is a representation of light intensity over a 2-dimensional (2-D) surface. It utilizes a sequential scanning procedure (Liff, 1979). During reproduction of a video signal by a monitor, a beam of electrons is swept sequentially through a 2-D surface (the television screen). The horizontal sweep rate (about 15 KHz) is much faster than the vertical (60 Hz), so that the electron beam is swept diagonally down the screen (Fig. 12). When the beam reaches the bottom, it is retraced vertically and started at near the center of the top. Each screen sweep is known as a video field, and two consecutive sweeps interlace but do not overlap each other. Only at a time interval of two consecutive fields (a video frame) will the beam reappear at the same spot on the screen. This particular spot will receive a beam every ⅟₃₀ s. A similar sweeping procedure is used during camera recording, so that the sampling frequency for a fixed spot in space is 30 Hz.

The temporal resolution, using the sampling theorem, is thus 15 Hz (half the sampling rate). Therefore, movements faster than 15 Hz, e.g., beating of the wings of an insect or hummingbird, will not be adequately sampled. This may be the limitation of the commercial video signal as opposed to filming. In terms of spatial resolution, there are 525 horizontal sweeps in one sweep or 525 vertical elements. The horizontal width is usually ⅘ × the vertical length, giving about 700 horizontal elements. However, retrace and blanking of the beam reduce the actual displayed elements. The transmission of the vertical and horizontal blanking and synchronizing pulses, together with the intensity signal during the sweeps, constitute the composite video signal. The transmission of 525×700 intensities once every ⅟₃₀ s gives an 11×10^6/s or a 5.5 MHz bandwidth (2 elements making a cycle). The television transmission standard (FCC) specifies a 4.2 MHz limit.

3.3. Analysis of the Video Signal

Since the video is a sequential scanning signal, a separation in space becomes a separation in time. Simple objects, e.g., spots of light, may be located by this method. In Fig. 13, a dark spot is encountered soon after the start of the frame (in the odd field during "AB" sweep from 1 to 2), whereas the bright spot is not encountered until near the end of the even field (sweep from 11 to 12). In the camera, the dark object gives a low intensity, and the

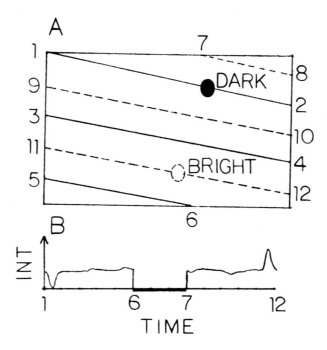

Fig. 13. (A) Illustration of video signal using 2 ½ interlaced horizontal sweeps/field. The temporal sequence of sweeping is 1–12, as shown.
The odd sweeps (field) are drawn as solid lines and the even sweeps as
dotted lines. (B) Intensity (INT) as a function of time. The dark spot is
crossed between 1 and 2, and the bright spot later (between 11 and 12)
during the sweep sequence. Theoretically, spatial positions of the bright
and dark spots can be estimated from the temporal intensity profile. The
time represented by the dark solid line between time points 6 and 7 is
taken up by vertical retrace and blanking.

bright one a high intensity. The actual location of each of the
objects and their separation in space can therefore be theoretically
extracted from the time the object's signal appears with respect to
frame start. The latter instant in time (the vertical synch pulse) may
be extracted from the video signal by special electronic circuitry. By
placing a small light on the head of a rat, its location may be
decoded from the video output. By automated recording of both
neuronal firing and the spatial position of the animal, cells with

place-specific firing (place cells) have been found in the hippocampus (Muller et al., 1987).

In some experiments, the locations of more than one part of the body or spot of light may be required. More sophisticated (but perhaps tedious) behavioral analysis may be made by using the complete video signal. This analysis is hindered by the high bandwidth (4.2 MHz) of the video signal. Complete digitization of this signal requires an expensive (flash) ADC operating at 8.4 MHz. A cheaper alternative is to digitize only the low-frequency part of the video signal, therefore giving a poorer spatial resolution.

Many circuit boards available for a microcomputer are capable of digitizing a video frame by means of 256×256 points in space with 6–8 bit intensity resolution (and probably in 3 colors). The spatial digitization represents about $1/4$ of the spatial information. Each of the spatial units is known as a pixel (picture element). An 8-bit intensity resolution means that 8 different shades of gray (black to white) are distinguishable. However, it may take seconds to digitize and store one video frame and, for many currently available frame-grabber boards, a complete sequence of frames cannot be digitized in real time. Once digitized, however, the video signal may be manipulated by the microcomputer. Positions of joints and limbs of the body may be manually detected and stored on the computer, and a complete profile of movements may then be displayed. Video tracking systems for gross body movements are available (Table 5).

3.4. Other Movement Analysis Systems

The video signal has been developed from television. Much of its design is catered for human vision, e.g., the 30 Hz sampling will be sufficient to cause flicker fusion, the number of horizontal lines is beyond human visual resolution when the screen subtends 1.5° at the retina, and the 4.2 MHz is fixed by transmission (FCC) standards. These specifications are certainly not ideal for scientific studies on precise spatial locations. The reason for using the video signal for movement analysis is the same as that for using a microcomputer in the laboratory—the system is economical and versatile.

In specific applications, the deciding factor may not be economics or versatility. Other systems may be equipped with data reduction at the input stage. Instead of the whole animal data, investigation may be principally interested in eye or limb position. For eye position, there are infrared devices that make use of reflected light in the location of the eye. For limb movements, contacts of a certain limb with a surface can be detected by a small current flowing from the animal to the ground surface (Chapin et al., 1980). Movement sensors have been briefly reviewed by Vanderwolf and Leung (1985).

One of the movement analysis systems on the market is called a WATSMART system (Vendor: Northern Digital, Waterloo, Ontario). It makes use of tiny LEDs that are activated in a sequence at a high frequency. Custom-made infrared cameras then observe the sequential active markers (e.g., on a moving limb), specialized hardware and software digitize the coordinates of each LED in space, and the data are stored on a microcomputer. Three-dimensional reconstruction may be made from a 2-D input. The digitizing rate is 8 KHz, and is much superior to that of the video camera. However, the system is developed for human kinematics and the LEDs (with wires attached) are not suitable for use in small animals or in cases where behavior cannot be revealed by LED positions alone.

Acknowledgments

Preparation of this chapter is supported by operating grants from Canadian NSERC and MRC. I would like to thank Dr. C. H. Vanderwolf, Dr. C. Y. Yim and Mr. J. Lemieux for comments on various parts of the paper.

References

Aertsen A. M. H. J. and Gerstein G. L. (1985) Evaluation of neuronal connectivity: Sensitivity of cross-correlation. *Brain Res.* **340,** 341–354.

Artwick B. A. (1980) *Microcomputer Interface* (Prentice-Hall, Englewood Cliffs, New Jersey).

Bagust J. (1985) Sample, analyse, and display (SAD)—A microprocessor data acquisition system for laboratory use, in *Microcomputers in the Neurosciences* (Kerkut G., ed.), Clarendon, Oxford, pp. 118–141.

Brown K. T. and Flaming D. G. (1977) New microelectrode techniques for intracellular work in small cells. *Neuroscience* **2,** 813–827.

Brown P. B., (ed.) (1976) *Computer Technology in Neuroscience.* (Wiley, New York).

Bureš J., Krekule I., and Brozek G. (1982) *Practical Guide to Computer Applications in Neurosciences* (Wiley, New York).

Chapin J. K., Loeb G. E., and Woodward D. J. (1980) A simple technique for determination of footfall patterns of animals during treadmill locomotion. *J. Neurosci. Methods* **2,** 97–102.

Cox D. R. and Lewis P. A. W. (1966) *The Statistical Analysis of Series of Events* (Wiley, New York).

Gerstein G. L., Bloom M. J., Espinosa I. E., Evanczuk S., and Turner M. R. (1983) Design of a laboratory for multineuron studies. *IEEE Trans. Systems, Man and Cybernetics,* **SMC-13,** 668–676.

Glaser E. M. and Ruchkin D. S. (1976) *Principles of Neurobiological Signal Analysis* (Academic, New York).

Hamming R. W. (1983) *Digital Filters* (Prentice-Hall, Englewood Cliffs, New Jersey).

Hearn E. D. (1986) Digitizers for Data Entry. *Byte* **1,** 261–266.

Hopt, H. P., Wu J. Y., Xiao C., Rioult M. G., London J. A., Zecevic D. and Cohen, L. B. Multisite optical measurement of membrane potential, this volume.

Jenkins G. M. and Watts D. G. (1968) *Spectral Analysis and its Application* (Holden Day, San Francisco).

Kerkut, G. (1985) *Microcomputers in the Neurosciences* (Clarendon, Oxford).

Leung L. S. (1985) Timing pulse and sampling programs implemented on a laboratory microcomputer. *Comput. Programs Biomed.* **19,** 143–150.

Leung L. S. and Borst J. G. G. (1987) Electrical activity in the cingulate cortex of the rat. I. Generating mechanisms and relations to behavior. *Brain Res.* **407,** 68–90.

Leung L. S. and Buzsaki G. (1983) Spectral analysis of hippocampal unit train in relation to hippocampal EEG. *Electroencephalogr. Clin. Neurophysiol.* **56,** 668–671.

Leung L. S., Harvey G. C., and Vanderwolf C. H. (1982a) Combined video and computer analysis of the relation between the interhemisphere response and behavior. *Behav. Brain Res.* **6,** 195–200.

Leung L. S., Lopes da Silva F. H. and Wadman W. J. (1982b) Spectral characteristics of the hippocampal EEG in the freely moving rat. *Electroencephalogr. Clin. Neurophysiol.* **54,** 203–219.

Liff A. A. (1979) *Color and Black and White Television Theory and Servicing* (Prentice-Hall, Englewood Cliffs, New Jersey).

Lopes da Silva F. H. (1982) EEG Analysis: Theory and Practice, in

Electroencephalography (Niedermeyer E. and Lopes da Silva F. H., eds.) Urban-Schwarzenberg, Baltimore, pp. 685–711.

McNaughton B. L., O'Keefe J., and Barnes C. A. (1983) The stereotrode: A new technique for the simultaneous isolation of several single units in the central nervous system from multiple unit records. *J. Neurosci. Methods* **8,** 391–397.

Mize R. R. (ed.) (1985) *The Microcomputer in Cell and Neurobiology Research* (Elsevier, New York).

Moreton R. B. (1985) Choosing a microcomputer system, in *Microcomputers in the Neurosciences* (Kerkut G., ed.), Clarendon, Oxford, pp. 29–89.

Muller R. U., Kubie J. L., and Ranck J. B., Jr. (1987) Spatial firing patterns of hippocampal complex-spike cells in a fixed environment. *J. Neurosci.,* **7,** 1935–1950.

Mullikan W. H. and Davis T. L. (1985) Real-time analysis of visual receptive fields using an IBM XT personal computer, in *The Microcomputer in Cell and Neurobiology Research* (Mize R. R., ed.), Elsevier, New York, pp. 435–445.

Osborne A. (1979) *An Introduction to Microcomputers* vol. 0, *The Beginner's Book.* vol. 1, *Basic Concepts.* vol. 2, *Some Real Microprocessors,* and vol. 3, *Some Real Support Devices.* (Osborne/McGraw-Hill, Berkely, California).

Otnes R. K. and Enochson L. (1972) *Digital Time Series Analysis* (Wiley, New York).

Park M. R. (1985) In a completely digital neurophysiological recording laboratory, in *The Microcomputer in Cell and Neurobiology Research* (Mize R. R., ed.) (Elsevier, New York), pp. 411–434.

Perkel D. H., Gerstein G. D., and Moore G. P. (1967a) Neuronal spike trains and stochastic point processes. I. The single spike train. *Biophys. J.* **7,** 391–418.

Perkel D. H., Gerstein G. D., and Moore G. P. (1967b) Neuronal spike trains and stochastic point processes. II. Simultaneous spike trains. *Biophys. J.* **7,** 419–439.

Poler S. M., Akeson S., and Flaming D. G. (1985) Selection of hardware and software for laboratory microcomputers, in *The Microcomputer in Cell and Neurobiology Research* (Mize R. R., ed.), Elsevier, New York, pp. 47–82.

Rudell A. P., Fox S. E., and Ranck J. B., Jr. (1980) Hippocampal excitability phase-locked to the theta rhythm in walking rats. *Exp. Neurol.* **68,** 87–96.

Sayers B. McA., Beagley H. A., and Henshall W. R. (1974) The mechanism of auditory evoked EEG responses. *Nature* **241,** 481–483.

Schmidt E. M. (1984) Computer separation of multi-unit neuroelectric data—a review. *J. Neurosci. Methods* **12,** 95–111.

Schwarz E. L., Ramos A., and John E. R. (1976) Single cell activity in chronic unit recordings: A quantitative study of the unit amplitude spectrum. *Brain Res. Bull.* **1,** 57–68.

Teyler T. J., Cauller L., and Mayhew W. (1985) The use of the 6502 microcomputer in neurophysiology, in *Microcomputers in the Neurosciences,* (Kerkut G., ed.), Claredon, Oxford, pp. 90–117.

Toyama K., Kimura M., and Tanaka K. (1981) Cross-correlation analysis of interneuronal connectivity in cat visual cortex. *J. Neurophysiol.* **46,** 191–201.

Vanderwolf C. H. and Leung L. S. (1985) The study of brain electrical activity in relation to behavior, in *Neuromethods,* vol. 1, *General Neurochemical Techniques* (Boulton A. A. and Baker G. B., eds.), Humana Press, Clifton, New Jersey, pp. 305–341.

Vibert J. F. and Costa J. (1979) Spike separation in multiunit records: a multivariate analysis of spike descriptive parameters. *Electroencephalogr. Clin. Neurophysiol.* **47,** 172–182.

Zaks R. (1980) *Your First Computer. A Guide to Business and Personal Computer* 2nd Ed., sybex Inc., Berkeley, California.

Appendix

Glossary and Acronyms

ADC	Analog-to-digital converter
Address	A location in memory, identified by a numerical value
Algorithm	A sequence of steps to obtain a solution to a problem
Alphanumeric	Containing both letters and numerals as characters
Analog	Having a continuous range of values
ANOVA	*Analysis of variance*
ANSI	American National Standards Institute
Arthmetic logic unit	A device used to perform arithmetic and logical functions in a processor (ALU)
ASCII	American Standard Code for Information Interchange, commonly used for data communications

ASSEMBLY language	A low-level, symbolic computer language that is one step away from using binary codes (0s and 1s)
BASIC	Beginner's All-purpose Symbolic Instruction Code, a popular computer language
BAUD	Bits per second
BCD	Binary-coded decimal, using 4 bits to represent a numeral from 0 to 9
Bit	A binary digit that can be either 0 or 1
Boolean algebra	Binary arithmetic rules that include logical operations, such as AND, OR, XOR (exclusive OR), and negation
Bootstrap	An initialization program that is used to start a computer
Buffer	An area of the memory where data are temporarily stored
Bug	A hardware or software error
Bus	Connections between or within a computer
Byte	Typically 8 bits in microcomputer usage
Chip	Monolithic integrated circuit
Clock	A timing device used to synchronize computer or ADC operations
CMOS	Complementary metal oxide semiconductor
Compiler	A program that translates high-level languages to assembly language or machine codes
Complement	The logical inverse of a signal or bit
Console	Control terminal in a computer system
Crash	Losing control of a computer
CRT	Cathode-ray tube, a vacuum tube with a viewing system using a electron beam
DAC	Digital-to-analog converter
Database	A collection of data files organized for access
Diskette	A flexible disk used for storage of program or data; also known as a floppy disk
DMA	Direct memory access, the process of transferring data to and from memory without going through the processor
Dot matrix	A square or rectangular grid of dots used to represent characters or graphics
Double density	High-density storage in a disk
Driver	A circuit that converts input signals into outputs capable of driving a peripheral device

Duplex	Bidirectional data communication
Dynamic memory	Memory that is transient and needs periodic refreshing
EBCDIC	Extended Binary-Coded Decimal Interchange Code, a character code widely used in larger computers
Editor	A program used for the input or editing of text or data
EIA	The Electronic Industries Association, an agency that sets standards
Emulate	The process of simulating a device or system in real time
EOF	End-of-file character
EPROM	Erasable programmable read-only memory
Fetch	Retrieve from memory
File	A unit of stored information (data or program)
Floating-point processor	A processor that is used for the multiplication and division of floating-point numbers, or numbers represented as two parts, a mantissa and an exponential
Formatting	The process of dividing a disk into blocks of storage
FORTRAN	*Formula Translation*, a computer language designed for scientific use
Handshaking	A data communication technique that depends on an acknowledgment of a transfer request
Hard copy	A physical printed or plotted record of computer output
Hardware	The electronics and physical connections of a computer
Hexadecimal	Numerical representation with base (radix) 16: 10–15 are represented as A,B,C,D,E, and F, respectively
IMSL	A library of subroutines for mathematical and statistical analysis
Interface	The connection between computer and device, or between devices
Interlace	The technique of raster-scanning using two nonoverlapping scanned fields
Interpreter	A program that translates a high-level program (typically BASIC) line-by-line in real time during execution

Interrupt	A signal to alert the computer of real-time changes in peripherals; subsequent computer actions will depend on the servicing programs
LCD	Liquid-crystal display
LED	Light-emitting diode
Light pen	A pen that is used to point at different locations of a display screen in order to send positional information to a computer
Linking loader	A program that loads different program segments that were assembled separately
LSB	Least significant bit
Machine language	A computer program in binary codes
Memory—mapped I/O	An interfacing method that assigns a memory address to each input/output port.
Microprocessor	A complete processor containing arithmetic and logical processing units on one or more chips
Modem	*Mo*dulation–*dem*odulation device, or a device that modulates signals for transmission through a telephone line; another device is needed for demodulation on the receiving end
MSB	Most significant bit
Multiplex	The act of channeling two or more signals through one source
Off-line	The acquisition or analysis of data after an experiment
On-line	The acquisition or analysis of data during an experiment
Operating system	A program that manages files and executes software
PASCAL	A high-level, block-structured language
Peripheral	An external device connected to a computer
Pixel	Picture element, or the fundamental graphic unit in a display
Port (input/output)	An input or output connection to the computer
Priority	A system of assigning importance to different interrupting devices; the higher priority device will be serviced first
PROM	Programmable read-only memory
RAM	Random-access memory: memory that can be accessed in any position without interrogating another memory location

ROM	Read-only memory
Sample-and-hold	A circuit that holds an output voltage at the level of the sampled input voltage
Sampling	The act of digitizing a continuous, analog signal
SCR	Silicon controlled rectifier
Sector	A pie-slice-shaped section of a disk
Serial communication	Sending of data sequentially through a single wire
Software	Programs for running a computer
Spreadsheet	A program that manipulates data, usually presented in tabular form
Static memory	Memory that retains its contents without refreshing
Synch pulse	Synchronizing pulse used, e.g., in aligning horizontal and vertical sweeps of a video monitor
Throughput rate	The rate at which data is processed by a device
Track	A concentric ring on the disk
Triac	A device consisting essentially of two back-to-back SCRs connected in parallel
Two's complement	A binary numbering system for the representation of positive and negative numbers; the negative of a number is formed by inverting all binary digits and adding 1
TTL	Transistor-transistor logic
Utility programs	Useful programs that are often used in a computer system
Video field	One complete scan down the video monitor
Video frame	Two video fields generating by interlacing scans
Word	A unit of computer processing; a microcomputer typically uses 8, 16 or 32-bit words
Word processing	The use of computers for text and manuscript editing

From: *Neuromethods, Vol. 15: Neurophysiological Techniques: Applications to Neural Systems* Edited by: A. A. Boulton, G. B. Baker, and C. H. Vanderwolf Copyright © 1990 The Humana Press Inc., Clifton, NJ

Index

Action potential(s), 280, 289, 290, 307, 308, 324, 338
ACF (*see* Autocorrelation function)
AEPs (*see* Auditory and Average evoked potentials)
ADCs (*see* Analog-to-digital converters)
Ag/AgCl electrodes (*see* Silver/silver chloride electrodes)
AI (*see* Auditory cortex)
Alcian blue, 19
Alvear tract, 297
Amplifier(s), 21, 34
Amygdala, 218
Analog-to-digital converters (ADCs), 159, 163, 318, 327–329, 333, 341, 361
Analog (continuous) control, 357
Analysis of variance (ANOVA), 162, 163, 165, 323
Anistropy, 296
ANOVA (*see* Analysis of variance)
Anterior commissure, 215
Atropine, 220
Auditory cortex (AI), 177, 180, 181
Auditory evoked potentials (AEPs), 176–178, 181
Autocorrelation function (ACF), 349, 350
Average evoked potential (AEP), 297
Averaging (AEP and PSTH), 346

BAEP (*see* Brainstem auditory EPs)

Basket cells, 308
Bereitschaftspotential, 192
BIC (*see* Brachium of inferior colliculus)
Bins, 344, 349
Boltzmann's constant, 20
Boolean algebra, 315
Brachial plexus, 182
Brachium of inferior colliculus (BIC), 178
Brainstem, 176, 177, 221, 223
Brainstem auditory EPs (BAEPs), 176, 177

CA1, 308
Calcarine cortex, 189
Calcium, 324
Carbon-fiber microelectrodes, 33
Cartesian coordinates, 296
Caudate, 218
CCF (*see* Cross-correlation function)
Cerebellar nuclei, 194
Cerebellum, 291
Chloramphenicol, 127
Cholinergic neurons, 220
Circumferential recording electrodes, 79
CN (*see* Cochlear nucleus)
CNVs (*see* Contingent negative variations)
Cochlear nucleus (CN), 178
Cognitive correlates of the P3, 205
Cognitive correlates of the N4, 202
Cognitive EPs, 200, 223, 225
Collision interval, 50

Common peroneal (CP) nerve,
99, 101, 104
Computed tomography (CT), 169,
224
Computer language, 322
Computer techniques in
neurophysiology, 313–369
the computer in a neurophy-
siological laboratory, 324–358
behavioral analysis using a
microcomputer, 358–362
Connectors, 74
Contingent negative variations
(CNVs), 169, 199, 202, 215–
220
Continuous cable representation,
282
Corpus collosum, 215
Cortex, 193, 194, 196, 197, 218,
220, 222, 324, 345, 351
CP (see Common peroneal)
Cranial nerves, 105
Cross-correlation function (CCF),
350, 351
CSDs (see Current-source-
densities)
CT (see Computer tomography)
Current-source-density(ies)
(CSD[s]), 277, 285, 287, 288,
290, 292, 293, 299, 301–306

DACs (see Digital-to-analog con-
verters)
Data acquisition, 330, 334
Dendrite(s), 1, 2, 8, 11, 12, 289,
292, 297, 305–308
DI operation, 329
Digital-to-analog converters
(DACs), 318, 357
Digital control (switching), 356
Digital filtering, 348
Dimensionality, 301

Dipole(s), 168, 172, 173, 184, 290
Dirac delta function, 286
Disk drive, 319
Distensible length transducers,
119, 120
Distinct generators, 153
Dorsal root ganglion (DRG), 70–
73, 94, 132
Dorsal spinocerebellar tract
(DSCT) neurons, 77, 78
DRG (see Dorsal root ganglion)
DSCT (see Dorsal spineocerebellar
tract)

ECoG, 4
EEG (see Electroencephalography)
Eighth nerve (EN), 178
EKG, 154, 156, 160
Electrical model of the membrane, 282, 283
Electro-oculogram (EOG), 161
Electrocorticogram, 289
Electrode pullers, 17
Electrodes, 3, 4, 16, 18, 20, 22,
23, 27, 29, 31, 32, 34, 38, 39,
65–114, 116, 133, 156, 173,
295, 324, 338
Electroencephalography (EEG), 4,
38, 147–149, 155, 157, 159,
161, 163, 166, 167, 170, 173,
179, 184, 187, 190, 221, 224,
291, 295, 341–343, 345, 355
Electrolytic capacitor, 26
Electromyography (EMG), 66, 73,
75, 77, 79, 82, 85, 86, 89, 91,
95, 100, 101, 103, 104, 107,
109–114, 117, 122–125, 133,
156, 159, 190, 191, 194, 196,
198
Electroneurogram (ENG), 78, 95,
106

Electroretinogram (ERG), 160, 291
EMG (*see* Electromyography)
EN (see Eighth nerve)
ENG (*see* Electroneurogram)
EOG (*see* Electro-oculogram)
EPs (*see* Evoked potentials)
EPSPs (*see* Excitatory postsynaptic potentials)
ERG (*see* electroretrinogram)
ERP, 165, 222, 223
Evoked potentials (EPs), 147–149, 152, 154–157, 159–164, 166–169, 173–175, 186, 189, 221
Excitatory postsynaptic potentials (EPSPs), 43, 47, 179, 182, 188, 189, 304, 305, 306
Extracellular field, 2, 3
Extracellular single-unit recording methods, 1–64
  definitions, 2, 3
  extracellular fields of single neurons, 3–16
  recording methods, 16–51
  sampling single-neuron activity, 51–58

Factor analysis, 165
Fast Fourier transform (FFT), 166, 362
Fast Green FCF, 19
FD, 129, 131
Femoral nerve, 83, 102, 108, 109, 114
Femoral nerve cuff (FNC), 102, 109, 114
FES (*see* Functional electrical stimulation)
FET amplifiers, 21, 34, 35
FET input amplifiers, 75
FFT (*see* Fast Fourier transform)

Field potentials in the central nervous system, 277–309
  field potential theory, 278–293
  interpretation of field potentials, 304–308
  techniques in field potential recording and analysis, 294–304
Filter(s), 158, 348, 349
Floating microelectrodes, 32, 65–78
FNC (*see* Femoral nerve cuff)
Forward problem, 168
Fourier (frequency domain) analysis, 335, 352
Fourier transform, 158, 166, 352, 362
FP, 129, 131
Freely moving animals, study of spinal cord, peripheral nerve, and muscle activity in, 65–136
  electrodes, 107–113
  floating microelectrodes, 66–78
  limitations of chronic reading techniques, 128–136
  muscle and tendon length transducers, 116–126
  peripheral nerve cuff electrodes, 78–107
  selection, training, and care of implanted animals, 126–128
  tendon force transducers, 113–116
Functional electrrical stimulation (FES), 135

Gaussian distribution, 338
Generator(s), 208, 217
Glia, 220, 290, 291
Glutamate, 351
Graded potentials, 324

Granule cells, 291
Ground loops, 160

Halothane, 72, 78
Hatpin microelectrode (HPE), 70,
    71, 112, 114
HC (see Hippocampal)
Hippocampal (HC) pyramidal
    cell, 209, 293
Hippocampal CA1 region, 297
Hippocampus, 208, 209, 214, 292,
    293, 297
Human evoked potentials, 147–
    228
    cognitive EPs, 200–223
    methodology, 154–176
    movement potentials, 190–200
    sensory EPs, 176–190
    uses of EPs, 223–227
HPE (see Hatpin microelectrode)
Hypothalamus, 218

IC (see Inferior colliculi and Inte-
    grated circuit)
Implanted venous catheter, 127
Inferior colliculi (IC), 178
Infraslow potentials, 217
Inhibitory postsynaptic potentials
    (IPSPs), 188, 304, 305, 307
Initial segment-somatic dendritic
    (IS-SD), 340
Input voltage range, 328
Integrated circuit (IC), 313
Interfaces, 320
Interrupts, 320
Interval and correlation analysis
    of spike trains, 349
Ion-sensitive electrodes, 324
IPSPs (see Inhibitory postsynaptic
    potentials)
Ir (see Iridium)

Iridium (Ir), 24, 32, 69, 71, 95,
    110
IS-SD (see Initial segment-somatic
    dendritic)

K$^+$ (see Potassium)

Laplacian-transformed EPs, 167,
    169, 170
Late positive component (LPC),
    201
Lateral lemniscus (LL), 178
Lidocaine, 99
LL (see Lateral lemniscus)
LLAEPs (see Long latency audi-
    tory EPs)
Long latency auditory EPs
    (LLAEPs), 176, 179, 180
LPC (see Late positive com-
    ponent)

Macroelectrode(s), 3, 4, 18, 324
Magnetic resonance imaging
    (MRI), 169, 173, 224
Magentoencephalogram (MEG),
    167, 168, 170–173, 180, 181,
    184, 187
Medial gastrocnemius (MG), 119
Medial geniculate nuclei (MGN),
    178
MEG (see Magnetoencephalo-
    gram)
Mesencephalic reticular formation
    (MRF), 218, 219
Methylene blue, 121
MG (see Medial gastrocnemius)
MGN (see Medial geniculate
    nuclei)
Microcomputer, 315
Microdrives, 36

Microelectode(s), 4, 16, 20, 22, 23, 27, 29, 31, 39, 67, 116, 133, 295, 324, 338
Micromanipulator, 67
Microprocessor, 313, 317
Middle latency auditory EPS (MLAEPs), 176, 178, 179
Mirror galvanometer, 313
MLAEPs (*see* Middle latency auditory EPs)
MODEM (*see* Modulator-demodulator)
Modulator-demodulator (MODEM), 318
Most significant bit (MSB), 327, 328
Motor potential, 191
Motorneuron, 9
Movement potentials, 190
MRF (*see* Mesencephalic reticular formation)
MRI (*see* Magnetic resonance imaging)
MSB (*see* Most significant bit)
MTL, 207–214, 221
Multiple-channel wave acquisition, 333
Multiple electrode arrays, 309
Multiple generators, 153
Muscle fiber length, 123

N1–P2, 180
N2, 208, 224
N4, 152, 202–206, 214, 215, 224
N4–P3, 223
Na$^+$ (*see* Sodium ion)
NCH (*see* Number of channels)
Nerve cuff recording electrode(s), 79, 83, 84, 87
Nerve patch recording electrodes, 86
NPTS (*see* Number of data points)

Nucleus basalis, 220
Number of channels (NCH), 333, 336, 343
Number of data points (NPTS), 332, 341, 344

Olfactory bulb, 291

P1, 180
P100, 188, 189
P3, 152, 205–213, 217, 219–221, 224
Parahippocampal gyrus, 214
Parylene, 26, 32, 72
PCA (*see* Principal components analysis)
Peripheral nerve blocking cuffs, 98
Peripheral nerve cuff electrodes, 78
Peripheral nerve stimulating electrodes, 93
Peristimulus time histograms (PSTHs), 307, 340, 341, 349, 350
PET (*see* Positron emission tomography)
Piezoelectric crystals, 121, 123–125
Pinnation angle, 123
Platinum (Pt), 24, 29, 32, 69, 95
Population study, 51
Positron emission tomography (PET), 214, 224
Postcentral gyrus, 184
Potassium ion (K$^+$), 220, 290, 324
Potassium-ferrocyanide Prussion Blue method, 19
Potential divider, 292
Precentral gyrus, 184
Premotion positivity, 191
Premotor positivity, 192

Principal components analysis (PCA), 165
Printed circuit electrodes, 33
Processing negativities, 200
Processors, 315
Procion brown, 19
PSTHs (*see* Peristimulus time histograms)
Pt (*see* Platinum)
PT neurons, 15, 54
Pulse registration, 338
Purkinje cells, 291
Pyramidal cell(s), 9, 11, 15, 16, 40, 48, 49, 168, 177, 179, 194, 195, 289, 297, 304, 305, 307, 308

Quantization, 327

RAM (*see* Random access memory)
Random access memory (RAM), 317
Read-only memory (ROM), 317
Readiness potential, 191, 192
Reafferente potentiale, 191, 192
Reference electrode(s), 156, 173
REM sleep, 180
Reticular system (RS), 177
Retina, 26, 291
Retinal ganglion cells, 26
RF motoneuron, 117
ROM (*see* Read-only memory)
RP, 196–199, 215, 217
RS (*see* Reticular system)
Runge-Kutta formulae, 292

S:N, 171, 173
S1, 216, 218
S1–S2 interval, 217, 218, 220
S2, 216, 218

Sampling of pulses, 340
Sandwich electrodes, 109, 110
SC (*see* Stellate cells)
Sciatic nerve, 104
SCRs (*see* Silicon-controlled rectifiers)
SCS (*see* Spinal cord segment)
SE operation, 329
Second-order gradiometer configuration, 170
Semantic incongruity, 202
Sensory EPs, 176, 223
SEPs (*see* Somatosensory evoked potentials)
Silicon-controlled rectifiers (SCRs), 357
Silver/silver chloride electrodes, 34, 38
Simultaneous pulse and wave recording, 341
Single generator, 153
Single unit, 3
Sink, 5, 7, 13, 290
Slow wave (SW), 152, 156, 217, 224
SMC, 197
SOC (*see* Superior olivary complex)
Sodium ion (Na^+), 279, 290
Soelus (SOL) muscles, 119–121
Software support, 321
SOL (*see* Soleus)
Somatosensory evoked potentials (SEPs), 181, 183, 184
Spatial interval of mapping, 301
Spectral analysis, 88, 166
Spike potential field, 3
Spinal cord, 65, 66, 77
Spinal cord ENG electrodes, 106
Spinal cord segment (SCS), 72, 73
Spinocerebellar tract neurons, 65

SQUIDS (*see* Superconducting quantum interference devices)
Stellate cell(s) (SC), 11, 13, 177
Stepping motor, 357
Storage oscilloscope, 45
Strata pyramidale, 308
Stratum oriens, 307
Superconducting quantum interference devices (SQUIDS), 170, 171
Superior olivary complex (SOC), 178
SW (*see* Slow wave)

Template-matching, 189
Tendon force signal recording, 115
Tendon force transducers, 113
Tendon length, 123
Thalamus, 218–222
Thiopental, 128
TSW (*see* Typical slow wave)

Tungsten, 24, 29, 32, 33, 39, 71
Typical slow wave (TSW), 213

V-shaped channel MOS-field effect transistor (VFET), 357
VA, 218
Ventral root (VR), 72, 73, 129–131
Ventral spinocerebellar tract (VSCT) neuron(s), 77, 78, 98, 100, 106
Vertex potentials, 224
VEPs (*see* Visual EPs)
VFET (*see* V-shaped channel MOS-field effect transistor)
Visual EPs (VEPs), 185, 187, 188
Volume conduction, 285
VOP, 218
VR (*see* Ventral root)
VR potentials, 129–131
VSCT potentials, 129–131

Wave A, 180
Wave registration, 325
Window discriminator, 44